Cancer Drug Discovery and Development

The Cancer Drug Discovery and Development series (Beverly A Teicher, series editor) is the definitive book series in cancer research and oncology, providing comprehensive coverage of specific topics and the field. Volumes cover the process of drug discovery, preclinical models in cancer research, specific drug target groups and experimental and approved therapeutic agents. The volumes are current and timely, anticipating areas where experimental agents are reaching FDA approval. Each volume is edited by an expert in the field covered and chapters are authored by renowned scientists and physicians in their fields of interest.

More information about this series at http://www.springer.com/series/7625

Marc Damelin
Editor

Innovations for Next-Generation Antibody-Drug Conjugates

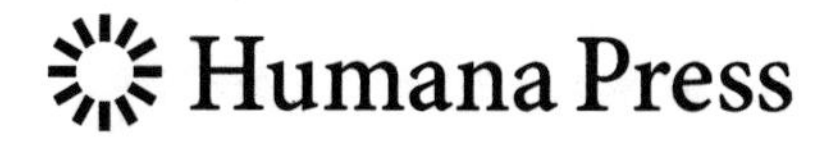

Editor
Marc Damelin
Mersana Therapeutics, Inc.
Cambridge, MA, USA

ISSN 2196-9906 ISSN 2196-9914 (electronic)
Cancer Drug Discovery and Development
ISBN 978-3-030-08627-5 ISBN 978-3-319-78154-9 (eBook)
https://doi.org/10.1007/978-3-319-78154-9

Softcover re-print of the Hardcover 1st edition 2018

Printed on acid-free paper

This Humana Press imprint is published by the registered company Springer International Publishing AG part of Springer Nature.
The registered company address is: Gewerbestrasse 11, 6330 Cham, Switzerland

Preface

Chemotherapy is good but not good enough: it is standard-of-care treatment for many tumor types, yet its efficacy is matched by and limited by toxicity. The concept of the antibody-drug conjugate (ADC) – to deliver chemotherapy preferentially to tumor tissue by conjugation to an antitumor antibody – has enticed scientists, clinicians, and drug developers to invest in ADCs for several decades. To date, the overall clinical success of ADCs has been modest, for which various explanations are offered throughout this volume. Nevertheless, there are many reasons to believe that the next generation of ADCs will command impressive success.

This volume is about the promise and excitement of the innovations that are enabling next-generation ADCs. The inherent complexities of ADCs were long appreciated as a general principle, and now with the data from preclinical studies and hundreds of clinical trials with ADCs, we can truly appreciate the challenges that are intertwined with the complexities. That understanding has brought us to an inflection point in the evolution of ADCs: new technologies have been developed to address specific observations and are beginning to emerge in the clinical space. This volume includes a critical assessment of the ADC field as a framework for contextualizing the innovations. As I wrote the Introduction (Chap. 1) in this mindset, the sequence of chapters came about rather organically, and the reader is encouraged to read them in order! It also became clear to me that this volume is much greater than the sum of its parts: each chapter is an independent, focused analysis, yet taken together, the chapters will allow the reader to integrate the complexities with the innovations, and ultimately to develop a holistic perspective on ADCs and devise thoughtful actions for future research.

A word about the volume's title: it includes two terms that suffer from overuse: "innovation" and "next-generation." In spite of their overuse, I chose these terms because they are incredibly powerful when used in a meaningful way. What is innovation? It is not just a new idea elevated by a trendy term – it is an idea that leads to a substantial change or improvement. For an inspirational read on this topic, I highly recommend "The Innovators" by Walter Isaacson (published by Simon and Schuster). What is "next generation"? It is not just what happens to come next and is elevated by a trendy term – it is a significant advance that reflects a new capability or approach. This volume describes a series of true innovations both in technology and thinking that, when considered critically, will enable true next-generation ADCs that promise to greatly improve the lives of patients with cancer (and other diseases – see Chap. 14).

I want to take this opportunity to thank many people who joined me in the journey of this project. The authors have shared my enthusiasm about the project since its inception; I thank them for their significant efforts that resulted in meaningful, consequential contributions. The anonymous peer reviewers are acknowledged for their extremely beneficial insights and suggestions. I thank the team at Springer, especially William Helms for guidance in the formative stages of the project, Maria David for effectively managing the project, and S. Suresh and the team who produced the book from the set of files that the contributors provided. I am very grateful to my many colleagues and collaborators over the past decade for all of the exciting work that we have done and are doing together on ADCs – with much more to come, of course. Finally, many thanks to my wife Sarah and our children Naomi, Leah, and Max for being supportive and accommodating while I worked on this project.

Cambridge, MA, USA Marc Damelin

Contents

Introduction: Motivations for Next-Generation ADCs

Marc Damelin

Abstract The new and emerging ADC technologies together with the field's cumulative experience provide new opportunities for ADCs and make them a more promising therapeutic modality than ever before. Despite a rapidly evolving clinical landscape in oncology, there is substantial unmet clinical need that could be addressed by next-generation ADCs. ADCs are also being explored to combat other diseases. This introductory chapter provides context for the key innovations of next-generation ADCs described throughout the volume. A framework for designing and interpreting preclinical pharmacology studies is proposed such that emerging technologies can be rigorously evaluated and molecules can be judiciously optimized.

Keywords Preclinical studies · In vivo · Pharmacology · Oncology · Challenge · Innovation · Tool · Technology · Patient-derived xenograft · PDX

The antibody-drug conjugate (ADC) is a therapeutic modality in which a small molecule is directly linked to an antibody or related biologic – thus marrying the potency of the small molecule (often called the "payload") with the tumor specificity of the antibody. The history of this modality and the current technologies, approaches and clinical molecules have been described [4–6, 9]. Tolcher's candid history of ADCs cautions against self-deception yet conveys optimism about next-generation ADCs [10]. This volume focuses on emerging ADC technologies, and in this chapter, I would like to provide context for how the reader might evaluate, integrate and ultimately act on the information. How will next-generation ADCs fit into the clinical landscape? What are the most pressing challenges? How can the emerging technologies be rigorously evaluated in the preclinical setting to maximize the chances of clinical success?

In the design of an ADC, not only are there seemingly endless possibilities for the small molecule and the antibody, but there are seemingly endless ways in which

M. Damelin (✉)
Mersana Therapeutics, Inc., Cambridge, MA, USA

M. Damelin (ed.), *Innovations for Next-Generation Antibody-Drug Conjugates*, Cancer Drug Discovery and Development,
https://doi.org/10.1007/978-3-319-78154-9_1

they can be combined – by various chemistries, in various ratios and with various linkers. While "antibody, payload and linker" are sometimes listed as the three components of the ADC, there is a fourth that cannot be ignored: the bioconjugation, in other words the way in which the first three components are assembled. Many emerging technologies have improved the bioconjugation aspect by engineering the antibody or enabling new chemistry. Three general principles have driven the improvements in bioconjugation. First, the biophysical properties – and thus the physiological disposition – of the ADC are defined by the molecule as a whole, not its components. A panel of ADCs comprised of the same antibody, linker and payload but generated with different bioconjugation methods will have distinct properties and likely distinct pharmacokinetic and pharmacodynamic profiles. Second, homogeneous preparations of ADCs are considered superior to heterogeneous preparations, due to enhanced manufacturing control over the ADC, including minimal or no occurrence of uncharacterized species. Third, an improved bioconjugation technique will theoretically serve as a platform and apply to many combinations of antibody, linker and payload.

The opportunity to continually tweak, improve and optimize ADCs is exciting to any scientist yet also forces the reality that we will not be able to evaluate all of them in the clinic (or even in preclinical experiments). We should not generate and evaluate ADCs simply because we can, because we have new technology, or because it's an intriguing or novel chemical possibility. We must be systematic and critical, while maintaining scientific exploration and its unanticipated benefits.

This Introduction includes a discussion of the common interpretations (and misinterpretations) of preclinical efficacy studies with ADCs in oncology. In order to critically evaluate new ADC technologies, we will need to design *and interpret* preclinical studies to be predictive of the clinic. More broadly, this Introduction highlights challenges, tools and innovations that are addressed in the other chapters. The chapters contain rich bibliographies of primary literature about the problems and the solutions.

Motivations for Next-Generation ADCs

What is the motivation for next-generation ADCs? Ultimately the motivation must be based in the clinic: the belief that the ADCs will offer superior benefits for cancer patients than current and emerging therapies. The oncology clinical landscape changed dramatically over the past decade with the demonstration that therapeutic molecules can successfully manipulate the patient's immune system to attack the tumor and achieve long-term (durable) responses. Investment in the preclinical and clinical space has shifted dramatically toward these "immuno-oncology" ("I-O") agents, and ADCs do not fall directly in this category – although mechanistic links and potential synergies have been characterized and are described in Chapter 2,"Combining ADCs with Immuno-Oncology Agents".

However, there are many limitations of I-O agents that clearly leave large patient populations in need of other therapies [2]. Serious immune-related adverse events are often associated with the manipulation of the patient's immune system, and even more so when multiple I-O agents are used in combination. Many patients do not respond at all to I-O agents, and successful strategies for patient selection are just beginning to emerge. Moreover, certain tumor types (such as acute myelogenous leukemia, AML) have extremely low response rates to I-O agents. AML is a good example of a clinical indication where I-O agents have not succeeded but many other therapeutic modalities have, including ADCs (e.g. gemtuzumab ozogamacin).

In chapter 2, "Combining ADCs with Immuno-Oncology Agents", Philipp Müller, Jonathan Rios-Doria, Jay Harper and Anthony Cao describe the integration of ADCs with the blossoming clinical landscape of immuno-oncology. Even first-generation ADCs can be appreciated in an innovative way: in a context where the ADCs stimulate the anti-tumor immune response and act in synergy with I-O agents. The authors describe multiple mechanisms by which ADCs can stimulate anti-tumor immunity. The discovery and development of next-generation ADCs must be guided by opportunities framed by I-O. The selection of ADC target (antigen), antibody, linker, payload and bioconjugation method, as well as the choice of clinical indication and the design of clinical trials, all must be optimized for the new clinical landscape.

Chemotherapy remains the standard-of-care treatment, or part of a combination of therapies in standard-of-care treatment, for many indications in clinical oncology. The original concept of ADCs, that antibody-mediated delivery will reduce the systemic toxicity of the payload and subsequently enhance the anti-tumor activity, remains the guiding principle. Where initial failures can be attributed to suboptimal technologies and a certain ignorance of the complexities of the ADC modality, the new and emerging ADC technologies together with the field's cumulative experience provide new opportunities for ADCs and make them a more promising therapeutic modality than ever before.

Challenges: Reality Versus Perception

There are undisputed challenges common to drug discovery across therapeutic modalities; this volume focuses on the challenges that are particular (though not necessarily unique) to ADCs. Many of the challenges that are more specific to this modality were not appreciated for several decades but have become strikingly clear with the field's collective experience.

In chapter 3, "Improving the Safety Profile of ADCs", Magali Guffroy, Hadi Falahatpisheh and Martin Finkelstein describe the preclinical and clinical safety profiles of ADCs. To date the safety profile of most ADCs has been defined by the technology platform, not the expression of the antigen in normal tissues. Platform-mediated toxicities, commonly referred to as "off-target" or "target independent," have been dose-limiting in most cases. Historically it was believed that "on-target" toxicity would be dose-limiting, since in theory the payload would be delivered only to target-expressing cells. In practice, due to the instability of payload attachment to the antibody (especially with older technologies) and various mechanisms of antigen-independent ADC internalization into cells, some payload is delivered where it is not wanted. The unanticipated limitation of off-target toxicities drove the development of several new ADC technologies described in this volume.

Understanding the anti-tumor activity of ADCs in preclinical models and predicting the activity in patient populations have proven to be major challenges, if only because they demand a rigorous and objective evaluation. Preclinical anti-tumor activity must be evaluated deeply in terms of pharmacology, pharmacokinetics and pharmacodynamics, as well as an understanding of the utilities versus limitations of each tumor model, in order to make appropriate predictions about clinical activity. Testing the activity at various dose levels and measuring the various ADC components (e.g. antibody, conjugated payload and unconjugated payload) provide a much broader perspective than for instance observing regressions at the one and only dose level tested. When the antibody does not react with the murine antigen, or the murine and human antigens have different patterns of normal tissue expression, the biodistribution of the ADC in mice (efficacy studies) may differ from in humans, with consequences for anti-tumor activity: the observed preclinical activity might be exaggerated. Testing dose levels not attainable in the clinic does not provide useful information even if impressive regressions are achieved; this issue is common to all drug discovery, but ADCs actually may have an *advantage* in that clinical information gleaned from an earlier ADC can inform preclinical studies with a new ADC based on the same or similar technology. In chapter 4, "Utility of PK-PD Modeling and Simulation to Improve Decision Making for Antibody-Drug Conjugate Development", Aman Singh and Dhaval Shah compare and contrast several modeling and simulation methods that can integrate the body of preclinical data to make predictions about the clinic.

Are the preclinical tumor models really as bad as everyone says? Agreed, many compounds have exhibited robust activity against subcutaneous xenografts of BxPC3 pancreatic cancer cells (for example) but have failed or would fail miserably in clinical trials against this disease. Given the unique desmoplastic stroma of pancreatic tumors [11], how could a subcutaneous xenograft of BxPC3 or any other cancer cell line constitute a physiological model of the disease? However, when the limitations of the models are understood, the preclinical models may be helpful after all. For example, the BxPC3 model might be useful for certain aspects of pharmacology, such as selection of lead molecules – as long as the data is not interpreted to be predictive of clinical success in pancreatic cancer. Patient-derived xenografts (PDXs) have become very popular and are generally considered better disease models than cell-line xenografts, but even so, careful assessment of the limitations of PDXs and associated pharmacology data is required.

More generally, Tolcher [10] suggests that when activity is achieved in preclinical models of a tumor type that historically has not been responsive to the related chemotherapy (i.e. related by payload class or mechanism), it is not appropriate to infer that the ADC will be active in that tumor type in the clinic. This discussion reflects the longstanding debate about whether ADCs can sensitize a tumor type to

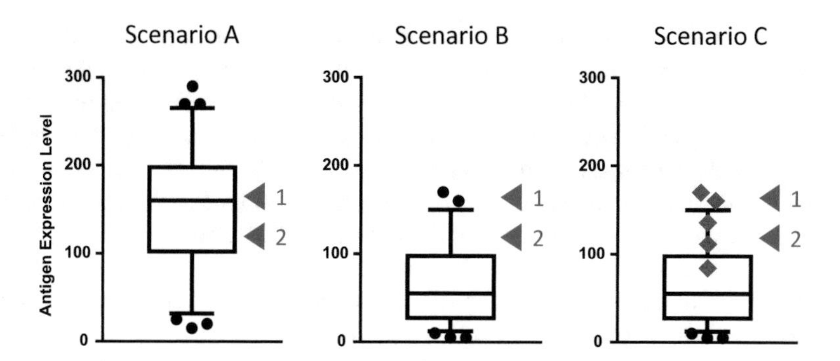

Fig. 1 Contextualizing preclinical models with clinical data. The schematics represent hypothetical distributions of antigen expression in clinical samples of a defined tumor type. The box spans the 25th–75th percentiles with median, and the whiskers demarcate the 5th–95th percentiles. In Scenario C, the red diamonds indicate a subset of tumors that are distinguished e.g. by mutation or other feature. The arrowheads marked "1" and "2" represent specific preclinical models that were evaluated with an ADC. While the preclinical models and pharmacology data are equivalent across the scenarios, the data should be interpreted differently in these scenarios as described in the text

a chemotherapy that has not shown clinical activity in that tumor type (while it has in other tumor types), or whether ADCs simply improve the therapeutic index of chemotherapy in validated tumor types. It is possible though not concluded that the former represents an original philosophy on ADCs and the latter is consistent with actual observations to date.

A notable, recurring observation is that depending on the preclinical tumor model and the ADC technology, some degree of anti-tumor activity may be observed with a non-binding "control" ADC (built with the same ADC technology as the ADC of interest, but using an antibody that does not bind any antigen in the tumor or host species). There can be various underlying reasons for this phenomenon depending on the specific case. Regardless, it is imperative to design and interpret efficacy studies with this observation in mind. The implications for combination studies and comparisons of ADCs to "standard-of-care" small molecules should also be considered.

It is commonly observed, consistent with the therapeutic hypothesis of ADCs, that higher antigen expression correlates with greater efficacy; but what can easily be overlooked is how the expression level in preclinical models compares with the expression level in patient populations. The same pharmacology data should be interpreted very differently based on this comparison. Consider the scenarios presented in Fig. 1, where an ADC has induced sustained tumor regressions in two preclinical models (indicated by the blue arrowheads "1" and "2"). In Scenario A, the level of antigen expression in the models is representative of primary tumors in the corresponding indication, and there is confidence that the preclinical data predicts clinical feasibility. In Scenario B, the level of antigen expression in the preclinical models is higher than the large majority of primary tumors; thus despite the preclinical achievement of sustained tumor regressions, Scenario B does not confidently predict meaningful clinical activity. As a side note, preclinical models generated by the exogenous overexpression of antigen typically result in Scenario B and should be avoided. In Scenario C, a subset of the tumors indicated by red diamonds share a genetic background or other distinguishing feature with the two preclinical models; with this feature considered in addition to antigen expression level, Scenario C is similar to Scenario A in that the preclinical models are representative of a defined patient population (regardless of population size). The most striking aspect of this example is that the levels of antigen expression and anti-tumor activity for each model are identical in the three scenarios, and the interpretation depends on the contextualization of the models relative to patient populations.

All the scenarios in Fig. 1 would benefit from a larger preclinical dataset. A recent trend in ADC discovery is to test the compound in a large panel of preclinical models – typically PDXs – to generate hypotheses about tumor types and subtypes that are more likely to respond, and about the threshold of antigen expression in those tumor types and subtypes that is required for ADC activity. In some cases, these studies employ fewer mice per group and fewer dose levels to make it feasible to evaluate a large panel of models; this approach is sometimes referred to as "clinical trial in a mouse." The clinical development of several ADCs has been informed by evaluating large panels of PDXs [1, 3, 7, 8].

Patient selection for ADC therapies presents logistical challenges that can be broken down into two broad categories: predicting the patient population from preclinical studies, and developing the early-phase assays and companion diagnostics. The concept of patient selection for ADCs is straightforward (and theoretically an advantage of the modality) since the premise of the ADC is to deliver payload via an anti-tumor antibody, and thus tumors with higher antigen levels should generally exhibit better response. Such correlations have been observed across many preclinical and clinical studies with ADCs. But consider the contrasts to the selection strategy for a tyrosine kinase inhibitor (TKI) where a genetic mutation confers sensitivity: (1) selection for the TKI is binary (mutation vs. wildtype) while selection for the ADC is on a spectrum that requires a threshold to be defined; (2) the TKI employs DNA-based assays that do not depend on tumor type, while the ADC typically employs immunohistochemical assays that must be calibrated for each tumor type. The cost of developing patient selection assays for ADC can be high and might require early investment to support expedited development plans. Regulatory considerations and aspects of companion diagnostics for ADCs are discussed in chapter 5, "Regulatory Considerations and Companion Diagnostics" by Elizabeth VanAlphen and Omar Perez.

Beyond challenges of preclinical pharmacology, the complexity of ADCs has yielded a large degree of molecular heterogeneity in the clinical materials of most ADCs including multiple ADCs approved for marketing. While the technical challenge of achieving a homogeneous preparation has long been apparent, the potential advantages of homogeneous preparations have become increasingly appreciated. The tendency to simplify the description of heterogeneous ADC preparations, for example with "average drug-to-antibody ratio (DAR) of 4," has the effect of trivializing the existence of typically uncharacterized species at the extremes of the distribution; the properties of such species may diverge significantly from the average. Many of the emerging technologies will add complexity to the ADC molecule and thus add challenges to the manufacturing processes, as discussed in chapter 6, "ADC Process Development and Manufacturing" by Olivier Marcq.

These challenges are far from insurmountable. In fact, the ADC field has reached an inflection point: the challenges of a technical nature are being addressed by many innovations, and the challenges of a human nature are addressed by rigor and diligence informed by our collective experience. We have developed the tools and the perspective to overcome the challenges, and are poised for success.

Innovations in ADC Discovery and Development

The innovations described in this volume span the broad spectrum from target/antigen selection to clinical development and from antibodies to payloads and bioconjugation methods. In many cases, preclinical and/or clinical proof of concept has been sought with the HER2 (ERBB2) antigen, and many next-generation ADCs employ trastuzumab or an engineered variant. In chapter 7, "HER2-Targeted ADCs: At The Forefront Of ADC Technology Development", Kevin Hamblett provides background on HER2 and the approved HER2-targeted ADC (T-DM1, Kadcyla®) as a framework for describing next-generation HER2-targeted ADCs built on many of the emerging technologies.

The next two chapters address novel payloads and technologies to deliver more of it. In chapter 8, "Next Generation Payloads for ADCs", Nathan Tumey discusses the expanding repertoire within the two most common mechanisms-of-action for ADC payloads, tubulin binding and DNA damaging, as well as the exploration of other mechanisms-of-action including inducers of apoptosis; inhibitors of splicing, topoisomerase I or RNA polymerase; and novel cytotoxic mechanisms. Tumey concludes with a discussion of payloads that would apply to other therapeutic areas such as infectious disease and inflammation.

In chapter 9, "Delivering More Payload: High DAR ADCs", Natalya Bodyak and Alexander Yurkovetskiy present advancements that have achieved the longtime goal of loading more payload on each antibody molecule. Early attempts to increase potency in this manner revealed challenges to maintain adequate pharmacokinetic profiles with negative consequences for both efficacy and tolerability. These obstacles have been addressed by various approaches, several of which are used in clinical-stage ADCs. Bodyak and Yurkovetskiy also discuss the related technologies of antibody- or antibody fragment-targeted nanotherapeutics, which incorporate dramatically (orders of magnitude) more payload than most ADCs but have not yet demonstrated the same capability for targeted delivery as ADCs.

Chapters 10-12, "Site-Specific Antibody Drug Conjugates", "Bispecific and Biparatopic Antibody-Drug Conjugates", and "Targeting Drug Conjugates to the Tumor Microenvironment: Probody Drug Conjugates" provide insights on antibody engineering technologies to improve ADCs by various mechanisms. In chapter 10,

"Site-Specific Antibody Drug Conjugates", Feng Tian, Dowdy Jackson and Yun Bai describe a multitude of approaches to achieve site-specific conjugation with the overall goal of producing a homogeneous ADC preparation that is hypothesized to have increased therapeutic index and other advantages. Most methods for site-specific conjugation involve engineering the antibody. Site-specific conjugation has been applied broadly over the past decade in both preclinical and clinical settings.

Bispecific and biparatopic ADCs are discussed in chapter 11, "Bispecific and Biparatopic Antibody-Drug Conjugates" by Frank Comer, Changshou Gao and Steve Coats. These ADCs can be designed to internalize more efficiently and thus increase potency, or to exhibit improved tumor selectivity, depending on the molecular format. Some of these concepts have gained support from preclinical studies but there is limited clinical experience with this type of ADC. The authors discuss considerations of selection of antigen(s)/target(s) and selection of molecular format.

In chapter 12, "Targeting Drug Conjugates to the Tumor Microenvironment: Probody Drug Conjugates", Jason Sagert and Jack Lin describe two antibody engineering strategies to improve tumor selectivity by exploiting the tumor microenvironment. In one strategy, the antibody is engineered for enhanced binding in the tumor microenvironment, for example lower pH than normal tissue. In the other strategy, exemplified by the probody-drug conjugate (PDC), antigen binding is restricted by a peptide mask that is cleaved from the PDC in the tumor microenvironment, for example by tumor-associated proteases.

The tumor microenvironment can be exploited in another way – for targeting the ADC – as described by Alberto Dal Corso, Samuele Cazzamalli and Dario Neri in chapter 13, "Antibody-Drug Conjugates: Targeting the Tumor Microenvironment". This approach defies the conventional wisdom that ADCs must bind antigens on tumor cells and internalize into the tumor cell to deliver payload. Instead, ADCs could bind non-internalizing targets in the tumor microenvironment and release membrane-permeable payload in the extracellular space. A potential advantage highlighted here is that certain antigens in the tumor microenvironment are broadly expressed across and within many tumor types.

Many of the technological innovations described in this volume will in theory expand the ADC target space – on tumor cells and in the tumor microenvironment. Whether by masking antigen binding, loading more payload, or improving potency or selectivity with bispecific and biparatopic ADCs, these emerging technologies will rewrite the "rules" of ADC target selection in addition to increasing the therapeutic index for current ADC targets. It should also be noted that the technologies generally are not exclusive of the others, and multiple technologies could be combined into one ADC; theoretical examples are provided by Sagert and Lin in chapter 12, "Targeting Drug Conjugates to the Tumor Microenvironment: Probody Drug Conjugates". Of course, the goal is not to make the most complex ADC, but rather the opposite: to make the simplest ADC possible that will have robust clinical benefit.

Finally, in chapter 14, "Next Horizons: ADCs Beyond Oncology", Shan Yu, Andrew Lim and Matthew Tremblay describe the exploration of ADCs beyond oncology. The first non-oncology ADC is entering the clinic for infectious disease, and many other ADCs have been evaluated preclinically for inflammatory and autoimmune diseases, conditioning for hematopoietic stem cell transplants, and other applications. The authors compare and contrast the building blocks of these ADCs with those of oncology-based ADCs. Some of the payloads being explored for non-oncology ADCs are also described by Tumey in chapter 8, "Next Generation Payloads for ADCs". Thus, the innovations that are enabling next-generation ADCs for oncology are also paving the way for the use of this modality in many other therapeutic areas.

Conclusion

"Finally, we must raise our expectations" [10]. As described throughout this volume, as a field, we have substantial preclinical and clinical experience with ADCs, and we have developed innovative technologies to address the issues we encountered. With appropriate discipline and rigor, we can develop next-generation ADCs with the capacity to dramatically improve the lives of patients with cancer and other diseases.

References

1. Bialucha CU, Collins SD, Li X, Saxena P, Zhang X, Dürr C, Lafont B, Prieur P, Shim Y, Mosher R, Lee D, Ostrom L, Hu T, Bilic S, Rajlic IL, Capka V, Jiang W, Wagner JP, Elliott G, Veloso A, Piel JC, Flaherty MM, Mansfield KG, Meseck EK, Rubic-Schneider T, London AS, Tschantz WR, Kurz M, Nguyen D, Bourret A, Meyer MJ, Faris JE, Janatpour MJ, Chan VW, Yoder NC, Catcott KC, McShea MA, Sun X, Gao H, Williams J, Hofmann F, Engelman JA, Ettenberg SA, Sellers WR, Lees E (2017) Discovery and optimization of HKT288, a cadherin-6-targeting ADC for the treatment of ovarian and renal cancers. Cancer Discov 7(9):1030–1045. https://doi.org/10.1158/2159-8290.CD-16-1414. Epub 2017 May 19
2. Chen DS, Mellman I (2017) Elements of cancer immunity and the cancer-immune set point. Nature 541(7637):321–330. https://doi.org/10.1038/nature21349
3. Damelin M, Bankovich A, Bernstein J, Lucas J, Chen L, Williams S, Park A, Aguilar J, Ernstoff E, Charati M, Dushin R, Aujay M, Lee C, Ramoth H, Milton M, Hampl J, Lazetic S, Pulito V, Rosfjord E, Sun Y, King L, Barletta F, Betts A, Guffroy M, Falahatpisheh H, O'Donnell CJ, Stull R, Pysz M, Escarpe P, Liu D, Foord O, Gerber HP, Sapra P, Dylla SJ (2017) A PTK7-targeted antibody-drug conjugate reduces tumor-initiating cells and induces sustained tumor regressions. Sci Transl Med 9(372):pii: eaag2611. https://doi.org/10.1126/scitranslmed.aag2611
4. Damelin M, Zhong W, Myers J, Sapra P (2015) Evolving strategies for target selection for antibody-drug conjugates. Pharm Res 32(11):3494–3507. https://doi.org/10.1007/s11095-015-1624-3. Epub 2015 Jan 15
5. Gerber HP, Koehn FE, Abraham RT (2013) The antibody-drug conjugate: an enabling modality for natural product-based cancer therapeutics. Nat Prod Rep 30(5):625–639. https://doi.org/10.1039/c3np20113a

6. Lambert JM, Morris CQ (2017) Antibody-drug conjugates (ADCs) for personalized treatment of solid tumors: a review. Adv Ther 34(5):1015–1035. https://doi.org/10.1007/s12325-017-0519-6. Epub 2017 Mar 30
7. Mosher R, Poling L, Qin L, Bodyak N, Bergstrom D (2017) Relationship of NaPi2b expression and efficacy of XMT-1536, a NaPi2b targeting antibody-drug conjugate (ADC), in an unselected panel of human primary ovarian mouse xenograft models. Presentation at AACR-NCI-EORTC international conference, Philadelphia, 26–30 October 2017
8. Saunders LR, Bankovich AJ, Anderson WC, Aujay MA, Bheddah S, Black K, Desai R, Escarpe PA, Hampl J, Laysang A, Liu D, Lopez-Molina J, Milton M, Park A, Pysz MA, Shao H, Slingerland B, Torgov M, Williams SA, Foord O, Howard P, Jassem J, Badzio A, Czapiewski P, Harpole DH, Dowlati A, Massion PP, Travis WD, Pietanza MC, Poirier JT, Rudin CM, Stull RA, Dylla SJ (2015) A DLL3-targeted antibody-drug conjugate eradicates high-grade pulmonary neuroendocrine tumor-initiating cells in vivo. Sci Transl Med 7(302):302ra136. https://doi.org/10.1126/scitranslmed.aac9459
9. Sievers EL, Senter PD (2013) Antibody-drug conjugates in cancer therapy. Annu Rev Med 64:15–29
10. Tolcher AW (2016) Antibody drug conjugates: lessons from 20 years of clinical experience. Ann Oncol 27(12):2168–2172. https://doi.org/10.1093/annonc/mdw424. Epub 2016 Oct 11
11. Xu Z, Pothula SP, Wilson JS, Apte MV (2014) Pancreatic cancer and its stroma: a conspiracy theory. World J Gastroenterol 20(32):11216–11229. https://doi.org/10.3748/wjg.v20.i32.11216

Combining ADCs with Immuno-Oncology Agents

Philipp Müller, Jonathan Rios-Doria, Jay Harper, and Anthony Cao

Abstract Immuno-oncology (IO) has emerged as one of the most promising approaches to improve the therapeutic efficacy and durability of clinical responses in cancer patients. However, despite the clinical breakthroughs achieved with immuno-therapies, such as checkpoint blockade, the overall proportion of patients experiencing durable responses to single agent immuno-therapy remains relatively small. Therefore, the real promise for most cancer patients does not lie in mono-therapeutic approaches but in synergistic combination therapies, which combine the best of IO with the immune-promoting/supporting properties of other therapeutic modalities. The latter help to breach physical barriers, to overcome immunosuppressive networks within the tumor microenvironment and improve immune cell infiltration into tumors.

Certain classes of cytotoxic compounds as well as radiation have been shown to induce immunogenic cell death (ICD), which leads to potent stimulation of effector T-cell activation as well as their recruitment into tumors. It has been recently demonstrated that some ADC payloads are also able to elicit ICD. Furthermore, several cytotoxic warheads used in ADCs can directly induce dendritic cell activation and maturation. These previously unknown immune-stimulatory activities of ADCs therefore have the potential to boost anti-tumor immunity and indeed the synergistic activity of various ADC/IO combinations has been observed in preclinical tumor

P. Müller (✉)
Boehringer Ingelheim Pharma GmbH & Co. KG, Department of Cancer Immunology & Immune Modulation, Biberach an der Riss, Germany
e-mail: philipp_3.mueller@boehringer-ingelheim.com

J. Rios-Doria
MedImmune, Gaithersburg, MD, USA

Incyte Wilmington, DE, USA

J. Harper
MedImmune, Gaithersburg, MD, USA

A. Cao
Seattle Genetics, Inc, Bothell, WA, USA

M. Damelin (ed.), *Innovations for Next-Generation Antibody-Drug Conjugates*, Cancer Drug Discovery and Development,
https://doi.org/10.1007/978-3-319-78154-9_2

models. These preclinical data have supported the clinical evaluation of ADC/IO combinatorial approaches.

This chapter summarizes the current scientific knowledge on the immunomodulatory properties of cytotoxic warheads used in ADCs, the underlying molecular mechanisms and immunological as well as therapeutic benefits of combination regimens with immuno-therapies. It further provides an overview of the current clinical landscape of more than 20 clinical trials evaluating the therapeutic benefit of ADC/IO combinations for cancer patients.

Keywords Adcetris · ADC · ADC-IO combinations · Ado-trastuzumab emtansine · Ansamitocin P3 · Antibody drug conjugate · Antigen presentation · Auristatin · Atezolizumab · ATP · Brentuximab vedotin · Calreticulin · CD11c · CD27 · CD39 · CD4 · CD8 · CD73 · CD86 · CD91 · Cell death · Checkpoint inhibitors · Clinical development · Clinical trials · Combination therapy · Combo · CRT · CT26 · CTL-Cytotoxic lymphocyte · CTLA-4 · DCs · Dendritic cells · Dendritic cell activation · Dendritic cell maturation · Depolymerization · Destabilization · DM-1 · Dolastatin · EphA2 · ER stress · Fo5 · FoxP3 · GITR · GITRL · Her2 · HMGB1 · NHL · Non-Hodgkin Lymphoma · ICD · ICD hallmarks · IFN · IGF1R · Immunogenic cell death · Immuno-oncology · Immunotherapy · Interferon · Ipilimumab · Kadcyla · Keytruda · MCA205 · MHC-I · MHC-II · Microtubule Depolymerization · Microtubule Destabilization · MMAE · MyD88 · Nivolumab · Opdivo · OX40 · PBD · PD-1 · PD-L1 · Pembrolizumab · Regulatory T cell · Synergy · TAA · T cells · T cell agonists · T cell activation · T-DM1 · Therapeutic index · Therapy · TLR-4 · Trastuzumab emtansine · Treg · Tubulysin · Tumor · Tumor associated antigen · Varlilumab · Warhead · Yervoy

Introduction

The burgeoning field of immuno-oncology (IO) has led to promising new therapies that have profoundly reshaped the way we look at cancer treatment. In a variety of cancers, the tumor microenvironment is quite immunosuppressive, preventing the immune system from mounting a sufficient anti-tumor response. Cancer cells evade immune recognition through a variety of mechanisms. The tumor microenvironment is often bathed in anti-inflammatory molecules, such as adenosine and TGFβ, that limit the potency and activity of immune cells in the tumor tissue as well as tumor-proximal lymphatics, and allow tumors to grow in an uncontrolled manner. Tumor cells can also modify surface expression of a number of immunomodulatory molecules to escape T cell recognition and dampen T cell effector function. Downregulation of major histocompatibility complex I (MHCI) further limits T cell detection of tumor (neo)-antigens, while increased programmed death-ligand 1 (PD-L1) expression and the presence of other inhibitory immune checkpoints can mediate T cell anergy and exhaustion, thereby neutralizing the immune response [1]. Several strategies have been developed to overcome this immunosuppression and allow cytotoxic T lymphocytes (CTLs) to unleash an effective anti-tumor response. Monoclonal antibodies that antagonize immune checkpoints that normally limit CTL activity have demonstrated clinical efficacy and have been approved for the treatment of various cancers: Ipilimumab (Yervoy®) that targets CTL-associated protein 4 (CTLA4), nivolumab (Opdivo®) and pembrolizumab (Keytruda®) that target programmed cell death protein-1 (PD-1) as well as atezolizumab that targets the PD-1 ligand, PD-L1 [2]. In addition, several IO agents targeting alternative pathways that stimulate an immune response, for example OX40, GITRL, CD73 and others, are currently being investigated in clinical trials [3, 4].

While checkpoint inhibitors have demonstrated striking efficacy in the clinic, their success is critically dependent on the strength of the immune response against the tumor, and only a subset of individuals exhibit durable responses. In the event of low mutational load/neoantigenicity, or poor immune infiltration into the tumor, monotherapy checkpoint inhibition has proven to be largely ineffective [5, 6]. Therapeutic agents that increase infiltration into these "immune-deserts" or so-called immunologically "cold" or "non-T cell-inflamed" tumors, or have the ability to convert the "cold" tumors into "hot" or "T cell-inflamed" tumors, increase the likelihood of generating effective, tumor antigen-specific immune responses [7]. Recently, a mode of apoptosis, referred to as immunogenic cell death, has been described, by means of which dying tumor cells are able to potently activate the immune system. Experimental evidence has been presented, that ADCs can induce changes that are consistent with ICD induction [8, 9], and that ADCs containing either microtubule-targeting or DNA-damaging payloads can both interact synergistically with current immunotherapies in a therapeutic setting [10, 11].

This chapter will (1) describe the mechanism of immunogenic cell death (ICD), (2) present a summary on the preclinical validation of DC maturation and induction of ICD by ADC warheads, (3) provide evidence that combining the immunomodulatory effects of ADCs with immunotherapies can result in enhanced anti-tumor activity and (4) summarize the clinical studies evaluating such ADC-IO combinations.

Immunogenic Cell Death

ICD is a specific type of cell death that is able to stimulate immune responses against antigens expressed by dying cells. The hallmark outcome of ICD in cancer therapy is the killing of cancer cells that subsequently induces anti-cancer immunity and formation of an immunological memory. ICD-mediated killing of cancer cells provides immune education, which is critical to resist secondary exposure/tumor challenge/relapse in the absence of any additional treatment [12]. The gold-standard functional assay for determining whether therapeutic agents can induce ICD is to treat tumor cells with these drugs in vitro and administer the dying cancer cells to immune competent mice as a vaccination [13]. Cells undergoing ICD elicit an immune memory response that protects mice from subsequent challenges with live tumor cells of the same type, in the absence of any adjuvant. In essence, cancer cells dying from ICD serve as an endogenous vaccine to stimulate tumor-specific immune responses against any residual disease, or in the event of relapse/recurrence.

Intrinsically, tumor cells undergoing ICD display a unique set of characteristics that potentiate their immunogenicity. While most commonly-used cytotoxic therapeutics induce apoptosis, only a few are able to induce ICD [14]. The long-term T cell memory associated with ICD induction requires both potent antigenicity and adjuvanticity in order to provoke efficient recognition of (neo)-antigens and stimulate appropriate immune responses, which include signal transmission via specific pathogen-associated molecular patterns (PAMPs) and damage-associated molecular patterns (DAMPs) [15, 16]. Resident and infiltrating immune cells become activated by cognate receptors that recognize inflammatory signals and promote anti-tumor immunity. Highlighting the importance of ICD in tumor immunity, patients whose carcinomas displayed increased ICD-related immune responses following treatment tended to have improved prognosis compared to patients whose carcinomas featured decreased expression of ICD-associated molecular hallmarks and immune effector genes post-treatment [17–19]. As such, tumor cells dying from ICD appear to have the unique capability to establish a pro-inflammatory environment that promotes anti-tumor immune responses with clinically meaningful benefits.

The Hallmarks of ICD

Considerable biochemical work has revealed a number of distinctive hallmark properties of cells undergoing ICD: translocation of calreticulin (CRT) to the cell surface, secretion of ATP during apoptosis, release of the nuclear protein HMGB1, and secretion of IFNα from dying cells [13]. Satisfaction of all of these criteria in vitro leads to bona fide ICD induction, which can be confirmed by effective vaccination against live tumor challenges, via injection of the in vitro treated cancer cells into immune competent mice. Extensive work has revealed that lack of any of these characteristics leads to ineffective anti-tumor immunity [20].

CRT is a molecular chaperone involved in protein folding, which is typically found within the endoplasmic reticulum but becomes translocated to the cell surface as ecto-CRT during ER stress and ICD. Ecto-CRT functions as a potent phagocytosis signal when exposed on the surface of stressed and dying cells. CRT engagement of CD91 on phagocytes results in phagocytosis of the dying cancer cell and the induction of proinflammatory responses [21]. Critically, uptake of CRT-expressing bodies from dying tumor cells likely facilitates differential processing of the phagocytosed material, such that the phagocytes are able to process their antigens and prime cognate immune responses [22]. Surface expression of CRT is required for optimal ICD induction, and labeling apoptotic bodies with CRT can restore some immunogenicity to agents unable to confer ICD [20, 23]. While CRT functions as a potent "eat-me" signal, tumor cell-expressed CD47 functions as an anti-phagocytic "don't-eat-me" signal, and the balance between CD47 and CRT helps dictate the fate of the tumor cell. Indeed, therapeutic targeting of CD47 with monoclonal antibodies has been shown to drive T cell-mediated tumor destruction, which is abrogated when calreticulin is blocked, highlighting the important role of CRT in tumor elimination [24, 25].

Treatment with ICD-inducing agents can tip the balance of signals towards increased CRT surface expression and potentiate phagocytosis and antigen-processing. Notably, high CRT on tumors has been associated with improved outcomes in non-small cell lung cancer (NSCLC) [26] and melanoma [15, 27], while low CRT was correlated with poor survival and T cell infiltration [28, 29]. Importantly, induction of ER stress and the unfolded protein response is required for the surface expression of CRT and other protein-folding chaperones to mediate ICD induction. As such, severe and chronic ER stress is found to be activated by ICD-inducing agents, which eventually results in immunogenic cell death [30].

ATP is utilized as the energy currency of living cells. Produced in the mitochondria, ATP is stored within vesicles throughout the cell. Given the critical role of ATP in cellular survival, active secretion of ATP out of the cell is a rather unusual phenomenon. Induction of ICD involves activation of various autophagy pathways, culminating in expression of pannexin channels in the cell membrane that actively pump out ATP into the extracellular space [30]. Inhibition of tumor cell autophagy prevents the secretion of ATP, and limits the immunogenicity of dying cancer cells. Consistently, presence of autophagosomes was correlated with increased immune infiltrate in various carcinomas [31–34]. Extracellular ATP functions as a strong chemoattractant, stimulating migration of innate immune cells to the tumor environment. ATP also has immune effector function by signaling through purinergic receptors P2X7 and P2Y2 on infiltrating immune cells, triggering inflammasome activation and IL-1β secretion, as well as enhancing costimulatory and antigen-presentation function [15, 30, 35]. However, normal and cancer cell microenvironments have ways of converting ATP into immunosuppressive molecules. While ATP has proinflammatory effects, its metabolites ADP, AMP and adenosine actually dampen the immune response. The release of ATP from cells undergoing ICD can stimulate enhanced proinflammatory reactions from the initial tumor infiltrating immune cells. However, the short half-life of ATP, and sequential processing of ATP into ADP, AMP, and adenosine by the CD39/CD73 pathway allow for subsequent anti-inflammatory responses elicited by AMP and adenosine to be triggered, thereby dampening the immune response as multiple waves of immune cells respond to the inflamed tumor environment. Numerous cancer types possess altered gene expression, that prevents ATP secretion through autophagy, or overexpress the ATP exonucleases CD39 and CD73, thereby converting any ATP that does get released from, e.g. dying cancer cells into anti-inflammatory AMP and adenosine [15]. The enrichment of these genes in cancer establishes an increasingly immunosuppressive and pro-tumor microenvironment. Notably, strategies to inhibit the exonucleases/receptors (CD39, CD73, A2R) that process ATP into AMP and adenosine are beginning to see utility in preclinical and clinical settings [3, 36].

HMGB1 is a chromatin-interacting protein found within the nucleus of all cells. As a nuclear protein, HMGB1 is released after membrane permeabilization during necrosis. As cancer cells die and undergo ICD, HMGB1 is released from the cancer cell although it remains unclear whether there is an active secretion of the protein, or whether there is passive release as the cell dies. Regardless, extracellular HMGB1 is highly proinflammatory, binding to toll-like receptor 4 (TLR4) or receptor for advanced glycation end-products (RAGE) on innate immune cells in the surrounding stroma. HMGB1 signaling through either TLR4 or RAGE elicits proinflammatory responses through the MyD88 and NF-κB pathways, resulting in activated immune cells [13]. Notably, signaling through TLR4/MyD88 promotes endosomal recycling compartment fusion with phagosomes, thus enabling tumor-antigen processing through both the MHCI and MHCII pathways, which is critical for presentation and recognition of tumor-associated neoantigenes [37–39]. Furthermore, breast cancer patients harboring a single-nucleotide polymorphism in TLR4 (Asp299Gly) have an increased likelihood of early relapse after anthracycline treatment, as a potential consequence of poor response to ICD induction [16].

The induction of type I interferon (IFN) has recently been identified as an important factor released during ICD and is critical for driving subsequent induction of protective anti-tumor immunity [40]. Normally secreted upon viral or bacterial infection, type I IFNs function to increase the resistance of neighboring cells to infection, by slowing cellular processes and restricting proliferation. Type I IFNs are a crucial host defense mechanism, as virtually all cells are able to secrete IFNα, thereby providing strong stimulation of innate immune cells and cytotoxic natural killer cells. IFNα release profoundly alerts the immune system to the presence of pathogens and infected cells. Within the tumor space, IFNα release is a newly-identified ICD hallmark and it is hypothesized that tumor cell-derived RNA is able to activate intracellular TLR3 in order to elicit IFN production. As such, polymorphisms or loss-of-function mutations in the TLR3 gene or IFN receptors are seen in many carcinomas and metastases [15]. Furthermore, enzymes responsible for RNA editing are found to be increased in a variety of tumors, likely leading to suppression of interferon signaling [41–43].

While fulfilling each of these characteristics is required to demonstrate bona fide ICD induction, it is likely that the subsequent immune activation and extent of conferred anti-tumor protection will vary based on the agent, tumor type, and individual treated. Furthermore, the relative contribution, that each of these molecular "ICD hallmarks" plays in the induction of protective immune responses is currently not yet fully resolved. Many of the compounds screened for bona fide ICD induction did not fulfill all of the required characteristics associated with induction of ICD when used individually. However, some combinations of non-ICD-inducing agents were able to convert immunologically silent cancer cell death into ICD by complementary activity and elicit all of the required characteristics when used in combination [20, 44]. Notably, adsorption of free calreticulin to apoptotic bodies, or addition of exogenous TLR4 ligands has been shown to restore ICD and adaptive immunity in preclinical tumor models [45].

In summary, the improved immune cell infiltration and antigen processing that is characteristic of ICD improves the likelihood of tumor recognition by both arms of the adaptive immune system. From this perspective, ICD induction strengthens the foundation of the adaptive immune response directed against tumor antigens. Subsequent follow-up with checkpoint inhibition or agonists of the TNF receptor superfamily further magnifies the amplitude and duration of the T cell response.

Consistent with this hypothesis are numerous reported studies that combine immunogenic forms of chemotherapy with checkpoint inhibition and observe increased anti-tumor efficacy. These include but are not limited to radiation therapy, oxaliplatin, and anthracyclines [46–49]. The next section of the chapter will highlight how small molecule cytotoxics, typically used as ADC warheads are capable of having direct effects on antigen presenting cells and how these warheads, as well as ADCs conjugated with these warheads, are capable of eliciting ICD.

ADCs, Anti-Tumor Immunity and ICD

Classic ICD inducers include anthracyclines, cardiac glycosides, and notable platinum agents; however, these drugs have not been successful as ADC payloads due to either an inability to chemically link them to an antibody or a lack of sufficient potency. Certain microtubule inhibitors (auristatins, maytansinoids, and tubulysins) and DNA-targeting agents (calicheamicin, pyrrolobenzodiazepines) have been shown to be exceptionally potent payloads for ADCs [50]. As will be described in the rest of this chapter, recent data provide striking evidence that ADCs conjugated with these microtubule-inhibitors or DNA targeting agents provoke strong innate and adaptive immune responses against syngeneic tumor models, and thereby confer anti-tumor protection via direct effects on antigen-presenting cells (APCs) and by inducing ICD [10, 11, 51]. In addition, these agents exhibit profound anti-tumor synergy with IO drugs with different mechanisms of action.

Expression of calreticulin on the surface of dying cells is a critical hallmark of ICD induction, and immune activation. While the mechanism of CRT translocation to the cell surface is not completely understood, the detection of misfolded/unfolded proteins in the endoplasmic reticulum (ER) and the ER stress response is required for ecto-CRT expression, and bona fide ICD induction [52, 53]. Mammalian cells express IRE1, PERK, and ATF6 in the ER, all 3 of which function as sensors of misfolded proteins by detecting exposed hydrophobic domains and free cysteine residues [54]. Activation of these sensors leads to the unfolded protein response, a transcriptional program focused on relieving the burden of unfolded proteins in the ER by attenuating *de novo* global transcription, and induction of protein-folding chaperones. However, severe or chronic ER stress leads to apoptosis when the stress burden cannot be overcome. The ER possesses elasticity to accommodate the proper environment to facilitate protein folding, and its flexibility is dependent on microtubule activity. Given the dependence on microtubule integrity, preliminary data has revealed that targeted disruption of microtubules can induce severe ER stress [8].

Brentuximab vedotin (BV, ADCETRIS®) is an antibody-drug conjugate (ADC) directed against CD30. It consists of an anti-CD30 monoclonal antibody conjugated to monomethyl auristatin E (MMAE), a microtubule-disrupting agent. BV is approved for the treatment of relapsed Hodgkin lymphoma (HL) and systemic anaplastic large cell lymphoma (sALCL). The anti-tumor activity of BV is due to the binding of the ADC to CD30-expressing cells, followed by internalization, and release of MMAE after proteolytic cleavage resulting in microtubule depolymerization and subsequently in apoptosis of cancer cells. While BV induced cell death has been extensively studied, its potential immune modulatory activity has yet to be explored. Treatment of $CD30^+$ lymphoma cells with BV led to a disrupted microtubule network, indicative of MMAE delivery [8]. Disruption of the microtubule network led to mislocalization of the ER and ER fragmentation, which resulted in ER stress responses marked by the phosphorylation of IRE1. Activation of ER stress and IRE1 was confirmed by the increase in phosphorylation of the downstream effector Jun N-terminal kinase (JNK). The expression of CRT and HSP70 (another ER chaperone) on the cell surface, prior to apoptosis, is concurrent with ER stress induction. Functionally, cells killed by BV were able to invoke proinflammatory immune reactions. Dendritic cells that were exposed to BV-killed cells expressed increased amounts of co-stimulatory molecules and cytokines. Importantly, these dendritic cells were capable of inducing inflammatory activity in cytotoxic T cells [8, 55]. These results indicate that auristatin-ADCs are capable of killing tumor cells in a manner that is consistent with ICD induction, and may prove potent partners for clinical combination therapies with IO agents. The following sections will enumerate the immune-modulating properties of ADCs (Fig. 1).

Direct Activation of Antigen-Presenting Cells by Tubulin-Depolymerizing ADC Payloads

In addition to eliciting ICD, a second, direct mechanism of immune cell activation, namely the maturation and activation of APCs such as dendritic cells (DCs), has recently been attributed to certain microtubule-destabilizing ADC warheads. Previously, the microtubule inhibitors vinblastine, colchicine and podophyllotoxin had been identified as direct inducers of DC maturation [56–58]. Further research was recently conducted to investigate whether additional inhibitors of microtubule assembly, including dolastatin 10, dolastatin 15, monomethyl auristatin E (MMAE), ansamitocin P3, DM1, vindesine, vincristine and combretastatin-A4 possessed similar activity [9, 10, 51]. Of all the agents tested, the dolastatins and their synthetic auristatin analogues, as well as the maytansinoids DM1 and ansamitocin P3 (a precursor in the synthesis of DM1) were by far the most potent inducers of functional DC maturation. Interestingly, such effects on DC maturation were only observed following treatment with microtubule-destabilizing cytotoxics, whereas microtubule-stabilizing compounds such as taxanes were not able to induce DC maturation. These data suggest that this may be a "class effect", common to microtubule-depolymerizing agents, and that depolymerisation of microtubules results in the induction of a maturational program in DCs.

Direct activation of antigen presenting cells, such as DCs, is highly attractive from an immunotherapy perspective and may provide a fertile ground for the induction of potent anti-tumor immunity. DCs are central players during the initia-

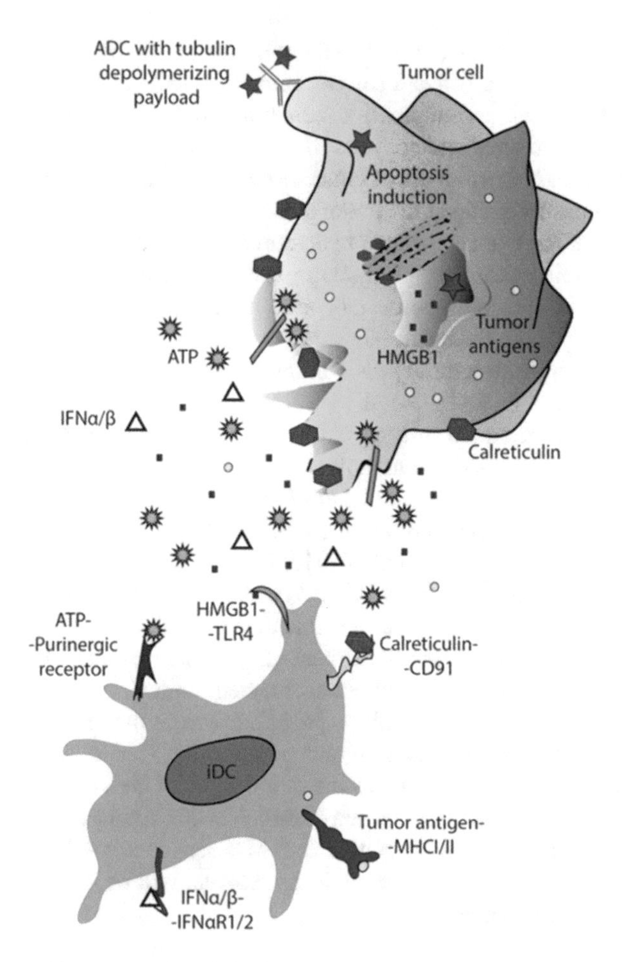

Fig. 1 Summary of immunogenic cell death and immune modulation. Certain chemotherapeutics and ADCs conjugated with specific warheads can induce immunogenic cell death (ICD) and modulate immune responses within the tumor. Induction of ICD requires the following characteristics to optimally confer anti-tumor immunity: (1) surface expression of calreticulin (CRT), (2) ATP secretion, (3) HMGB1 release, and (4) type I interferon (IFN) release. CRT is transported from the endoplasmic reticulum (ER) to the cell surface after induction of ER stress and the unfolded protein response. Surface CRT engages CD91 to provide a phagocytic signal and to facilitate tumor antigen processing and presentation. Induction of ER stress and ICD triggers autophagy, culminating in ATP secretion through pannexin channels of dying tumor cells. Extracellular ATP engages P2X7 and P2Y2 purinergic receptors and functions as a chemoattractant for immune cells, as well as eliciting inflammasome signalling. HMGB1 is released from membrane-compromised cells and nuclei and signals through TLR4 to activate immune cells. In addition, type I IFNs are produced by tumor cells and activates immune cells, after TLR3 activation through tumor derived RNAs, similar to what is observed during anti-viral immunity

tion of anti-tumor immunity, once they are fully matured. The vast majority of DCs found in solid tumors are dysfunctional immature DCs that are tolerogenic and contribute to the immunosuppressive tumor microenvironment. Any therapeutic approach, which matures and converts these cells into professional APCs will not only help to increase recruitment of tumor-reactive T cells but will also significantly reduce immunosuppression at the tumor site.

Further work has been conducted to determine how the auristatins and maytansinoids are capable of directly promoting maturation and activation of DCs. Data suggests that this DC maturation is independent of MyD88-dependent TLR signalling and unlikely to be the result of a direct triggering of other pattern-recognition receptors as all these structurally distinct inhibitors of microtubule polymerization exert similar effects on DC maturation and function. Microtubule depolymerizing compounds are for example able to activate the NF-κB and MAPK signalling pathways, which mediate cell death in rapidly dividing cancer cells on one had [59, 60] but on the other hand are an integral part of DC activation in response to pathogens [61–63]. Dolastatins, auristatins, ansamitocin P3 and DM1 all induced the upregulation of co-stimulatory molecules (CD40, CD80/CD86 and MHC-II) as well as pro-inflammatory cytokines (interleukins 1, 6 and 12) in mouse and human DCs [9, 10, 51]. These compounds were further able to induce functional DC activation in T cell:DC co-culture experiments. Treatment of syngeneic tumors with unconjugated dolastatins or maytansinoids in immunocompetent animals resulted in T cell- and DC-dependent tumor growth inhibition [9, 51]. It was further demonstrated that the treatment resulted in the activation of tumor-infiltrating T cells and synergized with immune checkpoint inhibition consisting of blockade of both CTLA4 and PD-1 [9, 10, 51]. Dolastatins/auristatins or maytansinoids are conjugated as payloads to tumor-selective antibodies to generate potent ADCs; as such, the translation of these findings into settings that are more clinically relevant will be the subject of the following sections of this chapter.

Activation of Anti-tumor Immunity by ADCs

Treatment of differentiated DCs in vitro, DC:tumor cell co-cultures, or DCs from primary human tumor resections with free cytotoxic compounds may produce effects different from delivering the same drug to tumors in vivo via an ADC. In vitro, free cytotoxic compounds are able to cross the plasma membrane barrier and reach their molecular target within multiple cell types, independent of the expression of an ADC target on tumor cells. Delivery of ADCs to tumors and release of the payload may follow completely different kinetics, and be heavily dependent on the antibody selectivity, functionalization (e.g. Fc), as well as linker chemistry and payload characteristics (e.g. membrane permeability). In addition, cleavage of the payload from the linker may result in altered payload metabolite structures and properties (e.g. polarity, target engagement and membrane permeability), as is the case for the cysteine adduct of DM1, which is generated upon proteolytic degradation of the antibody portion of the ADC within lysosomes.

The previously described experimental data demonstrated that two molecular classes of cytotoxic compounds that destabilize microtubules, auristatins/dolastatins and maytansinoids, not only induce cytotoxicity in rapidly dividing cancer cells, but are also exceptionally potent mediators of phenotypic and functional DC activation. However, it was critical to determine if these same effects were consistent when tumor cells or tumors were treated with ADCs conjugated with these same warheads. To this end, activation of DCs co-cultured with $CD30^+$ lymphoma cells required the binding and internalization of BV and subsequent release of the MMAE payload within lymphoma cells as DCs were not activated when co-cultured with $CD30^-$ tumor cells that were previously treated with BV [9]. To exclude the possibility that DC activation was solely due to indirect effects of BV-mediated apoptosis of lymphoma cells, tumor cells were exposed to and killed by a panel of free cytotoxic compounds prior to inclusion in the co-culture assays. As anticipated, these treatments did not result in elevated DC activation [9]. It therefore appears that, at least in this case, the ADC needs to be processed within tumor cells to free the payload and make it accessible to DCs. Whether the free payload can directly cross the plasma membranes of tumor-resident, immature DCs, or is taken up via phagocytosis of tumor cell debris by DCs may be different from ADC to ADC. Regardless of the mechanism of uptake, ADC payload-mediated activation of DCs may be critically important in priming the immune system.

BV has been reported to not only induce sustainable therapeutic responses in heavily pre-treated cancer patients but also to modulate the immune contexture and activation status, both in the periphery as well as locally at the tumor site. On one hand, BV counteracted immunosuppression through cytokine upregulation, reduction of regulatory T cells (T_{regs}) as well as immune cell recruitment and activation [9, 64, 65]. In the latter case, a lymphoma-specific increase in CD161-expressing T cells, an increase in activation marker-positive T cells as well as DCs and B-cells expressing elevated levels of co-stimulatory molecules was observed in the blood of BV-treated patients. Furthermore, a treatment-induced increase in tumor infiltrating CD4 and CD8 positive T cells was observed [9, 64, 65]. These ADC-based immune-activation data are further substantiated by the analysis of serial biopsies taken from treatment naïve breast cancer patients, who had received a single injection of another ADC, ado-trastuzumab emtansine (T-DM1 / Kadcyla®), conjugated with a DC-activating maytansinoid warhead, within the WSG-ADAPT trial. Comparison of pre- and post-treatment biopsies revealed a significant, therapy-induced infiltration of lymphocytes [10].

To further investigate these effects, an orthotopic, human Her2-driven allograft breast cancer model, Fo5, was utilized. Using this tumor model, which was originally developed and used to characterize ADCs such as T-DM1 [66], it was demonstrated that tumors treated with T-DM1 displayed an increased density of tumor infiltrating CD4 and CD8 positive T cells, which were highly activated, secreted interferon-γ (IFNγ), and upregulated inhibitory receptors, such as CTLA-4 and PD-L1 [10]. With regard to PD-1, it should be noted that its ligand, PD-L1, which is required for the induction of inhibitory signals within PD-1 expressing T cells was almost undetectable on myeloid cells in control tumors but highly upregulated after a single administration of T-DM1. It was also found that the therapeutic efficacy of T-DM1 was dependent on the presence of T cells as depletion of T cells in tumor models significantly reduced the anti-tumor activity of T-DM1 [10]. Together, these findings provided a clear rationale for the therapeutic combination of T-DM1 and checkpoint inhibitors.

Therapeutic Synergy of T-DM1 and Immune-Checkpoint Inhibition

The anti-tumor immunity mediated by ADCs indicates that there is a profound potential for synergies with IO drugs. Recently, published work demonstrated enhanced anti-tumor activity when T-DM1 was combined with checkpoint inhibitors targeting CTLA-4 and PD-1 [10]. Using the orthotopic Her2$^+$ Fo5 breast cancer models described in the previous section, it was shown that ADCs armed with tubulin depolymerizing warheads not only promote T cell immunity on their own, but display greatly enhanced therapeutic efficacy when combined with immune-checkpoint inhibition. The combination therapy resulted in almost universally complete responses (CRs) in tumor-bearing mice. These data argue for a synergistic combination effect, considering that this model is refractory to immune-checkpoint inhibition on its own. In addition, the combination therapy endowed the cured mice with a protective and long lasting immunological memory, making them resistant to a re-challenge with tumor cells of the same origin. Treatment with the combination therapy was accompanied by a significant T cell infiltration into the tumors (see Fig. 2), induction of cytokines (IL-1β, IL-4, IL-10 and IFN-γ), chemokines (MIP1α/β and CCL5), a pronounced Th1 polarization (Tbet upregulation in CD4 T cells) as well as an upregulation of the activation/proliferation markers CTLA-4, Granzyme B, Ki-67, PD-1 and Tim-3 [10].

The precise mechanism by which ADCs can synergize with IO drugs is unclear at this point, although it is likely a combination of the diverse effects induced by each single agent. As has been demonstrated, ADCs with these tubulin depolymerizing warheads are capable of direct tumor cell killing, induction of ICD and direct activation of tumor-resident antigen presenting cells, which most likely facilitates the presentation of tumor associated antigens and the induction of an anti-tumor T cell immunity. In addition, trastuzumab (the antibody component of T-DM1) contains a functional Fc domain, and may activate NK cells, capable of eliciting antibody-dependent cellular cytotoxicity (ADCC) against opsonized tumor cells. There are also hints that tumor-resident M2 polarized and tolerogenic macrophages may be repolarized by the ADC towards a M1-like, tumoricidal phenotype, as evidenced by the loss of arginase expression in these cells [10]. Taken together, ADCs appear to be able to leverage these factors in concert to convert the tumor

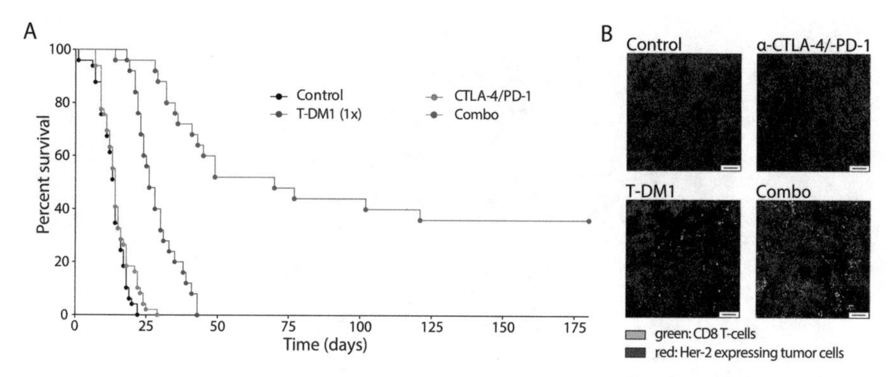

Fig. 2 Therapeutic Synergy of T-DM1 and α-CTLA4/-PD1. (**a**) Fo5 tumor-bearing mice were treated with the indicated reagents. T-DM1 in single dose Combo indicates a single dose of T-DM1 plus CTLA4 and PD-1 blocking antibodies. Once tumors reached an average volume of 80 mm^3 (day 0), mice were treated with T-DM1 (15 mg/kg) and/or anti-mouse PD-1 (10 mg/kg) and anti-mouse CTLA-4 (10 mg/kg). Anti–CTLA-4/PD-1 was given as monotherapy on days 0, 2, 4, 7, and 10 as well as in combination with 1× T-DM1 on days 7, 9, 11, 14, and 17. Mice were euthanized once the tumors exceeded a size of 1200 mm^3. (**b**) Tumors treated as indicated were stained for Her2 (red) and $CD8^+$ T cells (green). Both, panel A and B were modified from the original publication [10]

microenvironment into a T cell-inflamed milieu, which favours anti-tumor immunity and tumor rejection [67].

One of the rather unexpected findings in the described T-DM1 study was the massive increase in T_{reg} frequency amongst the tumor infiltrating $CD4^+$ T cells, since these cells have been associated with the dampening of CTL immunity [68]. The $CD8^+$ T cell to T_{reg} (CD8:T_{reg}) ratio even declined in the treatment group receiving the combination therapy, which is in contrast to the majority of reported cancer-immunotherapy studies employing cell line based, subcutaneous tumor models. An increase in the CD8:T_{reg} ratio is usually correlated with the therapeutic success of a given immunotherapy [69]. The activity of the combination therapy, despite the increased T_{reg} frequencies, is even more impressive given the demonstration that T_{regs} from these mice are immunosuppressive; T_{regs} from control and treated mice were equally potent in blocking in vitro T cell proliferation [10]. The crucial role of these cells only became apparent upon depleting $CD4^+$ and $CD8^+$ T cells from these mice. While the latter reduced the therapeutic efficacy as expected, deletion of T_{regs} (CD4 T cells) resulted in severe and in some cases lethal autoimmunity, a side-effect that was $CD8^+$ T cell-mediated as co-deletion of CTLs prevented the onset of autoimmunity. Therefore, it is clear that in this model T_{regs} are absolutely vital to protect the animals from hyperactivation of the immune system induced by the combination therapy. It will be important to be cognizant of this effect of ADC-IO combinations on T_{regs} as these are tested in the clinic, but as will be discussed later in this chapter, the impact of ADC-IO combos on T_{regs} may be influenced by the payload and/or cancer type (Fig. 3).

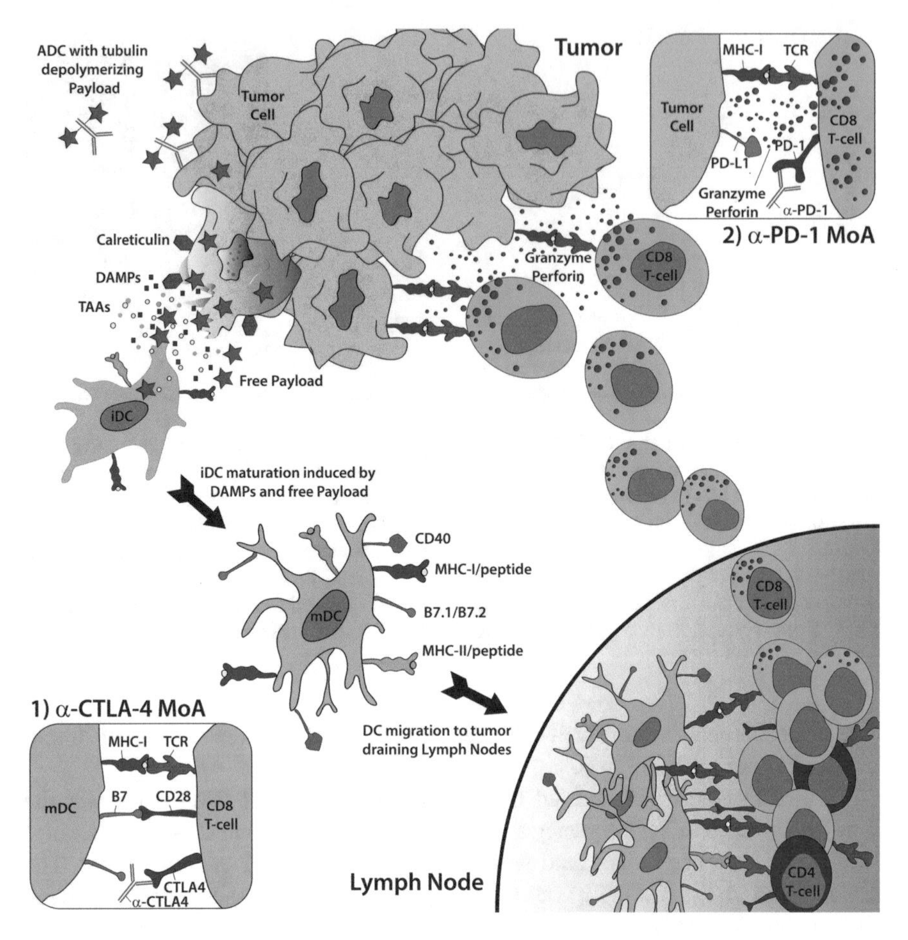

Fig. 3 DC activation by tubulin-depolymerizing ADC payloads, ICD and checkpoint inhibition. An ADC armed with a tubulin-depolymerizing warhead (e.g. DM1 or MMAE) engages tumor cells, gets internalized and kills the tumor cells; inducing immunogenic cell death (ICD) characterized by the hallmarks of ICD, such as extracellular calreticulin exposure, HMGB1 and ATP release. Tumor cell debris, tumor-associated antigens (TAAs) and ADC payload are engulfed by tumor resident, tolerogenic immature DCs (iDCs), which through exposure to damage associated molecular patterns (DAMPs) and the payload are induced to mature. At the same time these DCs upregulate co-stimulatory as well as MHC molecules, which are essential for the efficient presentation of TAAs within tumor draining lymph nodes, to which the DCs migrate upon activation. These mature DCs (mDCs) are very efficient APCs, able to induce potent anti-tumor T cell immunity. As a consequence activated, TAA specific T cells move back to the tumor and killing the tumor cells, which may have survived the initial ADC treatment

Additional Therapeutic ADC-IO Combinations

Aside from maytansinoids, in preclinical models other ADC payloads have been investigated for immunogenic properties, including auristatins, pyrrolobenzodiazepines (PBDs), tubulysins, calicheamicins and anthracyclines [70]. While anthracyclines are well-known to be classical inducers of ICD, early ADCs containing anthracyclines failed clinical trials due to immunogenicity, linker instability and insufficient potency [71]. To overcome these limitations, next-generation anthracycline-containing ADCs with significantly higher potency and site-specific conjugation have been recently developed and have been shown to possess immunostimulatory properties in preclinical models [72]. While there has been no data implicating immunostimulatory properties of calicheamicin-based ADCs as of yet, it has been recently shown that auristatin-containing ADCs induce ICD by mediating ER stress responses [8].

Two other ADC payload classes that have entered the clinic are PBDs and tubulysins. PBDs are derivatives of naturally occurring antibiotics that bind to the minor groove of DNA forming inter- and intra-strand cross-linked adducts [73]. Tubulysins are anti-mitotic agents that function to depolymerize microtubules [74]. Although their cytotoxic modes of action are well-understood, little is known about their effects on immune cells. Therefore, the immunomodulatory functions of these ADC payloads were studied in syngeneic mouse tumor models in a recent study [11]. To test whether tubulysin or PBD warheads could induce ICD, a vaccination/challenge experiment was conducted in immunocompetent BALB/c mice [14]. Mice were implanted with tumor cells pre-treated with either PBD or tubulysin in vitro, followed by implantation with live CT26 cells on the opposite flank 1 week later. Both PBD- and tubulysin-treated cells were able to serve as vaccines, leading to protective anti-tumor immunity and tumor rejection upon re-challenge with CT26 tumor cells, indicating that these warheads are able to induce ICD [11]. In order to investigate whether ADCs conjugated to either PBD or tubulysin payloads could induce protective anti-tumor immunity in vivo, ADCs were prepared targeting the tumor-associated antigen (TAA) EphA2, namely EphA2-PBD and EphA2-tubulysin [11, 75]. The antibody used in this ADC was selected for these studies in syngeneic mouse models as it cross reacts with mouse EphA2. EphA2 expression was observed in several commonly used mouse tumor cell lines including CT26, MCA205, 4T1, and Renca [11]. In both the CT26 and MCA205 tumor models, mice that were cured following treatment with either EphA2-PBD or EphA2-tubulysins rejected tumors when re-challenged with the same tumor cell line. Functional analyses of spleens from these mice demonstrated the presence of memory T cells, which likely contributed to the vaccination effect of ADC treatment. Taken together, these data demonstrated that PBD- and tubulysin-based ADCs induced anti-tumor immunity in vivo.

Given the observed effects of the ADCs on T cells, the relative anti-tumor activity of EphA2 ADCs in tumor models grown in immunocompetent vs. immunodeficient mice was explored, to determine the contribution of a functional immune system to the ADC activity. These studies demonstrated that both EphA2-PBD and EphA2-

tubulysin were more active in immunocompetent mice compared to immunodeficient mice in the CT26, MCA205, 4T1 and Renca tumor models, again highlighting the critical role of the immune system for the efficacy of these ADCs. Even more telling, depletion studies demonstrated that $CD8^+$ cytotoxic T-lymphocytes (CTLs) were required for full efficacy of the ADCs in the CT26 model; depletion of CTLs resulted in significantly diminished anti-tumor activity of the ADCs. Based on these results, the authors hypothesized that EphA2-tubulysin and EphA2-PBD ADCs could provide increased anti-tumor efficacy when combined with either immune checkpoint inhibitors or agonists of the TNF receptor (TNFR) family, both of which can modulate T cell function. Checkpoint inhibitors targeting the PD-1/PD-L1 pathway and agonists of TNFR members OX40 and glucocorticoid-induced TNFR-related protein (GITR), which are important co-stimulatory receptors on T cells, have been shown to control tumor growth in mouse models [49, 76]. In CT26 tumor-bearing mice, combining either EphA2-tubulysin or EphA2-PBD with multiple different immunotherapies including anti-PD-1 antibodies, anti-PD-L1 antibodies, OX40 ligand fusion protein (OX40L FP) or GITR ligand fusion protein (GITRL FP), resulted in synergistic anti-tumor activity. These data demonstrated that ADCs conjugated with PBD or tubulysin payloads can potentiate the activity of a diverse array of IO drugs with differing mechanisms of action.

In order to determine how the ADCs were affecting immune cells, immunophenotyping was performed on CT26 tumor-bearing mice treated with either EphA2-tubulysin or EphA2-PBD alone or in combination with PD-L1 or OX40 antibodies [11]. EphA2-tubulysin as a single agent increased the percentage of $CD45^+$ leukocytes, $CD8^+$ CTLs, $CD8^+Ki67^+$ proliferating CTLs, and $CD8^+CD69^+$ activated CTLs within the tumor, demonstrating a direct effect on these cells by ADCs armed with this particular payload. Although EphA2-PBD did not significantly increase the percentage of CTLs in CT26 tumors, it did increase the percent of activated CTLs ($CD8^+CD69^+$) within these tumors, suggesting differences in immunomodulatory effects by each payload. Interestingly, neither EphA2-PBD nor EphA2-tubulysin affected the percentage of infiltrating $CD4^+$ cells. In contrast to EphA2-PBD, EphA2-tubulysin increased the percentage of $FOXP3^+$ regulatory T_{regs} within the CT26 tumors slightly. However, due to the increased proliferation of $CD8^+$ CTLs, the CD8:T_{reg} ratio remained elevated following treatment with EphA2-tubulysin, providing one potential mechanism for the enhanced anti-tumor efficacy seen with this ADC in this tumor model. In combination studies, higher percentages of $PD\text{-}1^+$ expressing $CD4^+$ cells and $CD4^+Ki67^+$ proliferating cells within the splenic $CD45^+$ population were observed following treatment with either EphA2-PBD or EphA2-tubulysin and anti-PD-L1 as compared to anti-PD-L1 alone. These data suggest that peripheral activation and proliferation of $CD4^+$ cells in the spleen may be important for the observed increased therapeutic activity with ADC-IO combinations as compared to the single agent activity.

It was previously demonstrated that auristatins and maytansinoids are able to affect DC maturation [9, 10, 51]. Therefore, in addition to evaluating effects of PBD- or tubulysin-conjugated ADCs on various T cell populations, their effects on myeloid cell populations were examined. Immunophenotyping experiments evaluating DC maturation markers demonstrated that EphA2-tubulysin directly increased the percent of $CD86^+$ cells as well as $F4/80^+$ macrophages within the $CD45^+$ cell population in CT26 tumors. Importantly, both EphA2-tubulysin and EphA2-PBD increased the percentage of $CD86^+$ cells within the pool of mature dendritic cells ($CD11c^+MHCII^{hi}$) in CT26 tumors, which suggests higher co-stimulatory and most likely also antigen-presenting capacity of these cells. CD86 was also found to be significantly increased on splenic myeloid populations in mice treated with ADC-IO combinations compared to single agent therapy [11]. The observation of increased CD86 levels on splenic myeloid cells in preclinical models, may be mechanistically linked to the observed increase in peripheral, activated DCs in BV-treated cancer patients and could also be contributing to the increased anti-tumor efficacy in ADC-IO combinations compared to single agent therapy.

In order to determine if the enhanced activity of ADC-IO combinations would be observed in tumor models with microenvironments distinct from CT26 tumors, similar efficacy and immunophenotyping experiments were carried out in the Renca syngeneic renal cell carcinoma model [11]. The Renca model was previously shown to be dependent on T_{regs} for growth, as depletion of $CD4^+$ cells resulted in tumor rejection [77]. Combining the EphA2-PBD with a CD4-depleting antibody resulted in greater anti-tumor activity than anti-CD4 alone in the Renca model. Examination of the TIL profile within Renca tumors following EphA2-PBD treatment showed a transient decrease in the number of $CD45^+$ and CD4+ T cells (including CD4 + FOXP3+ T_{regs}), which rebounded 12 days post-administration. Immunohistochemistry did not detect EphA2 expression on tumor-resident TILs, suggesting that $CD45^+$ TILs were not directly targeted by the ADC. Instead, the data suggest that $CD45^+$ cells were likely killed due to bystander effect of EphA2-PBD ADC, where free warhead released from target-positive tumor cells undergoing apoptosis is taken up by and induces apoptosis in neighboring cells in the tumor. Due to the lower expression of EphA2 in Renca tumors, a relatively high dose of EphA2-PBD was required for efficacy in this model, which may explain the transient decrease in $CD45^+$ cells as compared to using a lower dose of the ADC, where this deleterious effect was not observed [11].

Given the negative impact of EphA2-PBD on T_{regs} and the dependency of the Renca tumors on T_{regs}, studies were carried out to determine if combining EphA2-PBD with GITRL FP, a molecule that has been shown to deplete T_{regs} [78], could enhance anti-tumor efficacy. Indeed, co-administration of EphA2-PBD and GITRL FP in the Renca model resulted in synergistic efficacy with 9/10 animals achieving complete remissions (CRs) while 0/10 and 3/10 CRs were observed with either EphA2-PBD and GITRL FP administered as single agent therapies, respectively. Immunophenotyping demonstrated that mice that received the combination had a higher CD8:T_{reg} ratio in the tumor compared to mice treated with either GITRL FP or EphA2-PBD alone. The data suggest that the transient decrease in T_{regs} by EphA2-PBD complements the T_{reg} depletion mediated by GITRL FP, resulting in the recruitment of higher levels of $CD8^+$ cells into the tumor.

PBD-conjugated ADCs targeting EphA2 and other TAAs were investigated further in additional tumor models. Contrary to its effects in CT26 tumors, EphA2-PBD induced robust infiltration of CTLs in the MCA205 model (Fig. 4a). Next, an

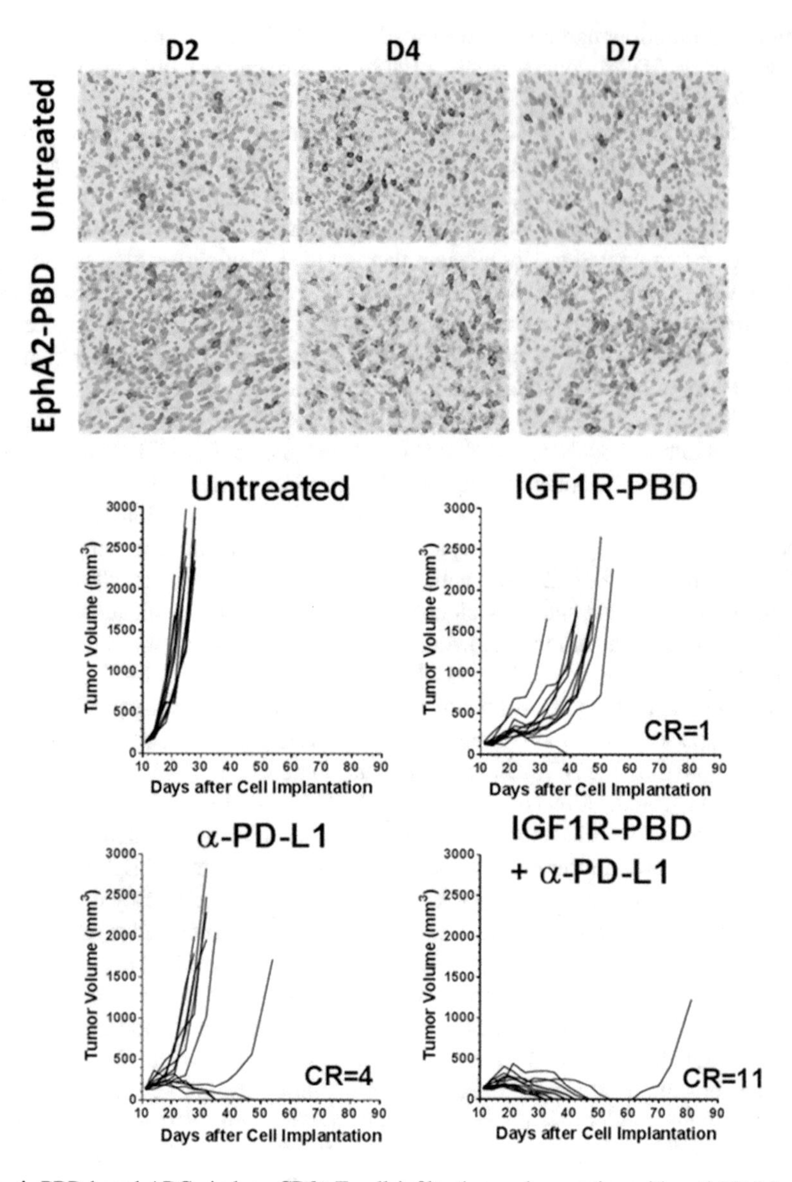

Fig. 4 PBD-based ADCs induce CD8⁺ T cell infiltration and synergize with anti-PD-L1. (**a**). EphA2-PBD induced CTL infiltration in MCA205 tumors. (**b**) Combining IGF1R-PBD with anti-PD-L1 resulted in striking synergy in the CT26 model, suggesting that the increased efficacy of ADC-IO combinations is likely to be independent of target antigen. (Reprinted with permission from AACR: Rios-Doria et al. [11])

ADC targeting the mouse IGF1 receptor was constructed with the PBD payload as this receptor was found to be overexpressed on CT26 tumors. Even though an antibody to a different TAA was used, the mIGF1R ADC also synergized with anti-PD-L1 (Fig. 4b), demonstrating that the combination effects seem to be dependent on the delivered warhead rather than on the target antigen. In summary, the preclinical data suggest that each ADC payload may have different effects on the immune microenvironment and that these effects may also be tumor-dependent. It will be important in the future to identify tumor biomarkers that may indicate sensitivity to ADC immunomodulation, which in turn may identify tumor types in which to combine ADCs with immunotherapy.

Taken together, the preclinical data with ADCs conjugated with various payloads including the microtubule-inhibiting auristatins, maytansinoids and tubulysins, as well as the DNA cross-linking PBD dimers, suggest several possible mechanisms for the observed enhanced anti-tumor activity of ADC-IO combinations. Such increased activity appears to be due to ADC-mediated direct maturation of dendritic cells and induction of ICD that leads to enhanced recruitment and/or activation of $CD8^+$ CTLs, payload-dependent effects on T_{regs} and bystander killing activity against immunosuppressive cells within the tumor microenvironment. Regardless of the mechanism(s) involved, it is clear that the preclinical data provide a strong rationale for assessing the therapeutic potential of these combinations in a clinical setting.

The Current Clinical Landscape of ADC-IO Combinations

This chapter has so far demonstrated that certain ADC payloads including auristatins, maytansinoids, PBD dimers and tubulysins are capable of eliciting immunomodulatory responses, and enhanced anti-tumor activity is possible when combining various IO agents with ADCs conjugated with these warheads [70]. However, all of the data and mechanisms discussed so far have been based on preclinical research. Several clinical trials investigating ADC-IO combinations are currently being evaluated and this section will summarize the rationale for these as well as available data.

Rationale for ADC-IO Combinations

While immunotherapies have generated significant efficacy as monotherapies in the clinic, many patients treated with these therapeutics do not respond. Certain cancers, such as prostate and colorectal carcinomas tend to be quite refractory to monotherapy IO agents, whereas cancers with high mutational burdens, including melanoma, NSCLC and bladder cancer seem to be the most likely to respond [79–81]. However, even in these more responsive indications CR's with durable survival benefits are only observed in approximately 20–30% of patients regardless of the IO agent being tested and approximately a quarter of those patients who initially respond will develop acquired resistance [79–81]. There have been some increased successes when combining multiple immunotherapies, with improved response rates as well as overall survival [79], however, there is still significant room for improvement. Therefore, there is substantial interest to combine IO drugs with other treatment modalities to improve upon the response rates of single agent immunotherapies [79], including ADCs [70]. As this chapter highlights, recent findings that ADCs and their warheads can have immunomodulatory effects above and beyond simply eliciting cytotoxicity in antigen-positive cancers [9–11, 51] have provided a rationale for and generated significant interest in combining ADCs with IO agents and evaluating these in the clinic. Treatment with ADCs conjugated with payloads that elicit ICD may not only debulk tumors by inducing cytotoxicity of target-positive tumor cells, but may do so in an antigenic manner thereby triggering a complementary immune response to further reduce tumor burden and perhaps eliminate residual disease. Based on the preclinical data demonstrating direct effects of certain ADC warheads on DC maturation and activation, such an immune response might further be enhanced by priming of the immune system via direct APC activation. If the enhanced efficacy and in many cases synergistic activity observed with ADC-IO combinations in preclinical tumor models translates to the clinic, such ADC-IO combinations would provide a very significant clinical benefit to patients.

Another potentially important aspect of these ADC-IO combinations could be the promise of improving the therapeutic index by lowering the required doses of therapeutics to see enhanced anti-tumor activity. As highlighted earlier, enhanced and even synergistic anti-tumor activity has been observed preclinically with non-curative doses of the ADC in syngeneic mouse tumor models [11]. It is known that both ADCs and IO agents can have significant and, in some cases, potentially fatal toxicities associated with their administration [82–84]. The possibility of combining these two classes of therapeutic agents at doses lower than those currently administered may decrease the risk of treatment-related adverse events while maintaining or even improving clinical efficacy. Whether such an improved therapeutic index will be observed in the clinic remains to be seen and the data from clinical trials combining ADCs and IO agents will be telling.

Clinical Trials Evaluating ADC-IO Agent Combinations

At the time of this writing, there are currently 27 trials, registered clinical trials evaluating ADC-IO combinations, 1x phase III, 9x phase II, and 17x phase I (Fig. 5, Table 1). All but one of these trials are testing ADCs combined with immunotherapies approved for various indications and the vast majority of these trials are combining ADCs with checkpoint inhibitors targeting either the PD-1 T cell co-receptor or its ligand, PD-L1. PD-1 is expressed on T lymphocytes and its ligand PD-L1 is typically found on the surface of antigen presenting cells [85]. PD-1/PD-L1 interactions lead to negative regulation of T cell activation and proliferation and even apoptosis of T cells, and also play a role in T cell exhaustion thereby promoting tolerance. This

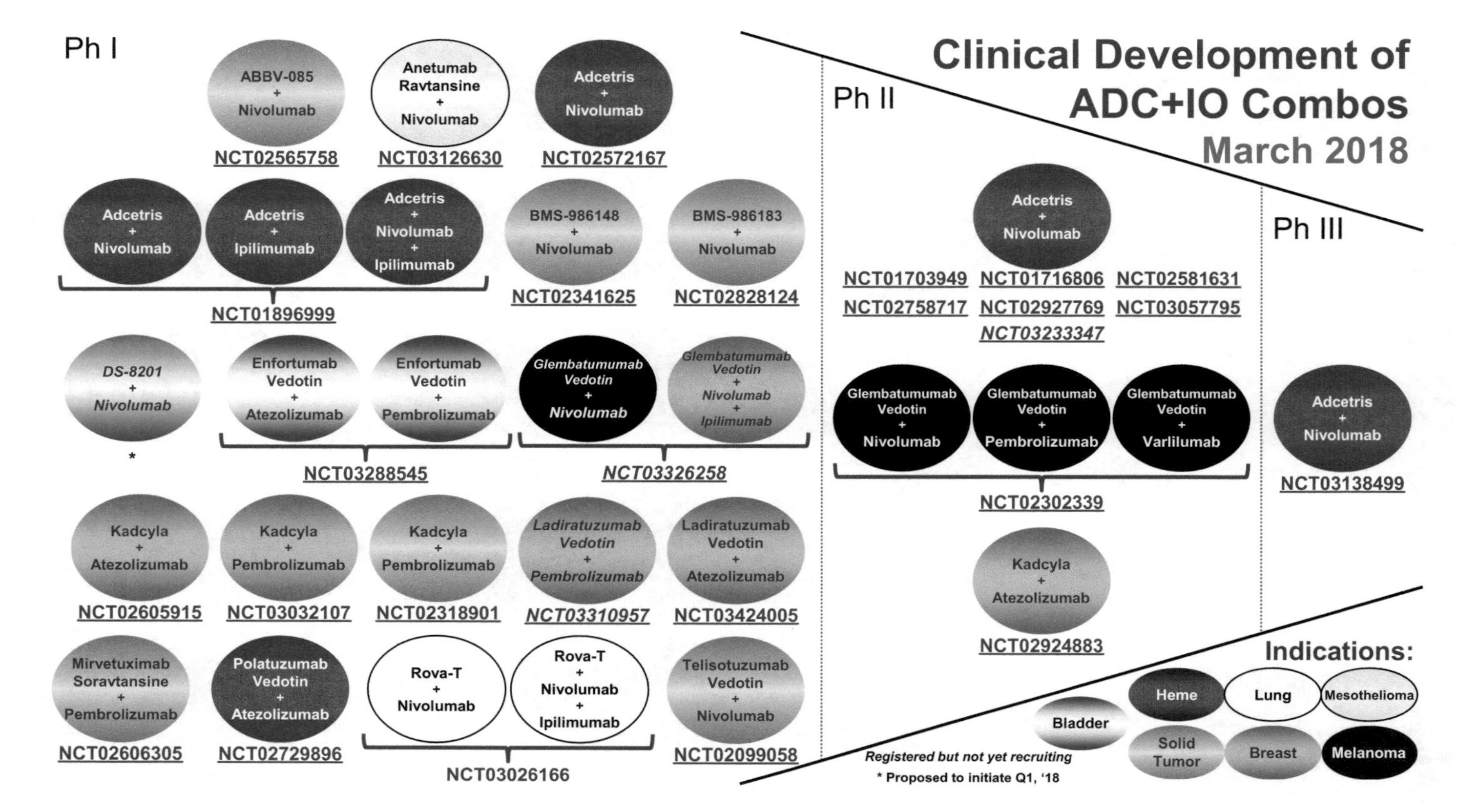

Fig. 5 ADC-IO combinations currently in clinical development (current as of September 2017)

Table 1 Clinical trials testing ADC-IO combinations (*Current as of March 2018*)

ADC	Target	Payload	IO Agent	Target	Phase/Indication	Clinical Trial Identifier
ABBV-085	LRRC15	MMAE	Nivolumab	PD-1	Ph I - Solid Tumors	NCT02565758
Anetumab Ravtansine	Mesothelin	DM4	Nivolumab	PD-1	Ph I - Mesothelioma	NCT03126630
BMS-986148	Mesothelin	DM4	Nivolumab	PD-1	Ph I/II - Meso, Gastric, PDAC, OvCa, NSCLC	NCT02341625
BMS-986183	Mesothelin	Unknown	Nivolumab	PD-1	Ph I/II - HCC	NCT02828124
Brentuximab Vedotin	CD30	MMAE	Ipilimumab	CTLA-4	Ph I - Relapsed or Refractory cHL	NCT01896999
			Nivolumab	PD-1		
			Ipilimumab + Nivolumab	CTLA-4 PD-1		
Brentuximab Vedotin	CD30	MMAE	Nivolumab	PD-1	Ph I/II - Relapsed or Refractory HL	NCT02572167
Brentuximab Vedotin	CD30	MMAE	Nivolumab	PD-1	Ph II – Relapsed / Refractory CD30+ HL	NCT01703949
Brentuximab Vedotin	CD30	MMAE	Nivolumab	PD-1	Ph II - Newly Diagnosed cHL in 60+yo Adults	NCT01716806
Brentuximab Vedotin	CD30	MMAE	Nivolumab	PD-1	Ph II - NHL	NCT02581631
Brentuximab Vedotin	CD30	MMAE	Nivolumab	PD-1	Ph II - Untreated cHL in 60+yo Adults	NCT02758717
Brentuximab Vedotin	CD30	MMAE	Nivolumab	PD-1	Ph II - cHL in Patients 5-30yo	NCT02927769
Brentuximab Vedotin	CD30	MMAE	Nivolumab	PD-1	Ph II - Relapsed / Refractory cHL (≥18yo Patients)	NCT03057795
Brentuximab Vedotin	CD30	MMAE	Nivolumab	PD-1	Ph II – HL Progressing after Dacarbazine + Vinblastine + Doxorubicin Therapy	NCT03233347
Brentuximab Vedotin	CD30	MMAE	Nivolumab	PD-1	Ph III – Advanced, Relapsed / Refractory cHL or ASCT Ineligible	NCT03138499
DS-8201	Her2	DXd	Nivolumab	PD-1	Ph Ib - Her2$^+$ mBrCa and UC	Not yet registered
Enfortumab Vedotin	Nectin-4	MMAE	Atezolizumab	PD-L1	Ph I - UC	NCT03288545
			Pembrolizumab	PD-1		
Glembatumumab Vedotin	gpNMB	MMAE	Nivolumab	PD-1	Ph II - Advanced Melanoma	NCT03326258
			Ipilimumab + Nivolumab	CTLA-4 PD-1		
Glembatumumab Vedotin	gpNMB	MMAE	Nivolumab	PD-1	Ph II - Advanced Melanoma	NCT02302339
Ladiratuzumab Vedotin	LIV-1	PBD	Pembrolizumab	PD-1	Ph I – BrCa	NCT03310957
Ladiratuzumab Vedotin	LIV-1	PBD	Atezolizumab	PD-L1	Ph I/II BrCa	NCT03424005
Mirvetuximab Soravtansine	FRα	DM4	Pembrolizumab	PD-1	Ph I - FRα$^+$ OvCa	NCT02606305
Polatuzumab Vedotin	CD79b	MMAE	Pembrolizumab	PD-1	Ph I - Relapsed or Refractory Follicular Lymphoma or DLBCL	NCT02729896
Rovalpituzumab tesirine	DLL3	PBD	Nivolumab	PD-1	Ph I - SCLC	NCT03026166
			Nivolumab + Ipilimumab	PD-1 CTLA-4		
Telisotuzumab Vedotin	c-Met	MMAE	Nivolumab	PD-1	Ph I - Solid Tumors	NCT02099058
Trastuzumab emtansine	HER2	DM1	Atezolizumab	PD-L1	Ph I - HER2$^+$ BrCa	NCT02605915
Trastuzumab emtansine	HER2	DM1	Pembrolizumab	PD-1	Ph I - HER2$^+$ mBrCa	NCT03032107
Trastuzumab emtansine	HER2	DM1	Pembrolizumab	PD-1	Ph I/II - HER2$^+$ mBrCa, Gastric, Esophagus, CRC	NCT02318901
Trastuzumab emtansine	HER2	DM1	Atezolizumab	PD-L1	Ph II - HER2$^+$ BrCa	NCT02924883

Abbreviations used: *BrCa* breast cancer, *cHL* classical Hodgkin lymphoma, *DLBCL* diffuse large B cell lymphoma, *HCC* hepatocellular carcinoma, *mBrCa* metastatic breast cancer, *Meso* mesothelioma, *NHL* non-Hodgkin's lymphoma, *NSCLC* non-small cell lung cancer, *OvCa* ovarian cancer, *PDAC* pancreatic ductal adenocarcinoma, *SCLC* small cell lung cancer, *UC* urothelial cancer immune checkpoint has evolved to resolve inflammation and prevent autoimmune attack during normal tissue homeostasis. However, tumors are thought to manipulate this pathway and inhibit anti-tumor immunity by expressing PD-L1, which can then essentially inactivate $CD8^+$ TILs expressing the PD-1 receptor. Strategies to block this PD-1/PD-L1 interaction have resulted in the development of antagonist antibodies that inhibit this immune checkpoint.

Several checkpoint inhibitors are approved for various indications and these are being combined with ADCs in the clinic. Nivolumab (Opdivo®) is an antibody targeting PD-1 and is FDA-approved for NSCLC [86], metastatic melanoma [87], advanced renal cell carcinoma as second-line therapy [88], relapsed or refractory squamous cell carcinoma of the head and neck (SCCHN) [89], classical Hodgkin lymphoma (cHL) that has recurred following autologous stem cell transplant followed by Adcetris [90], and for second-line therapy in advanced urothelial carcinoma (UC) [91, 92]. Pembrolizumab (Keytruda®) is another anti-PD-1 antibody and has been FDA-approved to treat PD-$L1^+$ advanced NSCLC [93], advanced melanoma [94, 95], platinum-insensitive SCCHN [96] as well as relapsed or refractory classical Hodgkin lymphoma [97]. Atezolizumab (Tecentriq®) is an FDA-approved antibody targeting PD-L1 for advanced UC [98] and previously-treated metastatic NSCLC (https://www.fda.gov/Drugs/InformationOnDrugs/ApprovedDrugs/ucm525780.htm). Ipilimumab (Yervoy®), an FDA-approved antibody for metastatic or unresectable melanoma, targets another checkpoint receptor, CTLA-4 which, like PD-1/PD-L1 interactions, transmits inhibitory signals to T cells to doampen an immune response [99–101].

The only non-checkpoint inhibitor and the only investigational IO agent being tested in combination with ADCs is varlilumab, an agonist monoclonal antibody that activates the tumor necrosis factor receptor (TNFR) family member CD27, which is a co-stimulatory molecule on T and B cells. Binding of varlilumab to CD27 results in activation of T cells and thus could potentiate anti-tumor immune responses in cancer patients [102].

The majority of clinical trials evaluating ADC-IO combinations are being conducted with the two clinically-approved ADCs, brentuximab vedotin (BV, Adcetris®) and ado-trastuzumab-emtansine (T-DM1, Kadcyla®). There are seven ongoing trials evaluating BV in combination with various IO agents. Five Phase 2 trials are currently evaluating BV combined with the PD-1-targeting nivolumab for either cHL or non-Hodgkin lymphoma (NHL). BV in combination with nivolumab and/or the anti-CTLA-4 antibody ipilimumab is being evaluated in a Phase 1 trial in patients with relapsed or refractory HL and another Phase 1 trial is also evaluating the BV plus nivolumab combination in patients with relapsed or refractory cHL.

The other approved ADC, T-DM1, is currently being evaluated with either the anti-PD-L1 antibody atezolizumab or with the PD-1-targeting antibody pembrolizumab in four trials. The combination of T-DM1and atezolizumab is being evaluated in patients with $Her2^+$ breast cancer in both a Phase 2 trial and a Phase 1 trial. Over the course of two Phase 1 trials, ado-trastuzumab emtansine in combination with pembrolizumab is being evaluated in several $Her2^+$ indications including metastatic breast, gastric, esophageal and colorectal cancer.

Several investigational ADCs have also incorporated combination arms with an IO agent into their trials. For example, rovalpituzumab tesirine, an ADC that targets DLL3-expressing tumor cells with a PBD payload, is currently in Phase 3 clinical trials as a single agent. Recently, a Phase 1/2 clinical trial that will test this ADC in combination with nivolumab or with nivolumab and ipilimumab in patients with small cell lung cancer (SCLC) was registered. Glembatumumab vedotin targets glycoprotein NMB (gpNMB)-expressing cells with the MMAE payload and is in Phase 3 clinical trials as a single agent but is also currently being evaluated in a Phase 2 clinical trial in combination with either nivolumab, pembrolizumab, or with the CD27 agonist varlilumab in patients with advanced melanoma. Mirvetuximab soravtansine, an ADC targeting folate receptor alpha (FRα) with a DM4 payload, is being evaluated as a single agent in a Phase 3 clinical trial enrolling patients with $FR\alpha^{+}$ ovarian cancer. In a Phase 1 study, the combination of mirvetuximab soravtansine plus pembrolizumab is being tested in patients with $FR\alpha^{+}$ ovarian cancer. Polatuzumab vedotin is an anti-CD79B ADC conjugated with MMAE that is currently in Phase 2 clinical trials in patients with diffuse large B cell lymphoma (DLBCL) or follicular NHL. It is also being tested in combination with atezolizumab in a Phase 1 trial in patients with relapsed or refractory follicular NHL or DLBCL. Enfortumab vedotin, a MMAE-conjugated ADC targeting Nectin-4 is currently being evaluated in urothelial cancer patients in a Phase 2 study and is also being tested in combination with either atezolizumab or pembrolizumab in urothelial cancer patients in a Phase 1 trial. Anetumab ravtansine, a mesothelin-targeting ADC currently in Phase 2 clinical trials in patients with mesothelioma or pancreatic cancer, is also being tested in patients with mesothelioma in a Phase 1 study in combination with nivolumab. Finally, an announcement was made recently about an upcoming study that will test the Her2-targeting ADC, DS-8201, with pembrolizumab in patients with $Her2^{+}$ breast or urothelial cancer.

While these ADCs had established Phase 1 trial data demonstrating a favorable safety profile before initiating clinical trials in combination with IO agents, there are others that have taken a different approach. There are a few clinical trials testing very early stage ADCs in combination with nivolumab as a separate arm of their initial Phase 1 clinical trials. For example, ABBV-085, an ADC conjugated with MMAE targeting LRRC15 [103], telisotuzumab vedotin (ABBV-399), an MMAE-conjugated ADC targeting c-Met, BMS-986148, an anti-mesothelin ADC conjugated with DM4, and BMS-986183, a GPC3-targeting ADC conjugated with an undisclosed warhead all initially began their Phase 1 trials as single agent therapies against various solid tumor types. However, over the course of the trials, separate arms were added to each trial as either expansion cohorts (for ABBV-085 and Telisotuzumab vedotin) or as a Phase 2 extension arm (for BMS-986148 and BMS-986183) evaluating the ADC in combination with nivolumab in solid tumors, presumably after some initial safety readouts were obtained. This approach, combining IO agents with early stage investigational ADCs, could represent a paradigm for ADC clinical development going forward, particularly with ADCs targeting cancer types where IO agents have demonstrated clinical efficacy such as lung cancer, melanoma and others.

Initial Data from ADC-IO Clinical Trials

While several clinical trials testing ADC-IO combinatorial therapies in cancer are currently ongoing, limited data is available at this time. However, the early readouts from a couple of these trials seem promising.

The first reported data from a clinical study of ADC-IO combinations was presented at the American Society of Hematology (ASH) meeting in December 2015 [104]. Preliminary safety and efficacy data was reported from a Phase 1 trial testing the combination of BV and ipilimumab in patients with relapsed/refractory HL. Based on data from twelve evaluable patients who received the combinatorial therapy, the clinical benefit rate was 83% (ten patients). Overall response rate was 67% (eight patients) with CRs observed in five of those patients (42%) and stable disease was reported for 2 patients (17%). The BV + ipilimumab combinatorial therapy was well tolerated with no dose-limiting toxicities observed. The most common adverse events (AEs) were diarrhea, rash and peripheral sensory neuropathy, while other observed AEs included alopecia, transaminitis and uveitis. Grade 3 AEs included infusion-related reactions, rash, vomiting and peripheral sensory neuropathy, while one case of Grade 4 thrombocytopenia was observed in a patient with pre-existing thrombocytopenia. Overall, the study authors concluded that the data suggested deepening of the clinical responses compared to historical monotherapy in this patient cohort. In addition, half of the CRs were observed in patients receiving a low dose of ipilimumab suggesting that low doses of the IO agent may still be highly active when combined with ADC therapy.

More recently, preliminary results from a Phase 1/2 study evaluating BV in combination with nivolumab were reported at the ASH meeting in December 2016 by Herrera et al. [105]. Forty-two patients with relapsed/refractory HL who failed frontline ABVD (adriamycin, bleomycin, vinblastine, dacarbazine) therapy enrolled on the study and received at least one dose of the combination therapy. Evaluable data was available from twenty-nine patients. Twenty-six patients (90%) had an objective response including 18 (62%) with a complete metabolic response and partial metabolic responses observed in eight patients. The remaining patients either had stable disease (1 patient; 3%) or progressive disease (2 patients; 7%). The safety profile of the combination was also favorable. The most common adverse events (AEs) occurring in more than 20% of patients included fatigue, nausea, infusion-related reactions, pruritus and rash. A serious AE was observed in one patient after the first cycle of BV and presented with Grade 3 dehydration, Grade 2 hypercalcemia and malaise, and Grade 1 asthenia and nausea. No patients had a dose reduction during treatment due to an AE though dose delays did occur for three patients with BV treatment and 4 patients with nivolumab treatment. Dose delays were due to urticaria, thrombosis, elevated lipase, chills and hypoxia. Pharmacodynamic analyses following the first cycle of combination therapy indicated an ADC-mediated decrease in regulatory T cells with no decrease in proliferating $CD8^+$ CTLs or $CD4^+$ Th1 cells, while nivolumab induced a robust expansion of T cells. Given the 90% objective response rate including a 62% CR rate, and acceptable safety profile, the study authors proposed further studies testing this promising ADC-IO combination as frontline therapy for patients with cHL as well as testing in patients with CD30-positive NHL.

Taken together these preliminary data from two of the eight studies evaluating ADC-IO combinations against hematological malignancies in the clinic suggest very promising results for such combinatorial therapies in these settings. In addition, ten trials are ongoing testing ADC-IO combinations in solid tumors. It will be interesting to see if the efficacy and tolerability in the hematological indications will also be observed in other trials and if a similar, promising efficacy is achieved in solid tumor indications as well.
In the BV plus ipilimumab trial, clinical responses were reported with low doses of ipilimumab. Based on the preclinical data it is possible that enhanced or synergistic activity may be achieved by combining ADCs and IO drugs at lower than standard of care doses. Therefore, it will be important to determine if administering an ADC and or the IO agent well below their respective MTDs could yield clinical benefits, while reducing toxicities associated with these combinations. Currently, this does not appear to be a strategy that is being investigated in ongoing clinical studies, but perhaps such lower dosing may be incorporated into ADC-IO clinical development plans as additional data from ADC-IO clinical trials become available. Another aspect of these ADC-IO combinatorial strategies that warrants further investigations is the timing of administration of each therapy. There is only limited preclinical data available, evaluating the effects of the timing of ADC and IO drug administration on the enhanced efficacy observed with these combinations. The clinical trials appear to be utilizing the same dosing regimen typically applied for each ADC or IO drug as a single agent, maintaining the same dosing cycles. While an enhanced benefit has been observed when ADCs and IO agents are administered simultaneously in preclinical models, perhaps even stronger effects could be observed by staggering the dosing regimens of these therapies. This of course could be dependent on the type of IO agent and its mechanism of action as well as the warhead conjugated to the ADC, used in these combinations. Again, further preclinical work is warranted in this area to guide clinical decision making, such as the application of staggered administration strategies.

Conclusions

Currently, there is a lot of excitement about the potential clinical benefit of ADC-IO combinations. The rationale for such promise is the growing literature of preclinical data demonstrating significant immunomodulatory effects of ADCs conjugated with auristatin, maytansinoid, PBD and tubulysin payloads. As discussed in this chapter, ADCs can directly activate DCs leading to greater recruitment to and activation of CTLs within tumors. They can also induce ICD of tumor cells leading to an enhanced immune response. One of the most surprising revelations of the preclinical studies was the critical role $CD8^+$ CTLs in the anti-tumor activity of ADCs. Depletion of $CD8^+$ T cells led to decreased activity of ADCs conjugated with different classes of warheads, thus clearly indicating that ADC-mediated anti-tumor immunity significantly contributes to the therapeutic ADC activity. Given these immunomodulatory effects of ADCs, one question that will need to be answered by both clinical and preclinical data is, in what settings ADC-IO combinations may be most effective. IO monotherapies are typically more effective in settings where there is significant infiltration of immune cells prior to therapy, so-called "immunologically hot" tumors, and less so in "immunologically cold" tumors that lack such infiltrates [7]. The available preclinical and clinical data demonstrating increased infiltration into and/or activation of $CD8^+$ T cells in tumors following treatment with ADCs suggests that it may be possible for ADCs to convert "cold" tumors into "hot" tumors, and thus may extend the clinical benefit of immunotherapies into currently refractory indications.

Another question that may be answered as the clinical data from ADC-IO combinations mature is how best to administer such combinatorial therapies. One could hypothesize that treatment with the ADC should be conducted first or perhaps concomitantly with IO therapy, such that the ADC can effectively begin to induce ICD of the tumor cells and stimulate antigen presentation, while simultaneous or subsequent IO therapy works to enhance and sustain the immune response to the treated tumor. Alternatively, and depending on the ADC warhead as well as the MoA of the IO therapy, the latter may be administered first to trigger anti-tumor immunity. Then the ADC can be administered second to eliciting ICD of the dying tumor cells and to further promote DC maturation, thereby providing additional stimulatory signals to the already activated immune system. Such decisions on timing will depend on many factors, including the immunomodulatory effects of the ADC warhead, the mechanism of action of the IO agent and the immunological status of the tumor itself at the time of treatment. Clearly more preclinical work needs to be done and more clinical data need to be collected to determine the proper sequence of ADC/IO administration for a particular warhead, IO therapy and cancer type.

With advances in antibody engineering and site-specific conjugation chemistries currently being applied to ADCs, it may be possible to load an antibody with multiple payloads all within one targeted therapeutic in order to most efficiently induce ICD. As such, modifying ADCs to deliver payloads that complement each other by eliciting ICD and/or direct immune stimulation may be a viable strategy to optimally engage the immune system.

Ultimately, the data from clinical trials currently evaluating ADC-IO combinations will reveal if the preclinical data indeed do translate to the clinic. In addition to an enhanced clinical benefit, the preclinical data thus far suggests that it may be possible to administer lower drug doses than those used currently in single agent regimens thereby decreasing the toxicities associated with these drugs as individual therapies. An increased overall therapeutic index of ADC-IO combinations is a very promising prospect, but again, the data from the clinic will be telling.

References

1. Mellman I, Coukos G, Dranoff G (2011) Cancer immunotherapy comes of age. Nature 480:480–489
2. Lonberg N, Korman AJ (2017) Masterful antibodies: checkpoint blockade. Cancer Immunol Res 5:275–281
3. Hay CM, Sult E, Huang Q, Mulgrew K, Fuhrmann SR, McGlinchey KA, Hammond SA, Rothstein R, Rios-Doria J, Poon E, Holoweckyj N, Durham NM, Leow CC, Diedrich G, Damschroder M, Herbst R, Hollingsworth RE, Sachsenmeier KF (2016) Targeting CD73 in the tumor microenvironment with MEDI9447. Oncoimmunology 5:e1208875
4. Moran AE, Kovacsovics-Bankowski M, Weinberg AD (2013) The TNFRs OX40, 4-1BB, and CD40 as targets for cancer immunotherapy. Curr Opin Immunol 25:230–237
5. Schumacher TN, Schreiber RD (2015) Neoantigens in cancer immunotherapy. Science 348:69–74
6. Snyder A, Makarov V, Merghoub T, Yuan J, Zaretsky JM, Desrichard A, Walsh LA, Postow MA, Wong P, Ho TS, Hollmann TJ, Bruggeman C, Kannan K, Li Y, Elipenahli C, Liu C, Harbison CT, Wang L, Ribas A, Wolchok JD, Chan TA (2014) Genetic basis for clinical response to CTLA-4 blockade in melanoma. N Engl J Med 371:2189–2199
7. Wargo JA, Reddy SM, Reuben A, Sharma P (2016) Monitoring immune responses in the tumor microenvironment. Curr Opin Immunol 41:23–31
8. Cao A, Heiser R, Law CL, Gardai S (2016) Auristatin-based antibody drug conjugates activate multiple ER stress response pathways resulting in immunogenic cell death and amplified T-cell responses. Cancer Res 76:Abstract-4914
9. Muller P, Martin K, Theurich S, Schreiner J, Savic S, Terszowski G, Lardinois D, Heinzelmann-Schwarz VA, Schlaak M, Kvasnicka HM, Spagnoli G, Dirnhofer S, Speiser DE, von Bergwelt-Baildon M, Zippelius A (2014) Microtubule-depolymerizing agents used in antibody-drug conjugates induce antitumor immunity by stimulation of dendritic cells. Cancer Immunol Res 2:741–755
10. Muller P, Kreuzaler M, Khan T, Thommen DS, Martin K, Glatz K, Savic S, Harbeck N, Nitz U, Gluz O, von Bergwelt-Baildon M, Kreipe H, Reddy S, Christgen M, Zippelius A (2015) Trastuzumab emtansine (T-DM1) renders HER2+ breast cancer highly susceptible to CTLA-4/PD-1 blockade. Sci Transl Med 7:315ra188
11. Rios-Doria J, Harper J, Rothstein R, Wetzel L, Chesebrough J, Marrero AM, Chen C, Strout P, Mulgrew K, McGlinchey KA, Fleming R, Bezabeh B, Meekin J, Stewart D, Kennedy M, Martin P, Buchanan A, Dimasi N, Michelotti EF, Hollingsworth RE (2017) Antibody-drug conjugates bearing pyrrolobenzodiazepine or tubulysin payloads are immunomodulatory and synergize with multiple immunotherapies. Cancer Res 77:2686–2698
12. Kroemer G, Galluzzi L, Kepp O, Zitvogel L (2013) Immunogenic cell death in cancer therapy. Annu Rev Immunol 31:51–72
13. Kepp O, Senovilla L, Vitale I, Vacchelli E, Adjemian S, Agostinis P, Apetoh L, Aranda F, Barnaba V, Bloy N, Bracci L, Breckpot K, Brough D, Buque A, Castro MG, Cirone M, Colombo MI, Cremer I, Demaria S, Dini L, Eliopoulos AG, Faggioni A, Formenti SC, Fucikova J, Gabriele L, Gaipl US, Galon J, Garg A, Ghiringhelli F, Giese NA, Guo ZS, Hemminki A, Herrmann M, Hodge JW, Holdenrieder S, Honeychurch J, Hu HM, Huang X, Illidge TM, Kono K, Korbelik M, Krysko DV, Loi S, Lowenstein PR, Lugli E, Ma Y, Madeo F, Manfredi AA, Martins I, Mavilio D, Menger L, Merendino N, Michaud M, Mignot G, Mossman KL, Multhoff G, Oehler R, Palombo F, Panaretakis T, Pol J, Proietti E, Ricci JE, Riganti C, Rovere-Querini P, Rubartelli A, Sistigu A, Smyth MJ, Sonnemann J, Spisek R, Stagg J, Sukkurwala AQ, Tartour E, Thorburn A, Thorne SH, Vandenabeele P, Velotti F, Workenhe ST, Yang H, Zong WX, Zitvogel L, Kroemer G, Galluzzi L (2014) Consensus guidelines for the detection of immunogenic cell death. Oncoimmunology 3:e955691
14. Obeid M, Tesniere A, Ghiringhelli F, Fimia GM, Apetoh L, Perfettini JL, Castedo M, Mignot G, Panaretakis T, Casares N, Metivier D, Larochette N, van Endert P, Ciccosanti F, Piacentini

M, Zitvogel L, Kroemer G (2007) Calreticulin exposure dictates the immunogenicity of cancer cell death. Nat Med 13:54–61
15. Galluzzi L, Buque A, Kepp O, Zitvogel L, Kroemer G (2017) Immunogenic cell death in cancer and infectious disease. Nat Rev Immunol 17:97–111
16. Inoue H, Tani K (2014) Multimodal immunogenic cancer cell death as a consequence of anticancer cytotoxic treatments. Cell Death Differ 21:39–49
17. Garg AD, De Ruysscher D, Agostinis P (2016) Immunological metagene signatures derived from immunogenic cancer cell death associate with improved survival of patients with lung, breast or ovarian malignancies: a large-scale meta-analysis. Oncoimmunology 5:e1069938
18. Ladoire S, Enot D, Andre F, Zitvogel L, Kroemer G (2016) Immunogenic cell death-related biomarkers: impact on the survival of breast cancer patients after adjuvant chemotherapy. Oncoimmunology 5:e1082706
19. Ladoire S, Senovilla L, Enot D, Ghiringhelli F, Poirier-Colame V, Chaba K, Erdag G, Schaefer JT, Deacon DH, Zitvogel L, Slingluff CL Jr, Kroemer G (2016) Biomarkers of immunogenic stress in metastases from melanoma patients: correlations with the immune infiltrate. Oncoimmunology 5:e1160193
20. Obeid M, Panaretakis T, Joza N, Tufi R, Tesniere A, van Endert P, Zitvogel L, Kroemer G (2007) Calreticulin exposure is required for the immunogenicity of gamma-irradiation and UVC light-induced apoptosis. Cell Death Differ 14:1848–1850
21. Gardai SJ, McPhillips KA, Frasch SC, Janssen WJ, Starefeldt A, Murphy-Ullrich JE, Bratton DL, Oldenborg PA, Michalak M, Henson PM (2005) Cell-surface calreticulin initiates clearance of viable or apoptotic cells through trans-activation of LRP on the phagocyte. Cell 123:321–334
22. Zitvogel L, Kepp O, Senovilla L, Menger L, Chaput N, Kroemer G (2010) Immunogenic tumor cell death for optimal anticancer therapy: the calreticulin exposure pathway. Clin Cancer Res 16:3100–3104
23. Panaretakis T, Joza N, Modjtahedi N, Tesniere A, Vitale I, Durchschlag M, Fimia GM, Kepp O, Piacentini M, Froehlich KU, van Endert P, Zitvogel L, Madeo F, Kroemer G (2008) The co-translocation of ERp57 and calreticulin determines the immunogenicity of cell death. Cell Death Differ 15:1499–1509
24. Chao MP, Jaiswal S, Weissman-Tsukamoto R, Alizadeh AA, Gentles AJ, Volkmer J, Weiskopf K, Willingham SB, Raveh T, Park CY, Majeti R, Weissman IL (2010) Calreticulin is the dominant pro-phagocytic signal on multiple human cancers and is counterbalanced by CD47. Sci Transl Med 2:63ra94
25. Liu X, Pu Y, Cron K, Deng L, Kline J, Frazier WA, Xu H, Peng H, Fu YX, Xu MM (2015) CD47 blockade triggers T cell-mediated destruction of immunogenic tumors. Nat Med 21:1209–1215
26. Fucikova J, Becht E, Iribarren K, Goc J, Remark R, Damotte D, Alifano M, Devi P, Biton J, Germain C, Lupo A, Fridman WH, Dieu-Nosjean MC, Kroemer G, Sautes-Fridman C, Cremer I (2016) Calreticulin expression in human non-small cell lung cancers correlates with increased accumulation of antitumor immune cells and favorable prognosis. Cancer Res 76:1746–1756
27. Stebbing J, Bower M, Gazzard B, Wildfire A, Pandha H, Dalgleish A, Spicer J (2004) The common heat shock protein receptor CD91 is up-regulated on monocytes of advanced melanoma slow progressors. Clin Exp Immunol 138:312–316
28. Liu R, Gong J, Chen J, Li Q, Song C, Zhang J, Li Y, Liu Z, Dong Y, Chen L, Jin B (2012) Calreticulin as a potential diagnostic biomarker for lung cancer. Cancer Immunol Immunother 61:855–864
29. Peng RQ, Chen YB, Ding Y, Zhang R, Zhang X, Yu XJ, Zhou ZW, Zeng YX, Zhang XS (2010) Expression of calreticulin is associated with infiltration of T-cells in stage IIIB colon cancer. World J Gastroenterol 16:2428–2434
30. Krysko DV, Garg AD, Kaczmarek A, Krysko O, Agostinis P, Vandenabeele P (2012) Immunogenic cell death and DAMPs in cancer therapy. Nat Rev Cancer 12:860–875

31. El-Mashed S, O'Donovan TR, Kay EW, Abdallah AR, Cathcart MC, O'Sullivan J, O'Grady A, Reynolds J, O'Reilly S, O'Sullivan GC, McKenna SL (2015) LC3B globular structures correlate with survival in esophageal adenocarcinoma. BMC Cancer 15:582
32. Koukourakis MI, Kalamida D, Giatromanolaki A, Zois CE, Sivridis E, Pouliliou S, Mitrakas A, Gatter KC, Harris AL (2015) Autophagosome proteins LC3A, LC3B and LC3C have distinct subcellular distribution kinetics and expression in cancer cell lines. PLoS One 10:e0137675
33. Ladoire S, Enot D, Senovilla L, Chaix M, Zitvogel L, Kroemer G (2016) Positive impact of autophagy in human breast cancer cells on local immunosurveillance. Oncoimmunology 5:e1174801
34. Ladoire S, Penault-Llorca F, Senovilla L, Dalban C, Enot D, Locher C, Prada N, Poirier-Colame V, Chaba K, Arnould L, Ghiringhelli F, Fumoleau P, Spielmann M, Delaloge S, Poillot ML, Arveux P, Goubar A, Andre F, Zitvogel L, Kroemer G (2015) Combined evaluation of LC3B puncta and HMGB1 expression predicts residual risk of relapse after adjuvant chemotherapy in breast cancer. Autophagy 11:1878–1890
35. Elliott MR, Chekeni FB, Trampont PC, Lazarowski ER, Kadl A, Walk SF, Park D, Woodson RI, Ostankovich M, Sharma P, Lysiak JJ, Harden TK, Leitinger N, Ravichandran KS (2009) Nucleotides released by apoptotic cells act as a find-me signal to promote phagocytic clearance. Nature 461:282–286
36. Allard B, Longhi MS, Robson SC, Stagg J (2017) The ectonucleotidases CD39 and CD73: novel checkpoint inhibitor targets. Immunol Rev 276:121–144
37. Mantegazza AR, Zajac AL, Twelvetrees A, Holzbaur EL, Amigorena S, Marks MS (2014) TLR-dependent phagosome tubulation in dendritic cells promotes phagosome cross-talk to optimize MHC-II antigen presentation. Proc Natl Acad Sci U S A 111:15508–15513
38. Nair-Gupta P, Baccarini A, Tung N, Seyffer F, Florey O, Huang Y, Banerjee M, Overholtzer M, Roche PA, Tampe R, Brown BD, Amsen D, Whiteheart SW, Blander JM (2014) TLR signals induce phagosomal MHC-I delivery from the endosomal recycling compartment to allow cross-presentation. Cell 158:506–521
39. Shiratsuchi A, Watanabe I, Takeuchi O, Akira S, Nakanishi Y (2004) Inhibitory effect of Toll-like receptor 4 on fusion between phagosomes and endosomes/lysosomes in macrophages. J Immunol 172:2039–2047
40. Sistigu A, Yamazaki T, Vacchelli E, Chaba K, Enot DP, Adam J, Vitale I, Goubar A, Baracco EE, Remedios C, Fend L, Hannani D, Aymeric L, Ma Y, Niso-Santano M, Kepp O, Schultze JL, Tuting T, Belardelli F, Bracci L, La Sorsa V, Ziccheddu G, Sestili P, Urbani F, Delorenzi M, Lacroix-Triki M, Quidville V, Conforti R, Spano JP, Pusztai L, Poirier-Colame V, Delaloge S, Penault-Llorca F, Ladoire S, Arnould L, Cyrta J, Dessoliers MC, Eggermont A, Bianchi ME, Pittet M, Engblom C, Pfirschke C, Preville X, Uze G, Schreiber RD, Chow MT, Smyth MJ, Proietti E, Andre F, Kroemer G, Zitvogel L (2014) Cancer cell-autonomous contribution of type I interferon signaling to the efficacy of chemotherapy. Nat Med 20:1301–1309
41. Han L, Diao L, Yu S, Xu X, Li J, Zhang R, Yang Y, Werner HMJ, Eterovic AK, Yuan Y, Li J, Nair N, Minelli R, Tsang YH, Cheung LWT, Jeong KJ, Roszik J, Ju Z, Woodman SE, Lu Y, Scott KL, Li JB, Mills GB, Liang H (2015) The genomic landscape and clinical relevance of A-to-I RNA editing in human cancers. Cancer Cell 28:515–528
42. Hartner JC, Walkley CR, Lu J, Orkin SH (2009) ADAR1 is essential for the maintenance of hematopoiesis and suppression of interferon signaling. Nat Immunol 10:109–115
43. Paz-Yaacov N, Bazak L, Buchumenski I, Porath HT, Danan-Gotthold M, Knisbacher BA, Eisenberg E, Levanon EY (2015) Elevated RNA editing activity is a major contributor to transcriptomic diversity in tumors. Cell Rep 13:267–276
44. Menger L, Vacchelli E, Adjemian S, Martins I, Ma Y, Shen S, Yamazaki T, Sukkurwala AQ, Michaud M, Mignot G, Schlemmer F, Sulpice E, Locher C, Gidrol X, Ghiringhelli F, Modjtahedi N, Galluzzi L, Andre F, Zitvogel L, Kepp O, Kroemer G (2012) Cardiac glycosides exert anticancer effects by inducing immunogenic cell death. Sci Transl Med 4:143ra99

45. Yamazaki T, Hannani D, Poirier-Colame V, Ladoire S, Locher C, Sistigu A, Prada N, Adjemian S, Catani JP, Freudenberg M, Galanos C, Andre F, Kroemer G, Zitvogel L (2014) Defective immunogenic cell death of HMGB1-deficient tumors: compensatory therapy with TLR4 agonists. Cell Death Differ 21:69–78
46. Chen DS, Mellman I (2017) Elements of cancer immunity and the cancer-immune set point. Nature 541:321–330
47. Golden EB, Apetoh L (2015) Radiotherapy and immunogenic cell death. Semin Radiat Oncol 25:11–17
48. Pfirschke C, Engblom C, Rickelt S, Cortez-Retamozo V, Garris C, Pucci F, Yamazaki T, Poirier-Colame V, Newton A, Redouane Y, Lin YJ, Wojtkiewicz G, Iwamoto Y, Mino-Kenudson M, Huynh TG, Hynes RO, Freeman GJ, Kroemer G, Zitvogel L, Weissleder R, Pittet MJ (2016) Immunogenic chemotherapy sensitizes tumors to checkpoint blockade therapy. Immunity 44:343–354
49. Rios-Doria J, Durham N, Wetzel L, Rothstein R, Chesebrough J, Holoweckyj N, Zhao W, Leow CC, Hollingsworth R (2015) Doxil synergizes with cancer immunotherapies to enhance antitumor responses in syngeneic mouse models. Neoplasia 17:661–670
50. Beck A, Goetsch L, Dumontet C, Corvaia N (2017) Strategies and challenges for the next generation of antibody-drug conjugates. Nat Rev Drug Discov 16:315–337
51. Martin K, Muller P, Schreiner J, Prince SS, Lardinois D, Heinzelmann-Schwarz VA, Thommen DS, Zippelius A (2014) The microtubule-depolymerizing agent ansamitocin P3 programs dendritic cells toward enhanced anti-tumor immunity. Cancer Immunol Immunother 63:925–938
52. Garg AD, Agostinis P (2014) ER stress, autophagy and immunogenic cell death in photodynamic therapy-induced anti-cancer immune responses. Photochem Photobiol Sci 13:474–487
53. Kepp O, Menger L, Vacchelli E, Locher C, Adjemian S, Yamazaki T, Martins I, Sukkurwala AQ, Michaud M, Senovilla L, Galluzzi L, Kroemer G, Zitvogel L (2013) Crosstalk between ER stress and immunogenic cell death. Cytokine Growth Factor Rev 24:311–318
54. Oslowski CM, Urano F (2011) Measuring ER stress and the unfolded protein response using mammalian tissue culture system. Methods Enzymol 490:71–92
55. Gardai SJ, Epp A, Law C-L (2015) Brentuximab vedotin-mediated immunogenic cell death. Cancer Res 75(15 Suppl):Abstract nr 2469
56. Mizumoto N, Gao J, Matsushima H, Ogawa Y, Tanaka H, Takashima A (2005) Discovery of novel immunostimulants by dendritic-cell-based functional screening. Blood 106(9):3082
57. Tanaka H, Matsushima H, Mizumoto N, Takashima A (2009) Classification of chemotherapeutic agents based on their differential in vitro effects on dendritic cells. Cancer Res 69:6978–6986
58. Tanaka H, Matsushima H, Nishibu A, Clausen BE, Takashima A (2009) Dual therapeutic efficacy of vinblastine as a unique chemotherapeutic agent capable of inducing dendritic cell maturation. Cancer Res 69:6987–6994
59. Huang Y, Fang Y, Wu J, Dziadyk JM, Zhu X, Sui M, Fan W (2004) Regulation of Vinca alkaloid-induced apoptosis by NF-kappaB/IkappaB pathway in human tumor cells. Mol Cancer Ther 3:271–277
60. Kolomeichuk SN, Terrano DT, Lyle CS, Sabapathy K, Chambers TC (2008) Distinct signaling pathways of microtubule inhibitors – vinblastine and Taxol induce JNK-dependent cell death but through AP-1-dependent and AP-1-independent mechanisms, respectively. FEBS J 275:1889–1899
61. Parola C, Salogni L, Vaira X, Scutera S, Somma P, Salvi V, Musso T, Tabbia G, Bardessono M, Pasquali C, Mantovani A, Sozzani S, Bosisio D (2013) Selective activation of human dendritic cells by OM-85 through a NF-kB and MAPK dependent pathway. PLoS One 8:e82867

62. Patil S, Pincas H, Seto J, Nudelman G, Nudelman I, Sealfon SC (2010) Signaling network of dendritic cells in response to pathogens: a community-input supported knowledgebase. BMC Syst Biol 4:137
63. Rescigno M, Martino M, Sutherland CL, Gold MR, Ricciardi-Castagnoli P (1998) Dendritic cell survival and maturation are regulated by different signaling pathways. J Exp Med 188:2175–2180
64. Theurich S, Malcher J, Wennhold K, Shimabukuro-Vornhagen A, Chemnitz J, Holtick U, Krause A, Kobe C, Kahraman D, Engert A, Scheid C, Chakupurakal G, Hallek M, von Bergwelt-Baildon M (2013) Brentuximab vedotin combined with donor lymphocyte infusions for early relapse of Hodgkin lymphoma after allogeneic stem-cell transplantation induces tumor-specific immunity and sustained clinical remission. J Clin Oncol 31:e59–e63
65. Theurich S, Wennhold K, Wedemeyer I, Rothe A, Hubel K, Shimabukuro-Vornhagen A, Holtick U, Hallek M, Scheid C, von Bergwelt-Baildon M (2013) CD30-targeted therapy with brentuximab vedotin and DLI in a patient with T-cell posttransplantation lymphoma: induction of clinical remission and cellular immunity. Transplantation 96:e16–e18
66. Lewis Phillips GD, Li G, Dugger DL, Crocker LM, Parsons KL, Mai E, Blattler WA, Lambert JM, Chari RV, Lutz RJ, Wong WL, Jacobson FS, Koeppen H, Schwall RH, Kenkare-Mitra SR, Spencer SD, Sliwkowski MX (2008) Targeting HER2-positive breast cancer with trastuzumab-DM1, an antibody-cytotoxic drug conjugate. Cancer Res 68:9280–9290
67. Belvin M, Mellman I (2015) Is all cancer therapy immunotherapy? Sci Transl Med 7:315fs48
68. Speiser DE, Ho PC, Verdeil G (2016) Regulatory circuits of T cell function in cancer. Nat Rev Immunol 16:599–611
69. Facciabene A, Motz GT, Coukos G (2012) T-regulatory cells: key players in tumor immune escape and angiogenesis. Cancer Res 72:2162–2171
70. Gerber HP, Sapra P, Loganzo F, May C (2016) Combining antibody-drug conjugates and immune-mediated cancer therapy: what to expect? Biochem Pharmacol 102:1–6
71. Stefan N, Gebleux R, Waldmeier L, Hell T, Escher M, Wolter FI, Grawunder U, Beerli RR (2017) Highly potent, anthracycline-based antibody-drug conjugates generated by enzymatic, site-specific conjugation. Mol Cancer Ther 16:879–892
72. Beerli RR (2017) Anthracycline-based antibody drug conjugates with potent immune-stimulatory functions. Cancer Res 77(13 Suppl):Abstract nr 66
73. Hartley JA (2011) The development of pyrrolobenzodiazepines as antitumour agents. Expert Opin Investig Drugs 20:733–744
74. Li JY, Perry SR, Muniz-Medina V, Wang X, Wetzel LK, Rebelatto MC, Hinrichs MJ, Bezabeh BZ, Fleming RL, Dimasi N, Feng H, Toader D, Yuan AQ, Xu L, Lin J, Gao C, Wu H, Dixit R, Osbourn JK, Coats SR (2016) A biparatopic HER2-targeting antibody-drug conjugate induces tumor regression in primary models refractory to or ineligible for HER2-targeted therapy. Cancer Cell 29:117–129
75. Jackson D, Gooya J, Mao S, Kinneer K, Xu L, Camara M, Fazenbaker C, Fleming R, Swamynathan S, Meyer D, Senter PD, Gao C, Wu H, Kinch M, Coats S, Kiener PA, Tice DA (2008) A human antibody-drug conjugate targeting EphA2 inhibits tumor growth in vivo. Cancer Res 68:9367–9374
76. Melero I, Hirschhorn-Cymerman D, Morales-Kastresana A, Sanmamed MF, Wolchok JD (2013) Agonist antibodies to TNFR molecules that costimulate T and NK cells. Clin Cancer Res 19:1044–1053
77. Teng MW, Swann JB, von Scheidt B, Sharkey J, Zerafa N, McLaughlin N, Yamaguchi T, Sakaguchi S, Darcy PK, Smyth MJ (2010) Multiple antitumor mechanisms downstream of prophylactic regulatory T-cell depletion. Cancer Res 70:2665–2674
78. Leyland R, Watkins A, Mulgrew K, Holoweckyj N, Bamber L, Tigue NJ, Offer E, Andrews J, Yan L, Mullins S, Oberst MD, Coates Ulrichsen J, Leinster DA, McGlinchey KA, Young L, Morrow M, Hammond SA, Mallinder PR, Herath A, Leow CC, Wilkinson RW, Stewart R (2017) A novel murine GITR ligand fusion protein induces antitumor activity as a monotherapy, which is further enhanced in combination with an OX40 agonist. Clin Cancer Res 23:3416–3427

79. Ott PA, Hodi FS, Kaufman HL, Wigginton JM, Wolchok JD (2017) Combination immunotherapy: a road map. J Immunother Cancer 5:16
80. Sharma P, Hu-Lieskovan S, Wargo JA, Ribas A (2017) Primary, adaptive, and acquired resistance to cancer immunotherapy. Cell 168:707–723
81. Sharma P, Retz M, Siefker-Radtke A, Baron A, Necchi A, Bedke J, Plimack ER, Vaena D, Grimm MO, Bracarda S, Arranz JÁ, Pal S, Ohyama C, Saci A, Qu X, Lambert A, Krishnan S, Azrilevich A, Galsky MD (2017) Nivolumab in metastatic urothelial carcinoma after platinum therapy (CheckMate 275): a multicentre, single-arm, phase 2 trial. Lancet Oncol 18:312–322
82. Donaghy H (2016) Effects of antibody, drug and linker on the preclinical and clinical toxicities of antibody-drug conjugates. MAbs 8:659–671
83. Hinrichs MJ, Dixit R (2015) Antibody drug conjugates: nonclinical safety considerations. AAPS J 17:1055–1064
84. Larkin J, Lao CD, Urba WJ, McDermott DF, Horak C, Jiang J, Wolchok JD (2015) Efficacy and safety of nivolumab in patients with BRAF V600 mutant and BRAF wild-type advanced melanoma: a pooled analysis of 4 clinical trials. JAMA Oncol 1:433–440
85. Balar AV, Weber JS (2017) PD-1 and PD-L1 antibodies in cancer: current status and future directions. Cancer Immunol Immunother 66:551–564
86. Kazandjian D, Suzman DL, Blumenthal G, Mushti S, He K, Libeg M, Keegan P, Pazdur R (2016) FDA approval summary: nivolumab for the treatment of metastatic non-small cell lung cancer with progression on or after platinum-based chemotherapy. Oncologist 21:634–642
87. Hazarika M, Chuk MK, Theoret MR, Mushti S, He K, Weis SL, Putman AH, Helms WS, Cao X, Li H, Zhao H, Zhao L, Welch J, Graham L, Libeg M, Sridhara R, Keegan P, Pazdur R (2017) U.S. FDA approval summary: nivolumab for treatment of unresectable or metastatic melanoma following progression on ipilimumab. Clin Cancer Res 23:3484–3488
88. Xu JX, Maher VE, Zhang L, Tang S, Sridhara R, Ibrahim A, Kim G, Pazdur R (2017) FDA Approval summary: nivolumab in advanced renal cell carcinoma after anti-angiogenic therapy and exploratory predictive biomarker analysis. Oncologist 22:311–317
89. Ferris RL, Blumenschein G Jr, Fayette J, Guigay J, Colevas AD, Licitra L, Harrington K, Kasper S, Vokes EE, Even C, Worden F, Saba NF, Iglesias Docampo LC, Haddad R, Rordorf T, Kiyota N, Tahara M, Monga M, Lynch M, Geese WJ, Kopit J, Shaw JW, Gillison ML (2016) Nivolumab for recurrent squamous-cell carcinoma of the head and neck. N Engl J Med 375:1856–1867
90. Ansell SM (2017) Nivolumab in the treatment of Hodgkin lymphoma. Clin Cancer Res 23:1623–1626
91 Sharma P, Retz M, Siefker-Radtke A, Baron A, Necchi A, Bedke J, Plimack ER, Vaena D, Grimm M-O, Bracarda S, Arranz JA, Pal S, Ohyama C, Saci A, Qu X, Lambert A, Krishnan S, Azrilevich A, Galsky MD (2017) Nivolumab in metastatic urothelial carcinoma after platinum therapy (CheckMate 275): a multicentre, single-arm, phase 2 trial. The Lancet Oncology 18(3):312–322
92. Poh A (2017) Nivolumab gets FDA nod for bladder cancer. Cancer Discov 7:OF7
93. Sul J, Blumenthal GM, Jiang X, He K, Keegan P, Pazdur R (2016) FDA approval summary: pembrolizumab for the treatment of patients with metastatic non-small cell lung cancer whose tumors express programmed death-ligand 1. Oncologist 21:643–650
94. Barone A, Hazarika M, Theoret MR, Mishra-Kalyani P, Chen H, He K, Sridhara R, Subramaniam S, Pfuma E, Wang Y, Li H, Zhao H, Fourie Zirkelbach J, Keegan P, Pazdur R (2017) FDA approval summary: pembrolizumab for the treatment of patients with unresectable or metastatic melanoma. Clin Cancer Res 23:5661–5665
95. Chuk MK, Chang JT, Theoret MR, Sampene E, He K, Weis SL, Helms WS, Jin R, Li H, Yu J, Zhao H, Zhao L, Paciga M, Schmiel D, Rawat R, Keegan P, Pazdur R (2017) FDA approval summary: accelerated approval of pembrolizumab for second-line treatment of metastatic melanoma. Clin Cancer Res 23:5666–5670
96. Bauml J, Seiwert TY, Pfister DG, Worden F, Liu SV, Gilbert J, Saba NF, Weiss J, Wirth L, Sukari A, Kang H, Gibson MK, Massarelli E, Powell S, Meister A, Shu X, Cheng JD,

Haddad R (2017) Pembrolizumab for platinum- and cetuximab-refractory head and neck cancer: results from a single-arm, phase ii study. J Clin Oncol 35(14):1542–1549. https://doi.org/10.1200/JCO.2016.70.1524

97. Colwell J (2017) Pembrolizumab approved for Hodgkin lymphoma. Cancer Discov 7:OF1
98. Inman BA, Longo TA, Ramalingam S, Harrison MR (2017) Atezolizumab: a PD-L1-blocking antibody for bladder cancer. Clin Cancer Res 23:1886–1890
99. Camacho LH (2015) CTLA-4 blockade with ipilimumab: biology, safety, efficacy, and future considerations. Cancer Med 4:661–672
100. Cameron F, Whiteside G, Perry C (2011) Ipilimumab first global approval. Drugs 71:12
101. Hodi FS, O'Day SJ, McDermott DF, Weber RW, Sosman JA, Haanen JB, Gonzalez R, Robert C, Schadendorf D, Hassel JC, Akerley W, van den Eertwegh AJ, Lutzky J, Lorigan P, Vaubel JM, Linette GP, Hogg D, Ottensmeier CH, Lebbe C, Peschel C, Quirt I, Clark JI, Wolchok JD, Weber JS, Tian J, Yellin MJ, Nichol GM, Hoos A, Urba WJ (2010) Improved survival with ipilimumab in patients with metastatic melanoma. N Engl J Med 363:711–723
102. Ramakrishna V, Sundarapandiyan K, Zhao B, Bylesjo M, Marsh HC, Keler T (2015) Characterization of the human T cell response to in vitro CD27 costimulation with varlilumab. J Immunother Cancer 3:37
103. Purcell J, Hickson J, Tanlimco S, Fox M, Chao D, Hsi E, Sho M, Powers R, Foster-Duke K, McGonigal T, Uziel S, Kumar T, Samayoa J, Longenecker K, Lai D, Hollenbaugh D, Afar D, Iyer S, Morgan-Lappe S, Gish K (2016) ABBV-085 is a novel antibody–drug conjugate (ADC) that targets LRRC15 in the tumor microenvironment. EJC 69(Supplement 1):S10. (Abstract)
104. Diefenbach CS, Hong F, Cohen JB, Robertson MJ, Ambinder RF, Fenske TS, Advani RH, Kahl BS, Ansell S (2015) Preliminary safety and efficacy of the combination of brentuximab vedotin and ipilimumab in relapsed/refractory Hodgkin lymphoma: a trial of the ECOG-ACRIN Cancer Research Group (E4412). Blood 126:4
105. Herrera AF, Bartlett NL, Ramchandren R, et al (2016) Preliminary results from a phase 1/2 study of brentuximab vedotin in combination with nivolumab in patients with relapsed or refractory Hodgkin lymphoma. In: 58th American Society of Hematology annual meeting, Abstract 1105

Improving the Safety Profile of ADCs

Magali Guffroy, Hadi Falahatpisheh, and Martin Finkelstein

Abstract Antibody–drug conjugates (ADCs) take advantage of the specificity of a monoclonal antibody to deliver cytotoxic agents directly into tumor cells. The plethora of ADCs investigated in clinical trials in recent years has enabled characterization of the major challenges faced by this therapeutic modality. With regard to safety, non-target-mediated toxicities, which are independent of the targeted antigens and similar for ADCs with the same linker-payloads, often drive dose-limiting events in patients and at the same time question the targeting efficiency of current ADCs. Development-limiting target-mediated toxicities have only been reported for a few ADCs. This manuscript will provide an overview of the major clinically relevant toxicities of ADCs with a presentation of key ADC attributes influencing these toxicities and discussion of potential mechanisms. Current research efforts to mitigate ADC-associated toxicities, including among others site-specific conjugation chemistry and prevention of normal tissue binding, will be presented and could be critical to future ADC endeavors.

Keywords Toxicology · Safety · Toxicity · Thrombocytopenia · Neutropenia · Off-target · On-target · Target · Dependent · Independent · Liver · Kidney · Peripheral neuropathy · Ocular · Dose-limiting · DLT · Auristatin · Microtubule inhibitor · Calicheamicin · Maximum tolerated dose · MTD · Therapeutic index

Introduction

Antibody-drug conjugates (ADCs) represent a distinct class of targeted agents that consist of cytotoxic drugs linked to monoclonal antibodies directed against tumor-associated antigens. These loaded antibodies were designed to allow targeted

M. Guffroy (✉) · M. Finkelstein
Pfizer Inc, Drug Safety Research and Development, Pearl River, NY, USA
e-mail: magaliguffroy@icloud.com

H. Falahatpisheh
Preclinical Safety Oncology, AbbVie Stemcentrx LLC, South San Francisco, CA, USA

M. Damelin (ed.), *Innovations for Next-Generation Antibody-Drug Conjugates*, Cancer Drug Discovery and Development,
https://doi.org/10.1007/978-3-319-78154-9_3

delivery of the cytotoxic agent to the tumor while sparing non-targeted normal tissues, thereby alleviating the systemic toxicity observed with conventional chemotherapies. ADCs were therefore conceptually anticipated to have low toxicity and to significantly widen the therapeutic index (TI; ratio between toxic and therapeutic dose) [1]. However, as most target antigens of interest were not tumor-specific but rather tumor-enriched with some degree of expression in normal tissues [2], the major initial safety concern was justifiably related to the potential for target-mediated toxicity in normal tissues and the TI was foreseen to be driven by the differential expression between normal tissues and tumor. This has typically not been the case for ADCs evaluated in clinical trials and normal tissue expression, although reported for many target antigens, has rarely been associated with adverse reactions and/or dose-limiting toxicities [3]. Major toxicities are in fact attributable to non-target-mediated effects [3, 4], which include premature extracellular release of the cytotoxic agent (in systemic circulation or particular tissues) and target-independent ADC internalization/uptake. The toxicities are therefore similar for ADCs with the same linker-cytotoxic agents (but distinct targeting antibodies), including affected organs, nature of toxicities and maximum tolerated dose (MTD) [3]. The fact that most dose-limiting toxicities are driven by non-target-mediated rather than target-mediated effects questions the targeting efficiency of ADCs and the limitations of current ADC constructs that require very high tumor antigen expression to demonstrate efficacy, as seen for HER2-targeting ado-trastuzumab emtansine (T-DM1, Kadcyla) [5–7]. Major efforts have therefore been undertaken by multiple research teams to alleviate non-target-mediated toxicities, increase the delivery of ADCs to tumors and improve the safety of ADCs. Innovations in linker technology and conjugation chemistry in particular are starting to yield promising results. ADCs were initially produced by random conjugation of the cytotoxic agents to lysine or cysteine residues on the antibodies with generation of chemically heterogeneous and variably toxic species [8]. A variety of more-controlled site-specific drug conjugation technologies have now been developed to control the sites of attachment of the cytotoxic agents to the antibodies and to yield homogeneous conjugates with improved plasma stability and exposure and reduced toxicity [8–10]. A handful of site-specific ADCs are currently undergoing clinical evaluation [11] that will inform us on the translation of the observed laboratory improvement in safety. With the expected alleviation of non-target-mediated toxicities accompanied by improved pharmacokinetics (manifested in particular as increased area under the plasma drug concentration-time curve [AUC]), target antigen expression by normal tissues may resurface as the major concern, and several approaches are currently evaluated to increase specific tumor targeting, such as prevention of binding of antibodies to normal tissues [12], conditional activation of antibodies in tumor microenvironment [13] or enhanced binding selectivity of antibodies to tumor cells [14]. These approaches will only provide meaningful benefit if we are concurrently able to efficiently mitigate non-target-mediated toxicities.

This manuscript will provide an overview of clinically relevant toxicities of ADCs and current and future approaches to mitigate them. We will first review key ADC attributes influencing toxicities and then present and discuss target-mediated and non-target-mediated toxicities with considerations regarding mechanisms.

ADC Determinants of Toxicity

ADC toxicities are influenced by the complex interplay of the three core elements of the molecules, the monoclonal antibody, the linker, and the covalently attached cytotoxic agent. Mechanistically, ADCs bind to target antigens on the cell surface and are internalized via receptor-mediated endocytosis, with subsequent trafficking to the endosome/lysosome compartment and release of the cytotoxic agent through proteolytic degradation of the antibody moiety or cleavage of the linker. Essential features of the ADC modality that affect toxicity will be reviewed and discussed.

Target Antigen

Identification and validation of suitable target antigens for ADCs are critical for the clinical success of this therapeutic modality and research teams have invested considerable efforts in understanding essential features of target antigens that will drive efficacy while ensuring acceptable toxicity profile. This has proven to be a challenging endeavor. Desired attributes of target antigens include: differential and sufficient expression in tumors versus normal tissues; accessibility to ADCs via systemic circulation; compatibility with intended pharmacology; and absence of downregulation with treatment [15]. Target expression in normal tissues and accessibility may influence the range of toxicities observed.

Evaluation of target expression usually starts with the comparative analysis of mRNA and/or protein expression in tumors and normal tissues in order to identify targets that are overexpressed in tumors and to recognize normal tissue expression of potential concern [2, 16]. Transcript information is available from a variety of sources including public mRNA expression databases such as The Cancer Genome Atlas (TCGA, tumors and matched normal tissues) [17], Genotype-Tissue Expression (GTEx, normal tissues) [18] and Illumina's Human BodyMap 2.0 (normal tissues) [19]. Resources are more limited regarding large-scale quantitative protein expression data; however the development of technologies such as mass spectrometry-based proteomics is starting to bridge the gap. The LC-MS/MS-based Human Proteome Map (HPM) for example already provides quantitative proteomic data from main normal human tissues [20]. Although these data provide valuable first tier information regarding total tissue concentrations of target transcript and/or protein, they do not provide any information regarding specific cell types and subcellular localization of target expression, thereby limiting inference about potential safety liabilities. Normal tissues are indeed composed of a variety of cell types and usually have a complex cytoarchitecture, so that total tissue concentrations of the target may fail to identify toxicologically significant high expression levels within specific cell types. Subcellular localization of expression may also inform on potential accessibility of the target antigen to the ADC.

These initial data should therefore be complemented by methods that will enable molecular detection with morphological context (i.e. tissue distribution and cellular localization), such as immunohistochemistry (IHC) and/or in situ hybridization (ISH) for protein and mRNA detection, respectively. IHC may be technically challenging but it is currently the preferred approach as it allows specific detection of the targeted antigen. The development of a rigorously validated IHC assay is critical for the generation of reliable data, and assay validation will include appropriate control materials and performance evaluation against orthogonal methods. A robust assay will allow accurate evaluation of target expression in tumors and normal tissues and will therefore inform not only of clinical indications but also of potential target organs of toxicity. For example, comprehensive characterization by IHC of the expression of the tumor-associated antigens ROR1 [21] and Trop2 [22] showed widespread normal tissue expression, with membrane expression seen in organs such as parathyroid, pancreatic islets and gastrointestinal tract for ROR1 and esophagus, skin, kidney, exocrine pancreas and salivary gland for Trop2. In addition, the intensity of staining in many normal tissues was overall similar to that seen in tumors for both targets, which raised concerns regarding potential for target-mediated toxicities [21, 22]. Prospective assessment of safety liabilities is however very complex and the various factors that may influence development of toxicities are still incompletely understood. Membrane expression and expression in highly proliferative compartments of normal tissues are strong indicators of potential liabilities. It is unclear however whether restricted membrane apical expression, as is often observed in differentiated epithelia, reduces toxicity concerns through limited accessibility of target antigen for ADC binding. There are a number of examples indicating that epithelial tight junctions, which are critical for separating apical and basolateral membrane domains, might not in fact prevent passage of antibodies between cells. For example, although ENPP3 expression was shown to be restricted to apical membranes in normal tissues such as kidney proximal tubules, bronchial epithelium and salivary gland, evaluation of an ENPP3-targeted biotherapeutic agent in monkeys showed toxicity consistent with accessibility of target antigen to the antibody construct [23]. The sensitivity of target-expressing cells to the pharmacological effects of the cytotoxic agents should also be considered in the assessment of potential safety risks as discussed in the following section.

In conclusion, IHC development efforts are critical for proper characterization of target expression in normal tissues and for inference about potential safety liabilities and, although target-mediated toxicity is currently not the major toxicity concern for ADCs, the situation should change with the improved stability and exposure of new generation ADCs leading to increased targeting efficiency.

Targeting Antibody

The targeting antibody component of the ADC can also influence the toxicity. The affinity (usually very high, sub-nanomolar) of the antibody for the target antigen will contribute to internalization efficiency of the ADC in target-expressing cells in both tumor cells and normal tissues. While the contribution of the cytotoxic agent to ADC activity is understood, it is still not clear whether intrinsic antibody activity is desirable and/or plays a part in anti-tumor activity and toxicity. Intrinsic antibody activity could originate from the modulation of the biological activity of the target antigen or from Fc-mediated immune effector functions, such as antibody-dependent cell-mediated cytotoxicity (ADCC) or complement-dependent cytotoxicity (CDC) that are in large part driven by the monoclonal antibody isotypes. Most ADCs in clinical development utilize IgG1 isotype antibodies [24] that have the potential to mediate strong ADCC and CDC effects, unlike IgG2 and IgG4 that have poor immune effector functions [25]. For example, ado-trastuzumab emtansine (T-DM1, Kadcyla, anti-HER2-SMCC-DM1) is a HER2-targeted ADC that maintains intrinsic trastuzumab antibody activity including HER2 function blocking and IgG1-driven ADCC effects [26]. Limited published data on evaluation of contribution of intrinsic antibody activity currently indicate that the majority of ADC efficacy and toxicity likely comes from the cytotoxic agent and not from the antibody activity. A panel of anti-CD70 antibodies of various IgG isotypes conjugated to the tubulin inhibitor monomethylauristatin F (MMAF) demonstrated comparable in vivo efficacy and toxicity between IgG1, IgG1 lacking FcγR binding, and IgG2 conjugates [27]. Additionally, an anti-CD30 diabody-MMAF conjugate lacking the Fc domain to support effector functions was shown to have similar in vivo anti-tumor activity in SCID mice as the parent anti-CD30 IgG1-MMAF conjugate [28]. Noteworthy also is that effector functions of antibodies require binding of their constant regions to various receptors and thus are possibly more limited for ADCs undergoing rapid internalization.

Cytotoxic Agent

The cytotoxic agent is the primary effector of the cytotoxic activity and as such is a key player in ADC-related toxicities. There are three main categories of cytotoxic agents currently utilized in ADCs [11, 24].

- Microtubule inhibitors. These are the most commonly used cytotoxic agents in ADC development [29]. They are mainly represented by maytansinoid and auristatin derivatives, which are potent inhibitors of tubulin polymerization. Although these microtubule disrupting agents are best known for their ability to interfere with the mitotic spindle and to induce cell cycle arrest in the G2/M phase with ensuing apoptosis, they can also affect non-dividing cells in interphase through interference with intracellular trafficking, cytoskeleton formation and/or cell motility [30, 31]. Microtubule disruption can therefore lead to toxicities in both rapidly proliferating tissues, such as bone marrow, gastrointestinal tract and testis through inhibition of mitosis, and also in more quiescent tissues, such as for example the peripheral nervous system through interference with axonal transport [32]. The potential effects on non-dividing cells should not be overlooked when evaluating toxicities of microtubule inhibitor-based ADCs and might contribute to the pathogenesis of unforeseen toxicities, such as for example the lung toxicity reported with site-specific conjugates of vc-MMAE [33].

- DNA-damaging agents. These include calicheamicin derivatives, duocarmycin analogs and pyrrolobenzodiazepine (PBD) dimers, which all bind in the minor groove of DNA thereby leading to DNA cross-linking or alkylation and blocking of DNA replication. Although the activity of these agents is usually considered to be cell-cycle independent, there is still increased susceptibility of dividing cells with most severe effects observed in rapidly dividing tissues.
- DNA topoisomerase I inhibitors under investigation consist of camptothecin derivatives and include SN38, the active metabolite of irinotecan, and exatecan mesylate with activity in MDR1-mediated multidrug-resistant cells. These agents are cell cycle-specific and induce double-strand DNA breaks in dividing cells culminating in apoptosis.

Although the specific mechanism of action of the cytotoxic agent may lead to distinct toxicities (e.g. peripheral neuropathy of microtubule inhibitors), ADC-related toxicities may be driven more by the potency of the cytotoxic moiety rather than the specific cell-killing mechanism. All cytotoxic agents used in ADCs are extremely potent with activity in the low nanomolar range for microtubule inhibitors and low to mid picomolar range for DNA-damaging agents [34]. The higher potency of DNA-damaging agents as compared with microtubule inhibitors may further explain some of the toxicities observed. LGR5 (Leucine-rich repeat-containing G protein-coupled receptor 5) is a stem cell antigen that is expressed on crypt base columnar cells in the intestinal tract and on putative cancer stem cells in colorectal cancer. The evaluation of 2 anti-LGR5 ADC constructs with different cytotoxic drugs conjugated via cleavable linkers demonstrated target-mediated intestinal toxicity in rats with the DNA-damaging anthracycline NMS818 and not with the microtubule inhibitor MMAE when given at similar intravenous doses [35]. While it is tempting to ascribe the toxicity to the activity of the DNA-damaging agent on non-dividing quiescent stem cells, bystander effects on neighboring crypt dividing cells would still be expected with both compounds and it is therefore a possibility that the increased potency contributed more to the intestinal toxicity than the specific mechanism of action of NMS818. Furthermore, the liver microvascular injury observed microscopically in monkeys dosed with antibody-calicheamicin conjugates [36] is not specific of this DNA-damaging cytotoxic agent and is also seen, although with a lower severity, in monkeys dosed with ADCs containing non-cleavable microtubule inhibitors (unpublished observations). The specific cell-killing mechanism of the cytotoxic agent is therefore not the decisive factor in the development of this liver toxicity.

The drug loading (drug-to-antibody ratio, DAR) is another important attribute of ADCs that may influence the toxicity. Both heterogeneity of DAR species and high DAR have been recognized to lead to faster clearance, lower plasma exposure, increased toxicity and lower therapeutic index [37]. The optimal drug loading is around 2–4 with PK generally comparable to the corresponding unconjugated antibody and slower clearance.

Linker Chemistry

The linker is a critical component of the ADC that dictates the mechanism of release of the cytotoxic agent and contributes to specific properties of the released moiety, both of which can influence ADC toxicity. Major considerations regarding linker design include plasma stability over several days and efficient release of active drug at the target site. Linkers for ADCs are generally broadly categorized into cleavable and non-cleavable linkers [38].

Cleavable linkers, which are currently the most commonly used linkers in ADCs, include:

- acid-labile linkers, such as hydrazone that undergoes hydrolysis in the endosomal and/or lysosomal acidic environment
- protease-cleavable linkers, such as valine-citrulline or valine-alanine dipeptide that are cleaved by lysosomal enzymes like cathepsin B
- disulfide linkers, such as N-hydroxysuccinimidyl-4-(2-pyridyldithio)butanoate (SPDB) that is cleaved through glutathione-mediated reduction.

Non-cleavable linkers require lysosomal catabolic degradation of the antibody for release of the cytotoxic agent and include moieties such as maleimidomethyl cyclohexane-1-carboxylate (MCC), succinimidyl-4-(N-maleimidomethyl) cyclohexane-1-carboxylate (SMCC) and maleimidocaproyl (mc).

Main safety considerations for cleavable linkers relate to plasma stability and bystander effect [38, 39]. Cleavable linkers are chemically or enzymatically labile and as such may be less stable in circulation than non-cleavable linkers, with potential premature release of cytotoxic drugs and associated systemic toxicity if the released drugs are able to cross cell membranes. Even low rate deconjugation of the ADC in circulation may be sufficient to induce significant toxicity given the very high potency of the cytotoxic drugs used in ADCs (100- to 1000-fold more potent than standard chemotherapeutic drugs). In addition, membrane-permeable drugs exacerbate target-mediated and non-target-mediated toxicities through bystander effects from killing of neighboring cells [39]. One such example of a cell-permeable drug with a cleavable linker is MMAE linked to the protease-cleavable valine-citrulline linker; the myelosuppression and peripheral neuropathy observed with this type of linker-cytotoxic agent will be discussed later. By contrast, non-cleavable linkers are very stable in circulation and antibody degradation releases amino-acid-capped cytotoxic drugs that are charged and non-membrane permeable, with no potential therefore for bystander killing [38]. Toxicities to non-target-expressing tissues with such ADCs are necessarily related to nonspecific internalization or uptake of the ADC with subsequent intracellular cytotoxic drug release.

Ongoing linker development efforts are largely focused on improvements in cleavable linker technology that yield better plasma stability and/or reduced clearance with associated improved safety, such as the enzyme-cleavable peptide linker Gly-Gly-Phe-Gly used in DS-8201a (anti-Her2-GlyGlyPheGly-DXd) [40], the enzyme-cleavable PEGylated glucuronide linker [41], or the acid-cleavable thiomaleamic acid linker [42].

Conjugation Technology

Improvement in conjugation technology, through site-specific conjugation and controlled cytotoxic drug stoichiometry (i.e. cytotoxic drug loading or DAR), has likely been the single most important factor with respect to safety improvement of ADCs.

Initial conjugation approaches were based on the random conjugation of the cytotoxic drugs to either lysine or cysteine residues of the antibody, which generated heterogeneous ADC products containing a mixture of species with different DARs, each with distinct in vivo pharmacokinetic, efficacy and safety profiles. An early experiment evaluated purified ADC species of anti-CD30-vc-MMAE with DARs of 2, 4 or 8 and demonstrated that the higher loaded species were more rapidly cleared and more toxic in tumor-bearing mice without a proportional increase in efficacy [37]. Noteworthy also is the vast number of potential conjugation sites for lysine-based conjugation that further influence the properties of the ADC species. As an example, 70 different sites of DM1 conjugation have been identified on the trastuzumab antibody of T-DM1 [43]. At this stage, the majority of ADCs that have been evaluated clinically are conventional (random) conjugates.

Significant research efforts were undertaken to generate homogeneous ADCs using site-specific conjugation methods, which demonstrated higher plasma exposure and improved therapeutic index and established the importance of the specific conjugation sites [10, 44]. A variety of site-specific conjugation methods have been developed to control attachment sites of cytotoxic agents to antibodies and are based on antibody modifications such as: engineering of reactive cysteine residues for conjugation with thiol-reactive linkers (e.g. THIOMAB); introduction of glutamine tags for enzymatic conjugation through transglutaminases; or incorporation of unnatural aminoacids with bioorthogonal handles through mutagenesis [9]. Site-specific ADCs contain precise numbers of cytotoxic molecules per antibody with DARs usually of 2 or 4. In a seminal paper, Junutula et al. evaluated anti-MUC16-vc-MMAE ADCs produced using conventional (DAR ~3.5) and site-specific THIOMAB (DAR = 2) conjugation methods [10]. The THIOMAB conjugate was shown to be as efficacious in tumor-bearing mice as the conventional conjugate despite the reduced drug loading, while demonstrating in both rats and cynomolgus monkeys slower plasma clearance and improved safety through reduced bone marrow and liver toxicity. In addition, further investigations showed that the locations of the conjugation sites on the antibodies may also influence linker stability and ADC pharmacokinetics [44, 45], underscoring the critical importance of conjugation site selection. The mechanisms underlying the improved pharmacokinetics and reduced toxicity of site-specific conjugates are not completely understood; the favorable conjugation sites may increase ADC stability through reduced linker accessibility in circulation and maintenance of antibody integrity preventing clearance.

However, site-specific conjugation has been reported to be associated with the potential unexpected development of new toxicities, likely related to the very high plasma exposures attained with these compounds. For example, lung toxicity characterized mainly by pulmonary alveolar edema and interstitial inflammation progressing to fibrosis was observed in cynomolgus monkeys after repeat-dose administration of a THIOMAB conjugated to vc-MMAE, irrespective of the targeting antibody [33]. Clinical relevance of this toxicity and potential safety margin in patients with regard to efficacious doses are uncertain at this stage.

There are currently few disclosed site-specific ADCs that are or have been evaluated clinically [11]. These include conjugates obtained using engineered cysteines such as SGN-CD33A (anti-CD33-ValAla-PBD), SGN-CD70A (anti-CD70-ValAla-PBD) and DMUC-4064A (anti-MUC16-vc-MMAE), or conjugates obtained using transglutaminase enzymatic conjugation such as RN927C (anti-Trop2-vc-0101). These are all DAR2 conjugates with cleavable linkers. More site-specific conjugates are poised to enter clinical development and aggregated patient data should soon provide information regarding clinical translation of their improved nonclinical therapeutic index.

This first section highlighted key ADC characteristics that influence development of toxicities and the complex interplay between the different ADC structural components. We will now review major toxicities observed clinically with ADCs with a discussion of possible mechanisms.

Target-Mediated Toxicities

Target-mediated toxicities, also referred to as on-target toxicities, are due to binding of the ADC to target antigen in normal tissues. Outside of ADCs developed for the treatment of hematological malignancies, which often induce blood cytopenias through the targeting of antigens that are present not only on neoplastic but also on normal hematolymphopoietic cells (e.g. CD33, CD19 and CD22), there are few reported cases of target-mediated toxicities with ADCs evaluated in clinical trials. Examples of such on-target toxicities include the skin toxicities observed with bivatuzumab mertansine and glembatumumab vedotin. Bivatuzumab mertansine (antiCD44v6-SPP-DM1) was evaluated in phase 1 trials in patients with squamous cell carcinoma of the head and neck or esophagus or with metastatic breast cancer [46, 47]. The clinical development was terminated early due to serious skin toxicity, which included maculopapular rashes, focal blister formation and skin exfoliation along with a fatal case of toxic epidermal necrolysis. Immunohistochemical evaluation of CD44v6 expression in normal human tissues showed expression that was largely confined to epithelial tissues, including squamous epithelium of the skin, esophagus and tonsils and lung airway epithelium [46, 48]. Dose-related non-severe and reversible skin toxicity was also observed in toxicity studies in cynomolgus monkeys [46]. As other ADCs containing DM1 have not shown similar toxicities in the clinic [49], the skin toxicity induced by bivatuzumab mertansine was considered related to CD44v6 expression on skin keratinocytes. Target-mediated skin toxicity was also observed with glembatumumab vedotin (anti-gpNMB-vc-MMAE) that has been investigated in patients with advanced melanoma and breast cancer, where skin rash was identified as one of the most common adverse events with 45–70% incidence across trials [50, 51]. Similar skin rash was not observed in patients treated with ADCs containing the same conjugated MMAE moiety and the skin toxicity was considered related to gpNMB (glycoprotein non-metastatic melanoma protein B) expression on epidermal melanocytes [52, 53]. Interestingly, development of rash within the first cycle was strongly predictive of clinical response to glembatumumab vedotin with higher overall response rate (ORR) and longer progression-free survival (PFS) in these patients. In the first melanoma trial for example, the association between rash and response was noticeable with ORR (rash) = 24% vs ORR (no rash) = 0% and PFS (rash) = 4.4 months vs PFS (no rash) = 1.3 months. The development of target-mediated rash may therefore be indicative of potential efficacy and understanding its mechanism may prove helpful in the benefit-risk assessment of the drug.

Noteworthy is that the potential for target-mediated toxicity can be difficult to predict and is not solely driven by target expression, as indicated by the number of ADCs with significant normal tissue expression that did not demonstrate target-mediated toxicities in the clinic. For example, although ado-trastuzumab emtansine (T-DM1, Kadcyla, anti-HER2-SMCC-DM1) targets HER2 that has significant normal tissue expression in epithelial cells of the gastrointestinal tract [54], skin and breast in particular, major dose-limiting toxicities observed in patients are non-target-mediated and consist of thrombocytopenia and elevated liver enzymes [55], as seen with other conjugates containing the same linker-payload, SMCC-DM1 [56]. Similarly, although DMOT4039A (anti-MSLN-vc-MMAE) targets mesothelin, which has high expression on mesothelial cells lining the peritoneal, thoracic and pericardial cavities, it did not induce any significant target-mediated toxicities up to the maximum assessed doses in a phase 1 trial in pancreatic and ovarian cancer patients and treatment-related grade 1 serositis (pleural effusion) was only seen in one patient [57]. A last noteworthy example relates to NaPi2b-targeting ADCs. NaPi2b (SLC34A2) is a sodium-dependent phosphate transporter protein normally expressed in epithelial cells of a variety of tissues, including lung, small intestine and kidney, and further characterization of NaPi2b expression specifically on lung type 2 pneumocytes was initially concerning [58, 59]. Evaluation of different ADC constructs, such as lifastuzumab vedotin (anti-NaPi2b-vc-MMAE) or XMT-1536 (anti-NaPi2b dolaflexin ADC), in patients or cynomolgus monkeys did not demonstrate target-mediated lung toxicity in either species [60, 61]. In particular, XMT-1536 is an anti-NaPi2b ADC with an auristatin cytotoxic agent (average of 15 auristatin molecules per antibody) and an enzymatically cleavable linker. XMT-1536 binds to cynomolgus monkey NaPi2b and its potential toxicity was evaluated in that species following a single XMT-1536 intravenous administration with necropsy after 1 and 3 weeks. There was no target-mediated toxicity up to the highest dose evaluated and in particular no evidence of lung toxicity from rigorous microscopic evaluation of tissue samples [61].

These previous examples provide evidence that target-mediated toxicities are not driven solely by target expression and that other factors, as indicated in the previous section, such as target antigen accessibility, proliferation rate of target expressing cells, mechanism of action and potency of the cytotoxic agent, may contribute to the development of toxicities. Furthermore, the infrequent observation of target-mediated toxicities points to poor targeting efficiency of current ADCs, which distribute broadly outside of target-expressing tissues. However, the next-generation ADCs are expected to distribute more specifically and selectively to antigen-positive tissues with an associated higher risk of target-mediated toxicities and the thorough characterization of target expression in normal tissues and in tumors for informed interpretation and decision cannot be overstated.

Non-Target-Mediated Toxicities

As indicated previously, most adverse reactions noted in patients treated with ADCs are currently attributable to non-target-mediated effects, which are independent of target expression and similar for ADCs with the same linker-cytotoxic agent and conjugation chemistry (Table 1). There are two main primary mechanisms for the development of these toxicities:

- Premature extracellular deconjugation of ADC and release of active cytotoxic agent in circulation
- Target-independent ADC internalization/uptake with subsequent intracellular release of cytotoxic agent. ADC ingestion by non-target-expressing cells can occur through receptor-mediated (e.g. FcγR or mannose receptors) or non-receptor-mediated (e.g. fluid phase endocytosis prior to FcRn binding) processes.

These toxicities can also be exacerbated by secondary bystander effects, whereby released membrane-permeable cytotoxic moieties can diffuse into neighboring cells to induce further cell killing.

We will now review major non-target-mediated toxicities with discussion regarding specific causative linker-cytotoxic agents and potential mechanisms.

Hematological Effects

We will exclude from this discussion target-mediated hematological toxicities, as seen with ADCs targeting hematopoietic antigens, such as for example CD33 that is expressed on the surface of both normal and malignant myeloid cells.

Neutropenia

Commonly reported adverse events (AEs) after administration of ADCs to patients include manifestations of myelosuppression characterized by decreases in circulating white blood cells, red blood cells and/or platelets. Neutrophils are most consistently and severely affected due to their short circulatory lifespan (1–2 days),

Table 1 Major nontarget-mediated toxicities of ADCs for the commonly used linker-cytotoxic agents

Class of cytotoxic agent	Microtubule inhibitors				DNA-damaging agents	
Cytotoxic agent	**MMAE**	**MMAF**	**DM1**	**DM4**	**Calicheamicin**	**PBD**
Linker	vc (valine-citrulline)	mc	SPP, SMCC	SPDB	Hydrazone	va (valine-alanine)
Conjugation chemistry	Conventional	Conventional	Conventional	Conventional	Conventional	Site-specific
Selected programs	Brentuximab vedotin Pinatuzumab vedotin Polatuzumab vedotin TAK-264 Glembatumumab vedotin DLYE5953A	SGN-75 Depatuxizumab mafodotin AGS-16C3F Denintuzumab mafodotin	Ado-trastuzumab emtansine Naratuximab emtansine (IMGN529) Cantuzumab mertansine AMG-595	SAR3419 Mirvetuximab soravtansine Cantuzumab ravtansine	Inotuzumab ozogamicin Gemtuzumab ozogamicin	Rovalpituzumab tesirine (Rova-T)
Clinical MTD	1.8–2.4 mg/kg iv, q3w	1.5–5.0 mg/kg iv, q2w or q3w	3.6–6.3 mg/kg iv, q3w	4.3–6.0 mg/kg iv, q3w	Variable dosing regimens iv	0.4 mg/kg iv, q3w
Major clinical toxicities	**Myelosuppression** (neutropenia, thrombocytopenia, anemia) **Peripheral neuropathy**	**Thrombocytopenia** **Ocular toxicity** **Liver toxicity** (increases in liver enzymes)	**Thrombocytopenia** **Liver toxicity** (increases in liver enzymes, NRH)	**Ocular toxicity** **Peripheral neuropathy**	**Liver toxicity** (increases in liver enzymes, SOS) **Thrombocytopenia**	**Serosal effusion** **Skin toxicity** **Thrombocytopenia**
References	[62–67]	[68–72]	[49, 55, 56, 73–75]	[76–78]	[36, 79, 80]	[81]

DM1 $N^{2'}$-deacetyl-$N^{2'}$- (3-mercapto-1-oxopropyl)-maytansine, *DM4* $N^{2'}$-deacetyl-$N^{2'}$- (4-mercapto-4-methyl-1-oxopentyl)-maytansine, *iv* intravenous route, *MTD* maximal tolerated dose, *mc* maleimidocaproic acid, *MMAE* monomethyl auristatin E, *MMAF* monomethyl auristatin F, *NRH* nodular regenerative hyperplasia, *PBD* pyrrolobenzodiazepine, *q2w* every 2 weeks, *q3w* every 3 weeks, *SMCC* succinimidyl-4-(N-maleimidomethyl)cyclohexane-1-carboxylate, *SOS* sinusoidal obstruction syndrome, *SPDB* N-hydroxysuccinimidyl 4-(2-pyridyldithio)butanoate, *SPP* N-succinimidyl 4-(2-pyridyldithio)pentanoate

while myelosuppressive effects on platelets and erythrocytes, which have longer lifespans (8–10 days and 120 days, respectively), are usually milder and manageable given the use of appropriate intermittent dosing regimens (e.g. drug administration every 3 weeks). Non-target-mediated dose-limiting neutropenia is mainly observed with conventional conjugate ADCs that contain cleavable linkers and release membrane-permeable cytotoxic agents.

The best known example of such linker-cytotoxic agent is the commonly used vc-MMAE (dipeptide protease-cleavable valine-citrulline linker and auristatin-derived MMAE cytotoxic drug), which is present in ADCs such as TAK-264 (anti-guanylyl cyclase C-vc-MMAE), glembatumumab vedotin (anti-gpNMB-vc-MMAE) or DLYE5953A (anti-Ly6E-vc-MMAE). Neutropenia was one of the major dose-limiting toxicities (DLTs) in the dose escalation phase I trials and/or one of the most frequent adverse reactions during later phases of clinical development for these ADC constructs, with maximal tolerated doses (MTDs) of 1.8–2.4 mg/kg across ADCs [62–64]. Nineteen patients with gastrointestinal malignancies were treated with TAK-264 once every 3 weeks at dose levels of 0.3–2.4 mg/kg in the dose escalation arm of a phase I trial [62]. Four of 19 patients experienced DLTs of grade 4 neutropenia during cycle 1 (onset on days 10–15), including 1/6 patients at 1.8 mg/kg, 2/4 patients at 2.1 mg/kg and 1/1 patient at 2.4 mg/kg. The MTD was determined as 1.8 mg/kg and additional patients were enrolled at this dose level in the expansion cohort. There were no grade ≥ 3 drug-related anemia and thrombocytopenia in this trial. Although DLTs in advanced melanoma patients treated with glembatumumab vedotin once every 3 weeks in a phase I trial were attributed to target-mediated skin toxicity with a MTD of 1.88 mg/kg [50], the most common grade ≥ 3 treatment-related AE in a subsequent phase II study conducted at the previously determined MTD was neutropenia (21/96 patients, i.e. 22%) while treatment-related grade ≥ 3 rash, thrombocytopenia and anemia were reported in only 4%, 1% and 0% of patients, respectively [63]. Neutropenia was similarly the most frequent grade ≥ 3 treatment-related AE reported in 12% of patients treated with DLYE5953A in a phase I dose escalation (0.2–2.4 mg/kg) and dose expansion (2.4 mg/kg) trial that had enrolled 57 patients at the time of initial data presentation [82].

Another example of linker-cytotoxic agent associated with myelosuppression and neutropenia is CL2A-SN38 that consists of a pH sensitive linker and the active metabolite of irinotecan. Sacituzumab govitecan (anti-Trop2-CL2A-SN38) was evaluated in patients with metastatic triple-negative breast cancer at 10 mg/kg on Days 1 and 8 of 3-week cycles and the most common grade ≥ 3 AE was neutropenia, which was reported in 39% of patients [83].

These hematological toxicities are similarly seen in nonclinical species and we performed investigations in Sprague-Dawley rats using vc-0101, a linker-cytotoxic agent closely related to vc-MMAE, to study the mechanism for this toxicity. As indicated above (see "Linker chemistry"), cleavable linkers may be less stable than other linkers in circulation and the objective of the study was to evaluate potential contribution to the toxicity of ADC deconjugation and release of cytotoxic agent in circulation. Sprague-Dawley rats (6 males/group) received a single intravenous bolus dose of a non-cross-reactive ADC carrying vc-0101 (anti-X-vc-0101) at a tolerated dose of 10 mg/kg or 72-h continuous intravenous infusion of the active cytotoxic moiety, Aur-0101, at variable dose levels over the interval to reproduce slow systemic Aur-0101 release from 10 mg/kg anti-X-vc-0101 [unpublished data]. All rats were euthanized and necropsied at 72 h after dosing initiation. Microscopic examination of the sternal bone marrow showed similar findings in both groups with marked decreased hematopoietic cellularity affecting similarly erythroid and myeloid cell populations in all animals. These observations confirm that bone marrow suppression is the primary mechanism for the hematological toxicity observed with these ADC constructs, likely from cytotoxicity to rapidly proliferating hematopoietic cells, and that bone marrow suppression can also be induced by Aur-0101 in circulation. In addition, although mean serum exposure data for Aur-0101 were approximately two-fold higher in the Aur-0101 group as compared to the ADC group, individual data do indicate that the bone marrow toxicity is due, at least in part, to ADC deconjugation in circulation. Potential contribution of ADC deconjugation locally in bone marrow microenvironment could not be ruled out. Noteworthy is that ADC deconjugation in circulation may also contribute to the clinical efficacy reported with some of these constructs.

As indicated above (see "Conjugation technology"), nonclinical data suggest that site-specific conjugation has the potential to alleviate the hematological toxicity of these ADC constructs. When cynomolgus monkeys were dosed on Days 1 and 22 with an anti-MUC16-vc-MMAE ADC at 5.9 mg/kg (DAR ~3.5) or a site-specific anti-MUC16-vc-MMAE THIOMAB at 12.8 mg/kg (DAR = 2), which corresponded to the same MMAE dose of 1200 mg/m^2, marked transient decreases in neutrophil counts were noted after ADC administration while there were no notable effects on neutrophil counts with the THIOMAB [10]. Decreases in neutrophil counts were recapitulated with the THIOMAB at higher doses of ≥2400 mg/m^2 MMAE. The reduced hematological toxicity of site-specific conjugates may be related to increased ADC stability and reduced levels of unconjugated cytotoxic drug in circulation. The translation of these observations to patients is currently explored clinically and could represent a quantum leap with respect to alleviation of non-target-mediated myelosuppression of these drugs.

Thrombocytopenia

Non-target-mediated adverse thrombocytopenia, in the absence of overt myelosuppression, is another common hematological toxicity of conventional conjugate ADCs, which is mainly observed with more stable ADCs containing non-cleavable linkers (e.g. maleimide linkers mc and SMCC) or more potent ADCs containing DNA-damaging cytotoxic agents (e.g. calicheamicin).

A well characterized example of a non-cleavable ADC associated with dose-limiting thrombocytopenia is ado-trastuzumab emtansine (T-DM1, Kadcyla, anti-HER2-SMCC-DM1), which is comprised of an anti-HER2 antibody linked to a potent maytansinoid agent DM1 through a non-cleavable SMCC linker. In a phase I dose escalation study, 24 patients with advanced HER2-positive breast cancer were treated with T-DM1 once every 3 weeks by intravenous infusion at dose levels of 0.3–4.8 mg/kg [84]. Two of 3 patients treated at 4.8 mg/kg experienced transient dose-limiting grade 4 thrombocytopenia and the MTD was determined as 3.6 mg/kg. The 3.6 mg/kg cohort was expanded to include a total of 15 patients. The 2 most commonly report AEs in the trial were thrombocytopenia (54.2% of patients) and elevated transaminases (41.7%). In a phase III randomized trial in the same patient population, T-DM1 was evaluated at the dose of 3.6 mg/kg administered every 3 weeks [85]. The most commonly reported grade ≥ 3 AEs with T-DM1 were thrombocytopenia (12.9%) and elevated aspartate aminotransferase (4.3%) and alanine aminotransferase (2.9%) activities. Effects on platelet counts with T-DM1 were of rapid onset (platelet decreases first noted as soon as 1 day after T-DM1 administration) and showed a consistent pattern of cyclic decline, with nadir by Day 8 and recovery before the next dose [82, 85]. In addition, slow downward drifts in predose platelet counts were seen in some patients over multiple T-DM1 cycles [82]. It is noteworthy that hematological effects with T-DM1 were quite selective for platelets and other hematological lineages were relatively unaffected.

Thrombocytopenia is also consistently reported with non-cleavable ADCs containing mc-MMAF [68–70]. In a phase I dose escalation study, 47 patients with relapsed or refractory non-Hodgkin lymphoma (NHL) or metastatic renal cell carcinoma were treated with SGN-75 (anti-CD70-mc-MMAF) once every 3 weeks by intravenous infusion at dose levels of 0.3–4.5 mg/kg [68]. The most common grade ≥ 3 AE was thrombocytopenia (19% of patients), with nadir typically occurring on Day 4 or 8 of cycle 1 and less pronounced effects during subsequent cycles. There were no grade ≥ 3 AEs of neutropenia or anemia. In addition, mild to moderate elevations in aspartate and alanine aminotransferases were seen in 70% and 40% of patients, respectively, and serious AEs of grade 4 hepatotoxicity were reported in 2 patients (4.2%).

Thrombocytopenia is also one of the major toxicities reported with calicheamicin-containing ADCs, such as the recently approved inotuzumab ozogamicin (Besponsa) that is comprised of an anti-CD22 antibody linked to a calicheamicin derivative through an acid-labile linker. In the expansion cohort of an initial phase I study in NHL patients, inotuzumab ozogamicin was evaluated at the MTD of 1.8 mg/m^2 administered every 4 weeks. Thrombocytopenia was the most frequent AE (63% patients with grade ≥ 3 thrombocytopenia) and was one of the most common reasons for dose delay, dose reduction or treatment discontinuation. In addition, increases in aspartate aminotransferase (AST), alanine aminotransferase (ALT) and bilirubin were noted in 41%, 18% and 22% of patients, respectively [79]. Thrombocytopenia in the absence of myelosuppression was also observed in monkeys dosed with a non-cross-reactive antibody-calicheamicin conjugate, PF-0259, which contains the same linker-cytotoxic agent as inotuzumab ozogamicin [36]. In that experiment, cynomolgus monkeys received PF-0259 intravenously at 6 mg/m^2 once every 3 weeks and hematology alterations consisted mainly of acute thrombocytopenia that was characterized by: decreases in platelet counts starting at 24 h after the first dose with nadirs (up to 86% decrease) at 48–72 h after the first dose; platelet count recovery by the end of cycle 1; and slow downward drifts in platelet counts with repeated administrations.

The non-target-mediated thrombocytopenia observed with these ADCs share common features, such as overall similar temporal characteristics and association with increases in liver enzymes.

The mechanism underlying these thrombocytopenia is not completely clear and is debated. Given the pharmacological activity of the cytotoxic agents, it is tempting to ascribe this toxicity to myelosuppression, and non-cleavable ADCs such as T-DM1 and AGS-16C3F (anti-ENPP3-mc-MMAF) have indeed been reported to be cytotoxic to differentiating megakaryocytes in vitro, through either FcγRIIa-mediated uptake or macropinocytosis-mediated internalization of the ADC and subsequent release of the cytotoxic agent [86, 87]. However, these mechanisms do not adequately or entirely explain the thrombocytopenia observed in vivo with these compounds. As indicated above, the thrombocytopenia with these ADCs is usually characterized by an acute onset (starting at 24 h after the first treatment) which, given the normal platelet lifespan of 8–10 days and the magnitude of the effect, is not consistent with decreased production by the bone marrow and is more compatible with peripheral destruction or sequestration of platelets. We investigated the mechanism for the thrombocytopenia observed in monkeys dosed with the antibody-calicheamicin conjugate PF-0259 [36]. Monkeys received PF-0259 once every 3 weeks and were necropsied at 48 h (Day 3) after the first administration or 3 weeks after the 3rd administration. As indicated above, PF-0259 induced acute thrombocytopenia (up to 86% platelet reduction) with nadirs at 48–72 h after the initial PF-0259 dose. There were no appreciable histological or cytological alterations in the bone marrow (in particular megakaryocyte density and morphology were within normal ranges) and no evidence of platelet activation in peripheral blood. Microscopic evaluation of liver from monkeys necropsied on Day 3 (time of platelet nadir) showed degeneration and loss of sinusoidal endothelial cells associated with marked platelet sequestration in sinusoids (Fig. 1). The experimental data from this study suggest that liver injury may contribute in part to the thrombocytopenia observed with antibody-calicheamicin conjugates. Given the similarities in the characteristics of the non-target-mediated thrombocytopenia for calicheamicin-containing ADCs and non-cleavable ADCs and given that elevated liver function tests are consistently observed with all these ADCs, it is a possibility that liver injury is also contributing to the thrombocytopenia observed with non-cleavable ADCs through an initial sinusoidal endothelial damage. Thrombocytopenia is an important ADC-associated toxicity and we hope that these preliminary conclusions will stimulate additional investigations into the respective contributions of the liver and/or bone marrow injury to the platelet changes.

Liver Toxicity

Hepatic disturbances are mainly observed with more stable ADCs containing non-cleavable linkers (e.g. maleimide linkers mc and SMCC) or more potent ADCs containing DNA-damaging cytotoxic agents (e.g. calicheamicin). These are the same

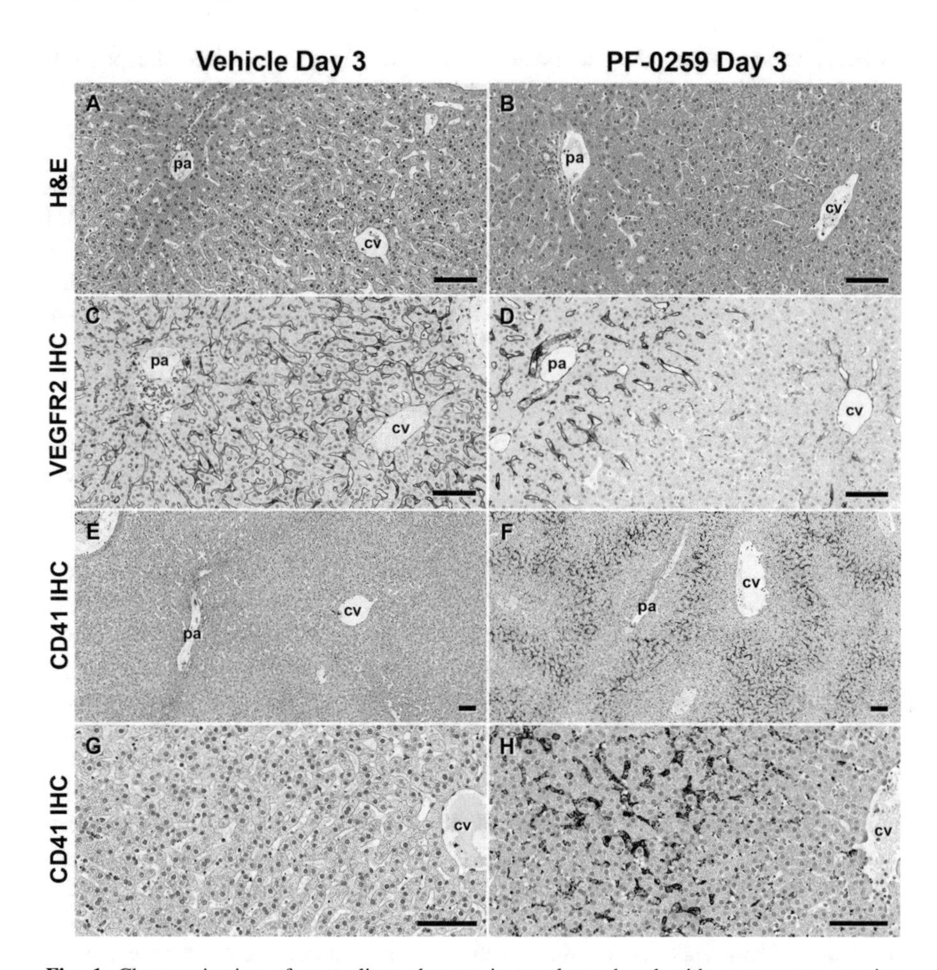

Fig. 1 Characterization of acute liver changes in monkeys dosed with a non-cross-reactive antibody-calicheamicin conjugate (PF-0259) demonstrated sinusoidal endothelial injury associated with marked platelet sequestration within sinusoids. Monkeys received a single intravenous administration of vehicle or PF-0259 at 6 mg/m^2 and were necropsied after 48 h on Day 3 (time of platelet nadir). Light microscopic evaluation of liver from vehicle control (**a**, **c**, **e**, **g**) and PF-0259-dosed (**b**, **d**, **f**, **h**) monkeys. There were no remarkable PF-0259-related liver changes at light microscopic examination of H&E-stained slides (**a**, **b**). VEGFR2 IHC showed delicate and diffuse staining of sinusoidal endothelial lining cells in control monkey (**c**) while there was staining disruption and marked loss of VEGFR2 immunoreactivity consistent with loss of endothelial cells in midzonal and to a lesser extent centrilobular regions in PF-0259-dosed monkey (**d**). CD41 IHC for platelets showed minimal scattered punctate staining in vascular spaces in control monkey (**e**, **g**) while there was abundant intrasinusoidal granular staining in midzonal regions throughout the liver sections in PF-0259-dosed monkey, consistent with platelet accumulation (**f**, **h**). The lower magnification (**f**) demonstrated the midzonal distribution and the higher magnification (**h**) the intrasinusoidal location of platelet sequestration. *pa* portal area, *cv* central vein. Scale bar = 100 μm

ADCs that are consistently associated with thrombocytopenia and the possible relationship between liver injury and thrombocytopenia was documented and discussed in the previous section, through presentation of effects on both platelet counts and liver function tests for selected ADCs.

Liver injury typically manifests as asymptomatic liver function abnormalities, such as elevations of transaminases and/or bilirubin. In the pivotal phase III T-DM1 trial in HER2-positive advanced breast cancer patients, hepatic disturbances in T-DM1-treated patients were characterized by elevations in AST and ALT (22% and 17% of patients, respectively), with low rates of grade $\geq$ 3 elevations (4% and 3% of patients for AST and ALT, respectively) [85]. In the pivotal phase III inotuzumab ozogamicin (Besponsa) trial in relapsed or refractory acute lymphoblastic leukemia (ALL) patients, liver-related laboratory abnormalities in inotuzumab ozogamicin-treated patients consisted mainly of increases in AST (23% of patients), ALT (15%), γ-glutamyltransferase (21%), bilirubin (21%) and alkaline phosphatase (13%), with grade $\geq$ 3 elevations noted in $\leq$5% of patients (except for increases in γ-glutamyltransferase grade $\geq$ 3 noted in 10% of patients) [80].

Although liver toxicity with these agents is often transient and reversible, it might progress and result in the development of specific liver diseases, such as nodular regenerative hyperplasia (NRH) or sinusoidal obstruction syndrome (SOS). Rare cases of biopsy-confirmed NRH have been reported in patients receiving a T-DM1-based regimen, and temporal association and absence of competing etiologies suggested a direct contribution of T-DM1 [73, 74]. NRH is a rare liver disorder that can lead to non-cirrhotic portal hypertension [88]. SOS is a known potential complication of therapy with antibody-calicheamicin conjugates, such as inotuzumab ozogamicin or gemtuzumab ozogamicin (Mylotarg). In the inotuzumab ozogamicin phase III trial in ALL patients, SOS was reported overall in 13% of patients and was more frequent in the subset of patients that proceeded to hematopoietic stem cell transplantation (HSCT) (22%) [80]. SOS, previously known as hepatic veno-occlusive disease, is a serious medical condition characterized clinically by jaundice, painful hepatomegaly, weight gain, and ascites. It is noteworthy that HSCT by itself is a recognized cause of SOS as a result of the conditioning myeloablative regimen [89].

NRH and SOS are both liver vascular disorders that are thought to result from initial insults to liver sinusoidal endothelial cells (SECs) [90, 91] and nonclinical investigation in monkeys with a non-cross-reactive antibody-calicheamicin conjugate demonstrated an initial and selective injury to liver SECs with recovery or progression to parenchymal remodeling and microscopic changes consistent with subclinical SOS [36].

The data presented here collectively indicate that ADC-associated hepatic disturbances likely originate primarily from liver endothelial injury. Liver endothelial cells are known to be involved in antibody recycling to the circulation via the neonatal Fc receptor (FcRn) pathway and we further hypothesize that liver endothelial toxicity may occur from deficient recycling and ADC clearance by endothelial cells. Definite demonstration of this mechanism has proven a challenging endeavor.

Peripheral Neuropathy

Peripheral neuropathy (PN) is predominantly reported after administration of conventional conjugate ADCs containing the linker-cytotoxic agent vc-MMAE. The clinical presentation, which is consistent with the PN observed with chemotherapeutic microtubule inhibitor drugs such as taxanes and vinca alkaloids, typically includes sensory symptoms, such as numbness, tingling or pain generally in the hands and/or feet ("stocking and glove" pattern), and less frequently motor symptoms, manifested for example as weakness [92, 93]. Although the exact mechanisms of the neurotoxic effects of microtubule inhibitors are not completely elucidated, the impairment of microtubule dynamics is likely to be a strong contributing factor through the disruption of microtubule-associated axonal transport that leads to axonopathy. This mechanism may further explain the preferential effects on sensory nerves due to the longer projections of axons in those nerves, making them more susceptible to neurotoxic effects.

In a pivotal phase II study of brentuximab vedotin (Adcetris, anti-CD30-vc-MMAE), 102 patients with relapsed or refractory Hodgkin's lymphoma were treated with brentuximab vedotin at 1.8 mg/kg by intravenous infusion once every 3 weeks [65]. The most common treatment-related AE was PN, with any grade PN occurring in 53% of patients and grade ≥ 3 sensory and motor PN occurring in 8% and 1% of patients, respectively. PN was the main reason for dose reduction (10% of patients) or treatment discontinuation (9%). PN is a cumulative toxicity and the median times to onset of any PN event, grade 2 PN and grade 3 PN were 12, 27 and 38 weeks, respectively. Neuropathy was largely reversible upon treatment completion, discontinuation, or dose reduction, as reflected by 80% of patients who had improvement, including 50% with complete resolution. Prior treatment with other neurotoxic chemotherapy agents might predispose patients to PN and it is noteworthy that 23% of patients had PN at the time of study entry [65]. PN was similarly a frequent AE in patients treated with other ADCs containing vc-MMAE, such as pinatuzumab vedotin (anti-CD22-vc-MMAE) or polatuzumab vedotin (anti-CD79b-vc-MMAE), which induced PN in 59% and 36% of NHL patients, respectively, when given as single agents at 2.4 mg/kg every 3 weeks [66, 67].

The PN observed with vc-MMAE ADCs is likely related to slight linker instability and ADC deconjugation in circulation with release of membrane-permeable free MMAE and subsequent axonal disruption of microtubules [Ref]. However, investigations of the specific mechanism and of potential mitigation strategies have been hampered by the absence of a relevant animal model, as this toxicity is not recapitulated in nonclinical species such as rat and monkey [94]. It is noteworthy that site-specific conjugation chemistry may mitigate this toxicity, through increased ADC stability and reduced levels of unconjugated cytotoxic drug in circulation, and we will have to wait for clinical data to confirm this hypothesis.

Ocular Toxicity

ADC-associated ocular toxicity has been well characterized clinically but its mechanism remains poorly understood. Ocular AEs are mainly reported after administration of ADCs containing SPDB-DM4 or mc-MMAF irrespective of the target antigens and can be dose limiting [95]. While the cytotoxins DM4 and MMAF are both microtubule inhibitors, the linkers are different with SPDB being a disulfide cleavable linker and mc a non-cleavable linker. Specific ocular findings reported with these ADCs are described below.

In a phase I dose escalation study, 39 patients with relapsed or refractory B-cell lymphoma were treated with SAR3419 (anti-CD19-SPDB-DM4) once every 3 weeks by intravenous infusion at dose levels of 10–270 mg/m^2 [76]. Drug-related ocular AEs were observed in 17 patients (44%), with grade $\geq$ 3 toxicities noted in 6 patients (15%). Findings occurred after the second or subsequent doses and consisted of blurred vision associated with microcystic corneal epitheliopathy, typically starting at the periphery of the cornea, which were reversible in all affected patients. Based on these ocular findings, the MTD was 160 mg/m^2. SGN-75 (anti-CD70-mc-MMAF) was evaluated in a phase I trial in 47 NHL or metastatic renal cell carcinoma patients treated intravenously every 3 weeks at dose levels of 0.3–4.5 mg/kg [68]. Ocular adverse events were generally observed after multiple doses of SGN-75 (medium time to onset of 44 days) and consisted of dry eye in 14 patients (30%), blurred vision in 5 patients (11%), microcystic corneal epitheliopathy in 7 patients (15%) and keratitis in 4 patients (9%). Grade $\geq$ 3 ocular AEs were reported in 21% of patients. Ocular events resolved or returned to grade 1 within 2–4 months. The use of artificial tears and steroid eye drops seemed to mitigate the duration and severity of ocular symptoms.

ADC-associated non-target-mediated ocular changes present similar features across ADCs with primary involvement of ocular surface and manifestation as blurred vision associated with reversible microcystic keratopathy. The findings are consistent with a primary damage to the proliferative compartment of the corneal epithelium, which starts peripherally at the corneo-scleral limbus and is mediated by the anti-mitotic activity of the cytotoxic agents. The corneal microcyst formation is likely related to corneal basal epithelial cell necrosis, as demonstrated for cytarabine-associated ocular toxicity [96, 97].

The mechanism underlying the selective toxicity to corneal epithelial cells is not understood. We can indicate however that the toxicity involves internalization of the intact ADC by epithelial cells, as it is observed with ADCs containing mc-MMAF that release non-membrane-permeable cytotoxic moieties.

Serosal Effusion

Serosal effusion and peripheral/generalized edema are emerging toxicities that are selectively observed with ADCs carrying DNA-damaging cytotoxic agents, such as PBD dimers or duocarmycin derivatives, via peptide cleavable linkers. These toxicities are independent of the target antigen and represent major safety issues for these ADCs.

In a phase I study of rovalpituzumab tesirine (Rova-T, anti-DLL3-ValAla-PBD), 74 patients with recurrent small-cell lung cancer were treated with Rova-T once every 3 or 6 weeks by intravenous infusion at dose levels of 0.5–0.8 mg/kg [81]. Treatment-related grade ≥ 3 serosal effusions were reported in 8 (11%) patients and included pleural effusion, pericardial effusion, ascites and capillary leak syndrome. Median onset of serosal effusion was 74 days (43–97 days) and median duration was 15 days (7–28 days). The serosal effusion prompted dose modification, delay or discontinuation in 8% of patients. Serosal effusion was also reported in acute myeloid leukemia patients treated with vadastuximab talirine (SGN-CD33A, anti-CD33-ValAla-PBD) in a phase I study by intravenous infusion once every 3 weeks at dose levels of 0.005–0.06 mg/kg. Adverse events of pleural effusion and peripheral edema were noted in 13% and 18% of patients, respectively [98]. Interestingly serosal effusion was also observed in patients treated with SJG-136, a small molecule PBD dimer. In a phase I dose escalation study in patients with advanced solid tumors, SJG-136 was administered intravenously once every 3 weeks and the major drug-related AE was delayed-onset vascular leak syndrome characterized by hypoalbuminemia, pleural effusion, ascites and peripheral edema [99].

Serosal effusion was also observed with an ADC carrying duocarmycin, a very potent cytotoxic DNA minor groove-binding alkylating agent. In a phase 1 dose escalation study, BMS-936561 (MDX-1203, anti-CD70-vc-MED2460) administered intravenously every 3 weeks led to delayed toxicities of pleural/pericardial effusion and facial edema in 38% of patients at the highest tested dose of 15 mg/kg [100].

Serosal effusion and peripheral/generalized edema were observed with both conventional (BMS-936561) and site-specific (Rova-T, SGN-CD33A) conjugates. The pathogenesis of these toxicities is uncertain but may involve endothelial damage to specific vascular beds.

Conclusion and Future Directions

Development of ADCs has proven much more challenging than originally anticipated and, although recent clinical approvals are a testimony of the progress of the science, research efforts are still needed to fulfill the larger promise of this technology.

Achievement of improved therapeutic index and clinical success are currently largely hampered by dose-limiting non-target-mediated toxicities. These toxicities may prevent reaching efficacious doses and also indicate broad distribution of ADCs outside of target-expressing tissues and associated limited tumor targeting efficiency. Significant research efforts are therefore currently focused on understanding and mitigating these target-independent toxicities, with particular emphasis on site specific-conjugation chemistry that is starting to yield promising data. Demonstration of successful alleviation of these toxicities in the clinics will likely be critical to future ADC endeavors.

Other current research areas include approaches to increase selective tumor targeting. Probody™ therapeutics for example are designed to remain inactive until they are activated by tumor-specific proteases, which leads to selective tumor binding and prevents binding to normal target-expressing tissues [12]. Enhanced binding selectivity of antibodies to tumor cells may also be achieved by engineering bispecific antibodies capable of binding two different epitopes on the same or different antigens/cells, with the rationale that normal tissues express only one or low levels of both targeted epitopes [14].

The previous approaches, if successful, should reduce nonspecific or specific healthy tissue targeting and increase selective tumor targeting, thereby improving the therapeutic index of ADCs and confirming the well-suited name of "guided missiles" for these drugs.

Acknowledgements All procedures performed on animals were conducted in accordance with regulations and established guidelines and were reviewed and approved by an Institutional Animal Care and Use Committee or through an ethical review process.

References

1. Schrama D, Reisfeld RA, Becker JC (2006) Antibody targeted drugs as cancer therapeutics. Nat Rev Drug Discov 5:147–159
2. Damelin M, Zhong W, Myers J, Sapra P (2015) Evolving strategies for target selection for antibody-drug conjugates. Pharm Res 32:3494–3507
3. Saber H, Leighton JK (2015) An FDA oncology analysis of antibody-drug conjugates. Regul Toxicol Pharmacol 71:444–452
4. Drake PM, Rabuka D (2015) An emerging playbook for antibody-drug conjugates: lessons from the laboratory and clinic suggest a strategy for improving efficacy and safety. Curr Opin Chem Biol 28:174–180
5. Gutierrez C, Schiff R (2011) HER2: biology, detection, and clinical implications. Arch Pathol Lab Med 135:55–62
6. Kim SB, Wildiers H, Krop IE, Smitt M, Yu R, Lysbet de Haas S et al (2016) Relationship between tumor biomarkers and efficacy in TH3RESA, a phase III study of trastuzumab emtansine (T-DM1) vs. treatment of physician's choice in previously treated HER2-positive advanced breast cancer. Int J Cancer 139:2336–2342
7. Stinchcombe T, Stahel R, Bubendorf L, Bonomi F, Villegas AE, Kowalski D et al (2017) Efficacy, safety and biomarker results of trastuzumab emtansine (T-DM1) in patients with previously treated HER2-overexpressing locally advanced or metastatic non-small cell lung cancer (mNSCLC). J Clin Oncol 35(suppl):abstr 8509
8. Sochaj AM, Świderska KW, Otlewski J (2015) Current methods for the synthesis of homogeneous antibody-drug conjugates. Biotechnol Adv 33:775–784
9. Jackson DY (2016) Processes for constructing homogeneous antibody drug conjugates. Org Process Res Dev 20:852–866
10. Junutula JR, Raab H, Clark S, Bhakta S, Leipold DD, Weir S et al (2008) Site-specific conjugation of a cytotoxic drug to an antibody improves the therapeutic index. Nat Biotechnol 26:925–932
11. Beck A, Goetsch L, Dumontet C, Corvaïa N (2017) Strategies and challenges for the next generation of antibody-drug conjugates. Nat Rev Drug Discov (5):315–337
12. Polu KR, Lowman HB (2014) Probody therapeutics for targeting antibodies to diseased tissue. Expert Opin Biol Ther 14:1049–1053

13. Chang C, Frey G, Boyle WJ, Sharp LL, Short JM (2016) Novel conditionally active biologic anti-Axl antibody-drug conjugate demonstrates anti-tumor efficacy and improved safety profile. In: Proceedings of the 107th annual meeting of the American Association for Cancer Research, 16–20 Apr 2016, New Orleans. Cancer Res 76 (14 Suppl): Abstract nr 3836
14. Mazor Y, Hansen A, Yang C, Chowdhury PS, Wang J, Stephens G et al (2015) Insights into the molecular basis of a bispecific antibody's target selectivity. MAbs 7:461–469
15. Bander NH (2013) Antibody–drug conjugate target selection: critical factors. In: Ducry L (ed) Antibody-drug conjugates. Methods in molecular biology (Methods and protocols), vol 1045. Humana Press, Totowa, pp 29–40
16. Carter P, Smith L, Ryan M (2004) Identification and validation of cell surface antigens for antibody targeting in oncology. Endocr Relat Cancer 11:659–687
17. Weinstein JN, Collisson EA, Mills GB, Shaw KM, Ozenberger BA, Ellrott K et al (2013) The cancer genome atlas pan-cancer analysis project. Nat Genet 45:1113–1120
18. The GTEx Consortium (2013) The genotype-tissue expression (GTEx) project. Nat Genet 45:580–585
19. www.illumina.com; ArrayExpress ID: E-MTAB-513
20. Kim MS, Pinto SM, Getnet D, Nirujogi RS, Manda SS, Chaerkady R et al (2014) A draft map of the human proteome. Nature 509:575–581
21. Balakrishnan A, Goodpaster T, Randolph-Habecker J, Hoffstrom BG, Jalikis FG, Koch LK et al (2017) Analysis of ROR1 protein expression in human cancer and normal tissues. Clin Cancer Res 23:3061–3071
22. Stepan LP, Trueblood ES, Hale K, Babcook J, Borges L, Sutherland CL (2011) Expression of Trop2 cell surface glycoprotein in normal and tumor tissues: potential implications as a cancer therapeutic target. J Histochem Cytochem 59:701–710
23. Nolan-Stevaux O, Fajardo F, Liu L, Coberly S, McElroy P, Nazarian A, et al (2016) Assessing ENPP3 as a renal cancer target for bispecific T-cell engager (BiTE) therapy. In: Proceedings of the 107th annual meeting of the American Association for Cancer Research, 16–20 Apr 2016, New Orleans. Cancer Res 76 (14 Suppl): Abstract nr 585
24. Kim EG, Kim KM (2015) Strategies and advancement in antibody-drug conjugate optimization for targeted cancer therapeutics. Biomol Ther (Seoul) 23:493–509
25. Salfeld JG (2007) Isotype selection in antibody engineering. Nat Biotechnol 25:1369–1372
26. Junttila TT, Li G, Parsons K, Phillips GL, Sliwkowski MX (2011) Trastuzumab-DM1 (T-DM1) retains all the mechanisms of action of trastuzumab and efficiently inhibits growth of lapatinib insensitive breast cancer. Breast Cancer Res Treat 128:347–356
27. McDonagh CF, Kim KM, Turcott E, Brown LL, Westendorf L, Feist T et al (2008) Engineered anti-CD70 antibody-drug conjugate with increased therapeutic index. Mol Cancer Ther 7:2913–2923
28. Kim KM, McDonagh CF, Westendorf L, Brown LL, Sussman D, Feist T et al (2008) Anti-CD30 diabody-drug conjugates with potent antitumor activity. Mol Cancer Ther 7:2486–2497
29. Chen H, Lin Z, Arnst KE, Miller DD, Li W (2017) Tubulin inhibitor-based antibody-drug conjugates for cancer therapy. Molecules 22(8):1281. https://doi.org/10.3390/molecules22081281
30. Dumontet C, Jordan MA (2010) Microtubule-binding agents: a dynamic field of cancer therapeutics. Nat Rev Drug Discov 9:790–803
31. Yang H, Ganguly A, Cabral F (2010) Inhibition of cell migration and cell division correlates with distinct effects of microtubule inhibiting drugs. J Biol Chem 285:32242–32250
32. Cashman CR, Höke A (2015) Mechanisms of distal axonal degeneration in peripheral neuropathies. Neurosci Lett 596:33–50
33. Schutten MM (2014) Antibody-drug conjugates: key challenges in safety assessment. Oral presentation at 2014 annual meeting of the American College of Veterinary Pathologists (ACVP). In: Industrial and toxicologic pathology focused scientific session II. Available via http://acvp2014.cmiav.com/schutten/

34. Tan C (2015) Payloads of antibody-drug conjugates. In: Wang J, Shen WC, Zaro J (eds) Antibody-drug conjugates, AAPS advances in the pharmaceutical sciences Series, vol 17. Springer, Cham
35. Junttila MR, Mao W, Wang X, Wang B-E, Pham T, Flygare J, Yu S-F, Yee S, Goldenberg D, Fields C et al (2015) Targeting LGR5[+] cells with an antibody-drug conjugate for the treatment of colon cancer. Sci Transl Med 7:314ra186. https://doi.org/10.1126/scitranslmed.aac7433
36. Guffroy M, Falahatpisheh H, Biddle K, Kreeger J, Obert L, Walters K et al (2017) Liver microvascular injury and thrombocytopenia of antibody-calicheamicin conjugates in cynomolgus monkeys – mechanism and monitoring. Clin Cancer Res 23:1760–1770
37. Hamblett KJ, Senter PD, Chace DF, Sun MM, Lenox J, Cerveny CG et al (2004) Effects of drug loading on the antitumor activity of a monoclonal antibody drug conjugate. Clin Cancer Res 10:7063–7070
38. McCombs JR, Owen SC (2015) Antibody drug conjugates: design and selection of linker, payload and conjugation chemistry. AAPS J 17:339–351
39. Li F, Emmerton KK, Jonas M, Zhang X, Miyamoto JB, Setter JR et al (2016) Intracellular released payload influences potency and bystander-killing effects of antibody-drug conjugates in preclinical models. Cancer Res 76(9):2710–2719
40. Nakada T, Masuda T, Naito H, Yoshida M, Ashida S, Morita K et al (2016) Novel antibody drug conjugates containing exatecan derivative-based cytotoxic payloads. Bioorg Med Chem Lett 26:1542–1545
41. Burke PJ, Hamilton JZ, Jeffrey SC, Hunter JH, Doronina SO, Okeley NM et al (2017) Optimization of a PEGylated glucuronide-monomethylauristatin E linker for antibody-drug conjugates. Mol Cancer Ther 16:116–123
42. Castañeda L, Maruani A, Schumacher FF, Miranda E, Chudasama V, Chester KA et al (2013) Acid-cleavable thiomaleamic acid linker for homogeneous antibody-drug conjugation. Chem Commun (Camb) 49:8187–8189
43. Kim MT, Chen Y, Marhoul J, Jacobson F (2014) Statistical modeling of the drug load distribution on trastuzumab emtansine (Kadcyla), a lysine-linked antibody drug conjugate. Bioconjug Chem 25:1223–1232
44. Strop P, Liu SH, Dorywalska M, Delaria K, Dushin RG, Tran TT et al (2013) Location matters: site of conjugation modulates stability and pharmacokinetics of antibody drug conjugates. Chem Biol 20:161–167
45. Shen BQ, Xu K, Liu L, Raab H, Bhakta S, Kenrick M et al (2012) Conjugation site modulates the in vivo stability and therapeutic activity of antibody-drug conjugates. Nat Biotechnol 30:184–189
46. Tijink BM, Buter J, de Bree R, Giaccone G, Lang MS, Staab A et al (2008) A phase I dose escalation study with anti-CD44v6 bivatuzumab mertansine in patients with incurable squamous cell carcinoma of the head and neck or esophagus. Clin Cancer Res 12(20 Pt 1):6064–6072
47. Riechelmann H, Sauter A, Golze W, Hanft G, Schroen C, Hoermann K et al (2008) Phase I trial with the CD44v6-targeting immunoconjugate bivatuzumab mertansine in head and neck squamous cell carcinoma. Oral Oncol 44(9):823
48. Fox SB, Fawcett J, Jackson DG, Collins I, Gatter KC, Harris AL et al (1994) Normal human tissues, in addition to some tumors, express multiple different CD44 isoforms. Cancer Res 54:4539–4546
49. Tolcher AW, Ochoa L, Hammond LA, Patnaik A, Edwards T, Takimoto C et al (2003) Cantuzumab mertansine, a maytansinoid immunoconjugate directed to the CanAg antigen: a phase I, pharmacokinetic, and biologic correlative study. J Clin Oncol 21:211–222
50. Ott PA, Hamid O, Pavlick AC, Kluger H, Kim KB, Boasberg PD et al (2014) Phase I/II study of the antibody-drug conjugate glembatumumab vedotin in patients with advanced melanoma. J Clin Oncol 32:3659–3666
51. Rose AAN, Biondini M, Curiel R, Siegel PM (2017) Targeting GPNMB with glembatumumab vedotin: current developments and future opportunities for the treatment of cancer. Pharmacol Ther 179:127–141

52. Tomihari M, Hwang SH, Chung JS, Cruz PD Jr, Ariizumi K (2009) Gpnmb is a melanosome-associated glycoprotein that contributes to melanocyte/keratinocyte adhesion in a RGD-dependent fashion. Exp Dermatol 18:586–595
53. Naumovski L, Junutula JR (2010) Glembatumumab vedotin, a conjugate of an anti-glycoprotein non-metastatic melanoma protein B mAb and monomethyl auristatin E for the treatment of melanoma and breast cancer. Curr Opin Mol Ther 12:248–257
54. Press MF, Cordon-Cardo C, Slamon DJ (1990) Expression of the HER-2/neu proto-oncogene in normal human adult and fetal tissues. Oncogene 5:953–962
55. Peddi PF, Hurvitz SA (2014) Ado-trastuzumab emtansine (T-DM1) in human epidermal growth factor receptor 2 (HER2)-positive metastatic breast cancer: latest evidence and clinical potential. Ther Adv Med Oncol 6:202–209
56. Stathis A, Freedman AS, Flinn IW, Maddocks KJ, Weitman S, Berdeja JG et al (2014) A phase I study of IMGN529, an antibody-drug conjugate (ADC) targeting CD37, in adult patients with relapsed or refractory B-cell non-Hodgkin's lymphoma (NHL). Blood 124:1760. [abstract]
57. Weekes CD, Lamberts LE, Borad MJ, Voortman J, McWilliams RR, Diamond JR et al (2016) Phase I study of DMOT4039A, an antibody-drug conjugate targeting mesothelin, in patients with unresectable pancreatic or platinum-resistant ovarian cancer. Mol Cancer Ther 15:439–447
58. Xu H, Bai L, Collins JF, Ghishan FK (1999) Molecular cloning, functional characterization, tissue distribution, and chromosomal localization of a human, small intestinal sodium-phosphate (Na+-Pi) transporter (SLC34A2). Genomics 62:281–284
59. Traebert M, Hattenhauer O, Murer H, Kaissling B, Biber J (1999) Expression of type II Na-P(i) cotransporter in alveolar type II cells. Am J Phys 277:L868–L873
60. Burris HA, Gordon MS, Gerber DE, Spigel DR, Mendelson SD, Schiller JH et al (2014) A phase I study of DNIB0600A, an antibody-drug conjugate targeting NaPi2b, in patients with non-small cell lung cancer (NSCLC) or platinum-resistant ovarian cancer (OC). J Clin Oncol 32:5s. (suppl; abstr 2504)
61. Bodyak N, Yurkovetskiy A, Yin M, Gumerov D, Bollu R, Conlon P, et al (2016) Discovery and preclinical development of a highly potent NaPi2b-targeted antibody-drug conjugate (ADC) with significant activity in patient-derived non-small cell lung cancer (NSCLC) xenograft models. In: Proceedings of the 107th annual meeting of the American Association for Cancer Research, 16–20 Apr 2016, New Orleans. Cancer Res 76 (14 Suppl): Abstract nr 1194
62. Almhanna K, Kalebic T, Cruz C, Faris JE, Ryan DP, Jung J et al (2016) Phase I study of the investigational anti-guanylyl cyclase antibody-drug conjugate TAK-264 (MLN0264) in adult patients with advanced gastrointestinal malignancies. Clin Cancer Res 22:5049–5057
63. Yardley DA, Weaver R, Melisko ME, Saleh MN, Arena FP, Forero A et al (2015) EMERGE: a randomized phase II study of the antibody-drug conjugate glembatumumab vedotin in advanced glycoprotein NMB-expressing breast cancer. J Clin Oncol 33:1609–1619
64. Modi S, Eder JP, Lorusso P, Weekes C, Chandarlapaty S, Tolaney SM et al (2016) A phase I study evaluating DLYE5953A, an antibody-drug conjugate targeting the tumor-associated antigen lymphocyte antigen 6 complex locus E (Ly6E), in patients with solid tumors. Ann Oncol 27(Suppl 6):abstract nr 3570
65. Younes A, Gopal AK, Smith SE, Ansell SM, Rosenblatt JD, Savage KJ et al (2012) Results of a pivotal phase II study of brentuximab vedotin for patients with relapsed or refractory Hodgkin's lymphoma. J Clin Oncol 30:2183–2189
66. Advani RH, Lebovic D, Chen A, Brunvand M, Goy A, Chang JE et al (2017) Phase I study of the anti-CD22 antibody-drug conjugate pinatuzumab vedotin with/without rituximab in patients with relapsed/refractory B-cell non-Hodgkin lymphoma. Clin Cancer Res 23:1167–1176
67. Palanca-Wessels MC, Czuczman M, Salles G, Assouline S, Sehn LH, Flinn I et al (2015) Safety and activity of the anti-CD79B antibody-drug conjugate polatuzumab vedotin in relapsed or refractory B-cell non-Hodgkin lymphoma and chronic lymphocytic leukaemia: a phase 1 study. Lancet Oncol 16:704–715

68. Tannir NM, Forero-Torres A, Ramchandren R, Pal SK, Ansell SM, Infante JR et al (2014) Phase I dose-escalation study of SGN-75 in patients with CD70-positive relapsed/refractory non-Hodgkin lymphoma or metastatic renal cell carcinoma. Investig New Drugs 32:1246–1257
69. Gan HK, Reardon DA, Lassman AB, Merrell R, van den Bent M, Butowski N et al (2017) Safety, pharmacokinetics and antitumor response of depatuxizumab mafodotin as monotherapy or in combination with temozolomide in patients with glioblastoma. Neuro Oncol. https://doi.org/10.1093/neuonc/nox202. [Epub ahead of print]
70. Thompson JA, Motzer R, Molina AM, Choueiri TK, Heath EI, Kollmannsberger CK et al (2015) Phase I studies of anti-ENPP3 antibody drug conjugates (ADCs) in advanced refractory renal cell carcinomas (RRCC). J Clin Oncol 33:2503
71. Reardon DA, Lassman AB, van den Bent M, Kumthekar P, Merrell R, Scott AM et al (2017) Efficacy and safety results of ABT-414 in combination with radiation and temozolomide in newly diagnosed glioblastoma. Neuro-Oncology 19:965–975
72. Fathi AT, Borate U, DeAngelo DJ, O'Brien MM, Trippett T, Shah BD et al (2015) A phase 1 study of denintuzumab mafodotin (SGN-CD19A) in adults with relapsed or refractory B-lineage acute leukemia (B-ALL) and highly aggressive lymphoma. Blood 126:1328
73. Force J, Saxena R, Schneider BP, Storniolo AM, Sledge GW Jr, Chalasani N et al (2016) Nodular regenerative hyperplasia after treatment with trastuzumab emtansine. J Clin Oncol 34:e9-12
74. Prochaska LH, Damjanov I, Ash RM, Olson JC, Khan QJ, Sharma P (2016) Trastuzumab emtansine associated nodular regenerative hyperplasia: a case report and review of literature. Cancer Treatment Commun 5:26–30
75. Gan HK, van den Bent M, Lassman AB, Reardon DA, Scott AM (2017) Antibody-drug conjugates in glioblastoma therapy: the right drugs to the right cells. Nat Rev Clin Oncol 14:695–707
76. Younes A, Kim S, Romaquera J, Copeland A, Farial S de C, Kwak LW et al (2012) Phase I multidose-escalation study of the anti-CD19 maytansinoid immunoconjugate SAR3419 administered by intravenous infusion every 3 weeks to patients with relapsed/refractory B-cell lymphoma. J Clin Oncol 30:2776–2782
77. Moore KN, Borghaei H, O'Malley DM, Jeong W, Seward SM, Bauer TM et al (2017) Phase 1 dose-escalation study of mirvetuximab soravtansine (IMGN853), a folate receptor α-targeting antibody-drug conjugate, in patients with solid tumors. Cancer 123:3080–3087
78. Mita MM, Ricart AD, Mita AC, Patnaik A, Sarantopoulos J, Sankhala K et al (2007) A phase I study of a CanAg-targeted immunoconjugate, huC242-DM4, in patients with Can Ag-expressing solid tumors. J Clin Oncol 25:3062
79. Advani A, Coiffier B, Czuczman MS, Dreyling M, Foran J, Gine E et al (2010) Safety, pharmacokinetics, and preliminary clinical activity of inotuzumab ozogamicin, a novel immunoconjugate for the treatment of B-cell non-Hodgkin's lymphoma: results of a phase I study. J Clin Oncol 28:2085–2093
80. Kantarjian HM, DeAngelo DJ, Advani AS, Stelljes M, Kebriaei P, Cassaday RD et al (2017) Hepatic adverse event profile of inotuzumab ozogamicin in adult patients with relapsed or refractory acute lymphoblastic leukaemia: results from the open-label, randomised, phase 3 INO-VATE study. Lancet Haematol 4:e387–e398
81. Rudin CM, Pietanza C, Bauer TM, Ready N, Morgensztern D, Glisson BS et al (2017) Rovalpituzumab tesirine, a DLL3-targeted antibody-drug conjugate, in recurrent small-cell lung cancer: a first-in-human, first-in-class, open-label, phase 1 study. Lancet Oncol 18:42–51
82. Bender BC, Schaedeli-Stark F, Koch R, Joshi A, Chu YW, Rugo H et al (2012) A population pharmacokinetic/pharmacodynamic model of thrombocytopenia characterizing the effect of trastuzumab emtansine (T-DM1) on platelet counts in patients with HER2-positive metastatic breast cancer. Cancer Chemother Pharmacol 70:591–601
83. Bardia A, Mayer IA, Diamond JR, Moroose RL, Isakoff SJ, Starodub AN et al (2017) Efficacy and safety of anti-Trop-2 antibody drug conjugate sacituzumab govitecan (IMMU-132) in heavily pretreated patients with metastatic triple-negative breast cancer. J Clin Oncol 35:2141–2148

84. Krop IE, Beeram M, Modi S, Jones SF, Holden SN, Yu W et al (2010) Phase I study of trastuzumab-DM1, an HER2 antibody-drug conjugate, given every 3 weeks to patients with HER2-positive metastatic breast cancer. J Clin Oncol 28:2698–2704
85. Verma S, Miles D, Gianni L, Krop IE, Welslau M, Baselga J et al (2012) Trastuzumab emtansine for HER2-positive advanced breast cancer. N Engl J Med 367:1783–1791
86. Uppal H, Doudement E, Mahapatra K, Darbonne WC, Bumbaca D, Shen B-Q et al (2015) Potential mechanisms for thrombocytopenia development with trastuzumab emtansine (T-DM1). Clin Cancer Res 21:123–133
87. Zhao H, Gulesserian S, Ganesan SK, Ou J, Morrison K, Zeng Z et al (2017) Inhibition of megakaryocyte differentiation by antibody-drug conjugates (ADCs) is mediated by macropinocytosis: implications for ADC-induced thrombocytopenia. Mol Cancer Ther 16:1877–1886
88. Hartleb M, Gutkowski K, Milkiewicz P (2011) Nodular regenerative hyperplasia: evolving concepts on underdiagnosed cause of portal hypertension. World J Gastroenterol 17:1400–1409
89. Dignan FL, Wynn RF, Hadzic N, Karani J, Quaglia A, Pagliuca A et al (2013) BCSH/BSBMT guideline: diagnosis and management of veno-occlusive disease (sinusoidal obstruction syndrome) following haematopoietic stem cell transplantation. B J Haematol 163:444–457
90. Wanless IR, Huang W-Y (2012) Vascular disorders. In: Burt A, Portmann B, Ferrell L (eds) MacSween's pathology of the liver, 6th edn. Churchill Livingstone/Elsevier, Edinburgh, pp 601–643
91. Rubbia-Brandt L, Lauwers GY, Wang H, Majno PE, Tanabe K, Zhu AX et al (2010) Sinusoidal obstruction syndrome and nodular regenerative hyperplasia are frequent oxaliplatin-associated liver lesions and partially prevented by bevacizumab in patients with hepatic colorectal metastasis. Histopathology 56:430–439
92. Younes A, Bartlett NL, Leonard JP, Kennedy DA, Lynch CM, Sievers EL et al (2010) Brentuximab vedotin (SGN-35) for relapsed CD30-positive lymphomas. N Engl J Med 363:1812–1821
93. Grisold W, Cavaletti G, Windebank AJ (2012) Peripheral neuropathies from chemotherapeutics and targeted agents: diagnosis, treatment, and prevention. Neuro-Oncology 14(Suppl 4):iv45–iv54
94. Stagg NJ, Shen BQ, Brunstein F, Li C, Kamath AV, Zhong F et al (2016) Peripheral neuropathy with microtubule inhibitor containing antibody drug conjugates: challenges and perspectives in translatability from nonclinical toxicology studies to the clinic. Regul Toxicol Pharmacol 82:1–13
95. Eaton JS, Miller PE, Mannis MJ, Murphy CJ (2015) Ocular adverse events associated with antibody-drug conjugates in human clinical trials. J Ocul Pharmacol Ther 31:589–604
96. Stentoft J (1990) The toxicity of cytarabine. Drug Saf 1:7–27
97. Hopen G, Mondino BJ, Johnson BL, Chervenick PA (1981) Corneal toxicity with systemic cytarabine. Am J Ophthalmol 91(4):500
98. Stein EM, Stein A, Walter RB, Fathi AT, Lancet JE, Kovacsovics TJ et al (2014) Interim analysis of a phase 1 trial of SGN-CD33A in patients with CD33-positive acute myeloid leukemia (AML). Blood 124:623. (abstract)
99. Hochhauser D, Meyer T, Spanswick VJ, Wu J, Clingen PH, Loadman P et al (2009) Phase I study of sequence-selective minor groove DNA binding agent SJG-136 in patients with advanced solid tumors. Clin Cancer Res 15:2140–2147
100. Owonikoko TK, Hussain A, Stadler WM, Smith DC, Kluger H, Molina AM et al (2016) First-in-human multicenter phase I study of BMS-936561 (MDX-1203), an antibody-drug conjugate targeting CD70. Cancer Chemother Pharmacol 77:155–162

Utility of PK-PD Modeling and Simulation to Improve Decision Making for Antibody-Drug Conjugate Development

Aman P. Singh and Dhaval K. Shah

Abstract Comprehension of the pharmacokinetics (PK) and pharmacodynamics (PD) of Antibody-drug Conjugates (ADCs) can be challenging as it requires integration of the information stemming from various moieties (i.e. the antibody, the drug, and the conjugate). Computational modeling provides an excellent tool to overcome these challenges by providing an opportunity to integrate all the available information within a mathematical framework. With an ever-increasing pipeline of more than 60 ADC molecules currently in the clinic, plenty of resources and time are invested towards discerning some key questions associated with PK, efficacy, and toxicity of the most promising candidates. In order to streamline the process of finding the answers to these questions and to expedite the development of ADCs, mathematical modeling and simulation (M&S) can be employed at different stages of ADC development. Successful application of this tool can not only enhance the scientific understanding of the processes underlying PK-PD of ADCs but can also provide comprehensive model-derived outcomes that can help accelerate the decision-making process. Within this book chapter, we have discussed an array of different PK-PD models and modeling strategies that could be employed at discovery, preclinical, or clinical stages, to make rational decisions for the development of ADCs. In addition, suitable examples from the literature are discussed where M&S has been utilized to make key go/no-go decisions.

Keywords PK-PD Modeling · Antibody-Drug Conjugate · Model-Based Drug Development · Preclinical-to-Clinical Translation · Decision Making · Population PK-PD Analysis

---

A. P. Singh · D. K. Shah (✉)
Department of Pharmaceutical Sciences, School of Pharmacy and Pharmaceutical Sciences, The State University of New York at Buffalo, Buffalo, NY, USA
e-mail: dshah4@buffalo.edu

M. Damelin (ed.), *Innovations for Next-Generation Antibody-Drug Conjugates*, Cancer Drug Discovery and Development,
https://doi.org/10.1007/978-3-319-78154-9_4

Introduction

Development of mathematical models to quantitatively characterize the exposure-efficacy and exposure-toxicity relationships have been widely recognized as a successful strategy for model-based drug development (MBDD) [1]. Such models can not only help facilitate go/no-go decisions while triaging lead candidates in early discovery stage, but can also influence late-stage clinical development and regulatory approvals. With increasing prevalence of late-stage clinical failures of drugs, especially for oncology therapeutics [2], application of PK-PD M&S can serve as a linchpin for effective utilization of time and resources in preclinical and clinical development processes. While there are several examples highlighting the applications of PK-PD M&S for both small and large molecule drug development, the use of these approaches for successful design and development of Antibody-Drug Conjugates (ADCs) [3] remains limited.

An ADC molecule is comprised of cytotoxic agents (payloads) conjugated to a monoclonal antibody (mAb) via a chemical linker. Presence of the mAb-backbone in these modalities facilitates targeted delivery of highly potent cytotoxic agents to antigen over-expressing tumor cells with the hope of achieving a wider therapeutic window compared to the conventional chemotherapeutic agents. The number of cytotoxic molecules attached on an antibody molecule constitutes the Drug: Antibody Ratio (DAR) of that molecule. Although the majority of the 1st generation ADCs were developed using random-conjugation method, where an ADC formulation is a mixture of different DAR species [4–6], recent advances have led to the development of ADCs with site-specific conjugation technology that yields a homogenous mixture of DAR species in a formulation [7]. Although the concept behind ADCs is simple, development of these molecules can be much more challenging, as it requires synchronous optimization of an antibody, linker, and cytotoxic agent [8].

The mechanism-of-action of an ADC entails binding to the antigen-expressing tumor cells followed by receptor-mediated internalization. Upon internalization, the drug or its metabolites are released in the endosomal/lysosomal space based on the nature of the linker chemistry. Released drug can either bind to its pharmacological target (microtubules or DNA) and elicit cytotoxic effects, or can efflux out of the cells [9]. Pharmacokinetic (PK) characterization of ADCs requires simultaneous understanding of the disposition of all three molecular species (i.e. the antibody, the cytotoxic drug/payload, and the conjugate), which are represented in the form of different bioanalytical measurements like total antibody, conjugated antibody, conjugated drug, or unconjugated drug [8, 10, 11]. Simultaneous integration of the exposure data for all these ADC analytes using a mathematical model can provide the key PK parameter estimates related to the antibody and small molecule components of the ADC (e.g. clearance and volume of distribution), and also the value of parameter related to the deconjugation rate of drug from the antibody. Utilization of an integrated multiple-analyte PK model can help with the characterization and prediction of plasma and tissue exposures of different ADC analytes, which can later serve as a driving force for making more mechanistic pharmacokinetic-pharmacodynamic (PK-PD) and pharmacokinetic-toxicodynamic (PK-TD) models [12].

To date various M&S approaches have been evaluated for ADCs, which range from data-driven models [13, 14], that are utilized to address specific drug developmental questions to more mechanistic models [3, 12, 15] that integrate the information from all phases of drug development to predict clinical behavior (e.g. progression-free survival (PFS), objective response rates (ORRs), toxicities) of ADCs. Once validated, these models can also be used to simulate untested scenarios, triage lead candidates, optimize different dosing regimens, and make key decisions during clinical development. With the advent of several guidelines issued by regulatory bodies (e.g. FDA) that highlights the significance of M&S in facilitating key decisions towards drug development [16], the focus of this chapter is to discuss key PK-PD modeling approaches that can be utilized at different stages of ADC development to make rational go/no-go decisions. In addition, examples from literature are also covered where PK-PD M&S has significantly impacted the understanding and development of ADCs.

Preclinical Development

The major objectives of early discovery and late preclinical stages are to identify the lead compounds to move forward to the clinic and to predict the first-in-human dose of most promising molecules, respectively [17]. Development of PK-PD models, and effective communication of the outputs from these models to other team members, can be of paramount importance in achieving these objectives efficiently. In a discovery setting, an array of different ADC molecules can be triaged based on key characteristics such as linker stability, intracellular delivery, potency, ability to exhibit bystander effect etc. Mathematical modeling can help estimate the values of these key parameters, which can in turn help in identifying the most promising ADC candidates. Additionally, during the preclinical stage system pharmacokinetic models (e.g. in vitro cell-disposition models and in vivo PBPK models, see Table 1) can also be used to evaluate clinical potential of different target antigens and select the most promising target that can maximize the chances of clinical success for the ADC moving forward. Later in the preclinical stage the in vivo PK, efficacy, and toxicity data can be further used to establish robust exposure-efficacy/toxicity relationships for ADCs, and choose the most promising ADC molecule for clinical development.

In Vitro PK-PD Models

An ideal ADC molecule should be stable in the extracellular space and should be able to effectively release the cytotoxic drug once internalized in a tumor cell. However, there are many determinants leading to successful intracellular delivery of ADC molecules, such as optimal linker chemistry, antigen-binding properties of

Table 1 A list of most prominent PK/PK-PD models for ADCs along with their description, proposed utility, and dataset requirements

Model figure	Model description	Proposed utility	Datasets required	Reference(s)
1a	Kinetic *in vitro* model to characterize stability of ADCs	Selection of stable mAb, ADC, and linker *in vitro*	Time-course measurements of total and conjugated antibody in media	[8]
1b	Single-cell disposition model for ADCs	Selection of feasible targets and lead ADC candidates based on desirable intracellular payload exposure	*In vitro* measurements of biomeasures and chemomeasures. Time-course measurements of multiple ADC-analytes in extracellular and intracellular spaces	[9, 12, 18]
2a, b	*In vitro* PD/PK-PD models to characterize cytotoxicity of ADCs	Triaging lead candidates based on model-derived parameters (e.g. $TSC_{invitro}$) and find out intracellular drug exposure needed for ADC efficacy	Time-course of cell-viability (model A &B), and availability of established cell-disposition model for ADC (model B)	[19]
3a	*In Vivo* plasma PK model for ADCs and released drugs	Selection of lead ADCs with optimal plasma PK of conjugate and released drug, and optimal linker stability	Time-course measurements of plasma concentrations of at least 3 ADC analytes (e.g. total antibody, unconjugated drug, and conjugated antibody/total drug)	[8, 10–12]
4a	*In Vivo* tumor disposition model for ADCs and released drugs	A priori prediction of tumor exposure of ADC and the released payload, development of systems PK/PD model for clinical translation	Time-course measurements of plasma concentrations of ADC analytes, and *In vitro* measurements of biomeasures and chemomeasures.	[12, 18, 20]
4b	*In Vivo* PBPK model for ADCs and released drugs	Prediction of tissue exposures of ADC and released drug, and evaluation of the effect of differential target expression on tissue and tumor exposure of analytes	Time-course measurements of plasma concentrations of ADC and released drug after ADC administration, and plasma and tissue concentrations of released drug after administration of just the drug.	[21, 22]

(continued)

Table 1 (continued)

Model figure	Model description	Proposed utility	Datasets required	Reference(s)
5a	*In Vivo* PK-PD model for ADCs to characterize tumor growth inhibition (TGI) data	Establish a concentration-response relationship and triage lead candidates based on model-derived parameters (e.g. TSC_{invivo})	Time course of plasma PK for relevant analyte and tumor volume measurements at multiple dose-levels in relevant mouse models	[8, 12, 23]
5b	*In Vivo* PK-TD model for ADCs to characterize mylosuppression/ neutropenia	Establish a concentration-toxicity relationship and triage lead candidates based on model-derived parameters. Optimize the clinical dosing regimen for maximum therapeutics index.	Time course of plasma concentrations of relevant analytes and continuous measurements of toxicity markers (e.g. neutrophils count)	[24–27]

antibody backbone, and the transport (diffusion/efflux) rate of released drug across a cell [9, 18]. Stability of a conjugate can be evaluated by incubating ADC in media, plasma, or other biological matrices, and quantifying different analytes such as total antibody and conjugated antibody at different time points. Generated datasets can be fitted to a model structure described in Fig. 1a. The parameter $\boldsymbol{K}_{\boldsymbol{ADC}}^{\deg}$ symbolizes the degradation rate of Antibody/ADC in media/plasma and the parameter $\boldsymbol{K}_{\boldsymbol{ADC}}^{\boldsymbol{dec}}$ symbolizes the non-specific deconjugation rate of cytotoxic agent/payload from ADC. For total antibody profiles, only $\boldsymbol{K}_{\boldsymbol{ADC}}^{\deg}$ is active whereas for ADC, both $\boldsymbol{K}_{\boldsymbol{ADC}}^{\boldsymbol{dec}}$ and $\boldsymbol{K}_{\boldsymbol{ADC}}^{\deg}$ are active. Simultaneous fitting of both total antibody and ADC profiles leads to estimation of each of these parameters. Once estimated, lead ADC candidates at the discovery setting can be triaged based on their in-vitro degradation and deconjugation rates. Of note, since this modeling approach accounts for antibody and linker stability separately, it helps prevent false negative triaging of a linker-drug combination due to instability of an antibody. The stability parameter can also be used to establish an in vitro-in vivo correlation (IVIVC) for ADC stability [8].

At the discovery stage it is also important to have mathematical models that can characterize the processes that leads to preferential exposure of cytotoxic agents (payload) within the tumor cells. Although, cellular disposition is at the center of the mechanism-of-action of ADCs, it is rarely quantified and mathematically characterized. Unlike small molecules, the exposure of the unconjugated drug in a tumor cell is driven by many ADC-specific characteristics, such as antigen-binding affinity, efficiency of linker cleavage, and physicochemical properties of released drug that determined retention vs. efflux of the drug outside the cell via passive or active routes. Additionally, many system-specific properties, such as antigen-density, intracellular cathepsin B levels, and presence/absence of efflux pumps, also influence the overall intracellular exposure of unconjugated drug. A theoretical approach

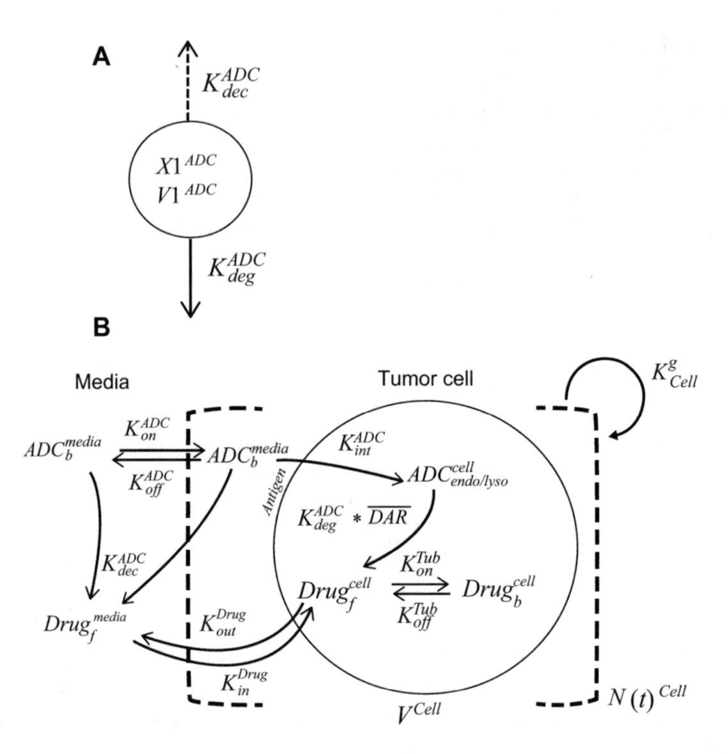

Fig. 1 In vitro pharmacokinetic models for ADCs. (**a**) Schematics of an in vitro model that can be used to characterize the stability of ADCs in buffer/plasma. (**b**) A single-cell pharmacokinetic model to characterize the disposition of ADC and the released drug in intracellular and extracellular space

to investigate the effect of these factors was presented by Sadekar et al. [28], who developed a general cell-level disposition model for ADCs and later integrated it with systemic pharmacokinetic model of ADCs. Using a set of simulations, authors highlighted the interplay of target abundance, internalization rate, payload elimination rate, and binding affinity of ADCs in sustaining the overall exposure of released drug (payload) within a tumor cell. Although conceptual, authors accentuated the utility of these early phase simulation exercises in target selection and optimal ADC design. A more experimental/mathematical modeling approach was undertaken by Maass et al. [29] for understanding the cellular disposition of trastuzumab-maytansoid conjugates. Using different HER2+ cell-lines and employing various cell-based assays, authors quantified key parameters, such as antigen-expression, binding affinities, intracellular degradation rates, and cell-efflux rates for the released drug, which can influence the exposure of drug within the cell. They integrated all these key determinants into a mathematical framework to predict cell-level pharmacokinetics of ADCs designed with smcc-DM1 based linkers. More recently a more detailed platform type cell-level PK model for ADCs has been presented [9, 18] (Fig. 1b), which can quantitatively characterizes the disposition of ADC and related analytes within a single cell. This model has been experimentally validated to describe the disposition of multiple analytes of both vc-MMAE and smcc-DM1 based conjugates. Main processes covered within the model are: (a) antigen-mediated binding and internalization, (b) intracellular ADC degradation, (c) binding of released cytotoxic drug (payload) to its pharmacological target, and (d) transport (efflux and influx) of payload across the tumor cells. Systems models like this one integrate known physiological parameters/biomeasures (e.g. receptor count, internalization rate etc.) in a mathematical framework and can validate the experimental PK measured in intracellular and extracellular spaces. Once validated, these models can be utilized to either triage lead ADC candidates on the basis of intracellular delivery, or identify the optimal PK parameters using local/global sensitivity analysis (e.g. binding affinity of an antibody, cytotoxic molecule efflux rates, binding affinity of cytotoxic agent to its pharmacological target) that can lead to successful ADC design [9, 18]. These models can also be used to evaluate the clinical potential of different target antigens by plugging in the target specific parameters (e.g. expression level, internalization rate etc.) in the model and predicting the intracellular exposure of ADC and the payload for each target.

In vitro efficacy of ADCs can be characterized using semi-mechanistic PK-PD models [19] like the one described in Fig. 2a. This model uses static media concentrations in the absence of cellular PK to drive the cell-killing in a concentration dependent manner using non-linear killing function. Efficacy parameters (such as maximal killing rate $\boldsymbol{K_{Kill}}$ and ADC potency $\boldsymbol{KC_{50}}$) obtained using mathematical modeling can then be utilized to triage lead ADC candidates at the discovery stage based on their ability to kill cancer cells. The delay in cytotoxicity, which is many times observed with ADCs, is incorporated into these models using transit compartments associated with signal transduction ($\boldsymbol{\tau_s}$) of the killing signal and/or cell distribution ($\boldsymbol{\tau_c}$) delay (i.e. shuttling of tumor cells from growing to non-growing phases). However, these models are empirical in nature and more mechanistic *in vitro* PK-PD models like the one described in Fig. 2b can also be developed for ADCs. In these models the cellular PK sub-model (same as Fig. 1b) governs the release of cytotoxic agent within the cancer cell, and intracellular occupancy of the pharmacological target (e.g. tubulin or DNA) by the released payload drives the killing function that leads to cell death. **A similar** but simplified experimental approach has been presented by Maass et al. [30] to predict the intracellular potency of an anticancer agent in different cancer cell-lines. Using naturally fluorescent doxorubicin as a model compound, authors determined the number of doxorubicin molecules required in the intracellular space to inhibit the proliferation of cancer cells. Incorporation of cellular PK in the in-vitro cytotoxicity models not only allowed them to develop a more mechanistic approach of characterizing the datasets, but also prevented addition of further signal transduction steps ($\boldsymbol{\tau_s}$). This is because the delay associated with attainment of certain target occupancy accounts for majority of the observed delay in the onset of ADC mediated cell-killing. The remaining delay in cell killing, as observed in many datasets, could then be accounted via cell distribution ($\boldsymbol{\tau_c}$) transit compartments. The growth ($\boldsymbol{K_g}$) and killing ($\boldsymbol{K_{Kill}}$ and $\boldsymbol{KC_{50}}$) parameters estimated using above described models can also be used to estimate a comprehensive efficacy parameter known as 'in vitro Tumor Static Concentration' ($\boldsymbol{TSC_{in\ vitro}}$), which is

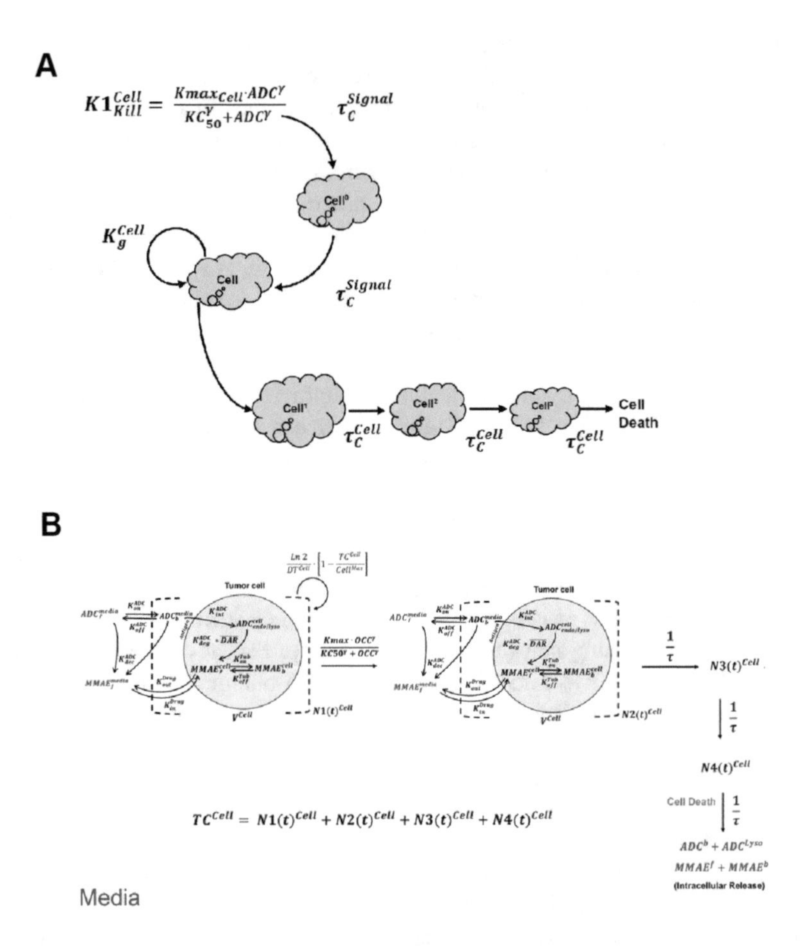

Fig. 2 In vitro PK-PD models for ADCs. (**a**) Schematics of an in vitro pharmacodynamic model that can be used to characterize the efficacy of ADCs. The model accounts for signal as well as cell-distribution delay. (**b**) Schematics of an in vitro PK-PD model for ADCs that incorporates cellular disposition of ADC and intracellular payload exposure driven cell killing

essentially a theoretical concentration of ADC that leads to steady-state tumor cell counts over time. $\boldsymbol{TSC_{in\ vitro}}$ is a better parameter compared to traditional efficacy parameters $\boldsymbol{IC_{50}/IC_{90}}$ because it takes into account the effect of the ADC over the period of time. The TSC values obtained in an in vitro setting can also be compared with the in vivo TSC values (described later) to establish In vitro-In vivo (IVIVC) correlation for ADC efficacy [8, 10]. Of note, selection of most promising ADC candidates based on such early phase in vitro PK-PD data could be more cost and time-effective compared to the use of *in vivo* tumor growth inhibition (TGI) studies to triage ADCs based on their efficacy at the late preclinical stage.

While discovering a novel ADC, it may be also beneficial to investigate one more favorable attribute of these molecules, which is their ability to demonstrate 'bystander effect'. In a heterogeneous tumor, only a fraction of the tumor cells generally expresses the antigen which is targeted using an ADC. However, drug released in antigen-positive (Ag+) cells can also efflux out and kill neighboring antigen-negative (Ag-) cells leading to additional efficacy known as the 'bystander effect' of ADCs. The main determinants leading to efficient bystander killing consists of: (a) optimal linker chemistry, which releases the drug in its pure form, and (b) appropriate cytotoxic agent/payload, which is capable of diffusing in and out of the cells and can cause bystander killing. We have performed in vitro experiments in the past to quantitatively characterize the bystander effect of ADCs using trastuzumab-vc-MMAE as a tool ADC in co-cultures of HER2 –ve (GFP-MCF7) and HER2 + ve (N87, BT474 and SK-BR3) cells. Using our model system a novel parameter 'bystander effect coefficient'($\boldsymbol{\varphi}^{BE}$) was coined, which quantifies the extent of bystander killing by an ADC in the presence of different % of antigen positive cells in a co-culture [19]. When triaging different ADC molecules, this parameter ($\boldsymbol{\varphi}^{BE}$) can be employed for comparing the extent of bystander killing induced by different candidates [19].

In Vivo PK-PD Models

Plasma/Serum Pharmacokinetics Models for ADCs

Once administered in the systemic concentration, an ADC yields different molecular species, such as unconjugated mAb, conjugated mAb/ADC and unconjugated drug. Each of these molecular species exhibits distinct disposition characteristics. In addition, the extent of drug loading on a mAb (i.e. DAR values) can also determines the clearance of ADC, where higher loading leads to faster elimination of ADC, mostly due to increased hydrophobicity. Thus, the PK analysis of ADCs is much more complex in comparison to traditional small and large molecule drugs.

Although plasma concentrations of ADC/mAb are not in rapid equilibrium with tissue concentrations, it is still the most accessible and routinely measured biological matrix. Thus, plasma PK of ADC is routinely used to triage these molecules. Mathematical modeling of the plasma PK data can be employed in deciding the lead ADC candidates that demonstrate favorable linker stability and plasma half-life. However, the type of the PK model that one can use to characterize the plasma PK data depend on the amount and nature of PK data available for analysis. Different ELISA methods can be developed to either measure total antibody levels (conjugated and unconjugated mAb) or antibodies conjugated to at least one drug molecule (conjugated mAb) in a biological sample. To analyze released drug/payload concentrations, LC-MS/MS methods can be developed, which can either quantify unconjugated drug or total drug (unconjugated and conjugated payload) in a biological sample. Additionally, relative abundance of different DAR species (DAR0-DAR8) within a sample can also be quantified using complex LC-MS/MS techniques. Decision on which measurements to make depends on available resources/time and questions at hand [3–6, 10, 17]. Figure 3a represents a PK model that integrates different analytes (i.e. total mAb, conjugated mAb, total drug, and unconjugated drug) and helps estimate primary PK parameters (e.g. clearances and volumes of distribution) for

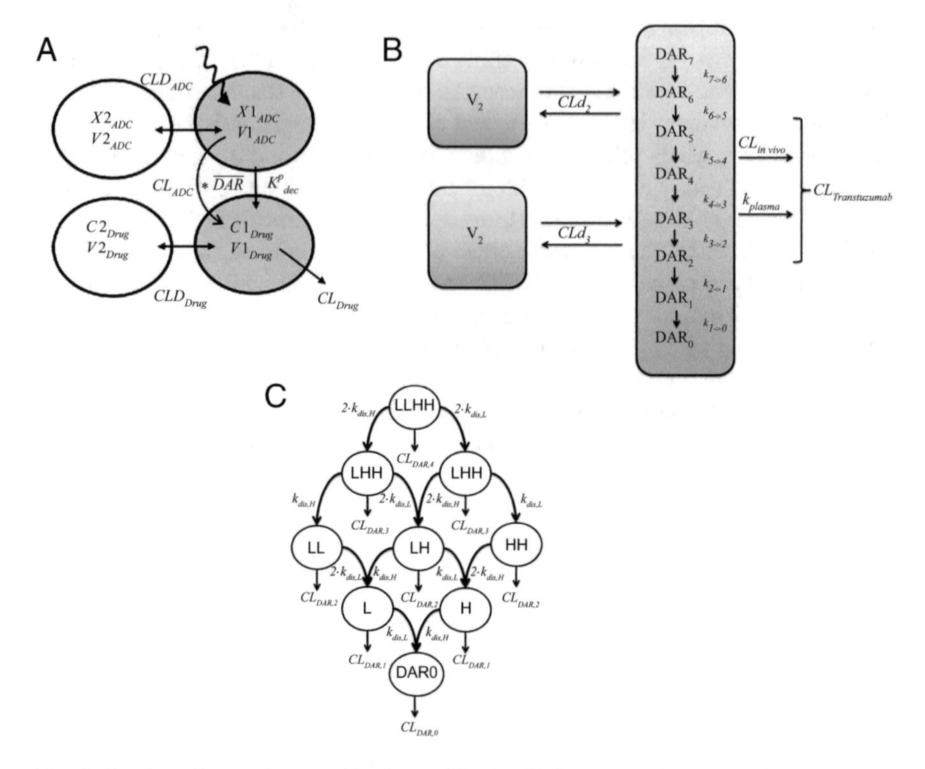

Fig. 3 In vivo plasma pharmacokinetic models for ADCs. (**a**) An integrated 2-compartment plasma PK model for ADC and the released drug [12]. (**b**) A plasma PK model for ADC that incorporates catenary deconjugation cascade in the central compartment of the model [31]. (**c**) A plasma PK model for site-specific ThioMAb-drug conjugates that accounts for the disposition of each DAR species [32]

ADC/mAb and the released drug, along with the estimation of average non-specific drug deconjugation rate (K_{dec}^{P}) in the systemic circulation. Bi-exponential profile of ADC/mAb is represented by a 2-compartment model followed by linear clearance from the central compartment. Disposition of the released drug is also characterized using a 2-compartment model where the two processes (i.e. non-specific deconjugation – K_{dec}^{P}, and proteolytic degradation of mAb/ADC -CL^{ADC}) serves as formation clearances for released drug/payload PK model. This model has been applied to characterize the disposition of an array of different ADC molecules (e.g. brentuximab-vedotin, T-DM1, inotuzumab-ozogamicin, and anti-5 T4 ADC A1mcMMAF) with varying linker chemistries and conjugated payloads [3, 12, 15, 18]. While selecting the lead candidate with desirable PK properties, comparison of these PK parameters across different molecules can be very beneficial. Some of the comparisons may include plasma half-life of conjugate and released drug, as well as deconjugation rate of different ADCs that represents the *in vivo* linker stability. ADCs with inferior half-life of the conjugate or with unusually high exposure of the released drug should be avoided for developmental purposes. Of note, the average non-specific deconjugation rate of drug from the ADC (K_{dec}^{P}) represents how the average DAR value of an ADC formulation is changing with time, and doesn't necessarily represents the deconjugation rate of each DAR species. Although, significant amount of resources and time are routinely spent in discerning the deconjugation rate for each DAR species in the formulation (where higher DAR species are usually observed to demonstrate faster deconjugation rate than lower DAR species), we still believe that there is some value in obtaining this average parameter since it may remain consistent across species [3]. In addition, as illustrated earlier, in vivo deconjugation rate (K_{dec}^{P}) value can also be compared with estimates obtained from *in vitro* experiments to establish an IVIVC for ADC stability [8].

As briefly explained earlier, characterization of more complex deconjugation process of ADCs within the body requires simultaneous measurement of the proportion of different DAR species in a biological sample. Although, determination of these complex bioanalytical measurements may require additional resources and time, development of such models can be very beneficial in elucidating the biological fate of different DAR species inside the body as well as their individual deconjugation rates. One such model has been presented by Bender et al. to characterize plasma PK of trastuzumab-emtansine (T-DM1) in rat and monkey (Fig. 3b). They constructed a catenary PK model to characterize deconjugation of ADC from higher to lower DAR species (DAR_7 to DAR_1), as well as overall stability of T-DM1 in an *in vitro* system of rat and monkey plasma. The catenary model was integrated within the central compartment of a 3-compartment mammillary PK model to characterize *in vivo* plasma PK of total trastuzumab and individual DAR species in rats and monkeys. While they assumed all DAR species have similar clearance from the systemic circulation, it may not be always true since it has been reported that higher DAR species are shown to eliminate faster due to increased hydrophobicity. Nonetheless, their modeling work revealed that deconjugation rate from higher DAR species (i.e. DAR_7 to DAR_3) was 34–40% faster than DAR_2 species (i.e. DAR_2 to $DAR_1 - K_{2\rightarrow1}$). In addition, the rate of deconjugation from DAR_1 ADC to naked trastuzumab ($K_{1\rightarrow0}$) was found to be the slowest with an estimate ~3.5 fold lower than $K_{2\rightarrow1}$ [31]. Similar catenary PK model structure has also been developed by Chudasama et al. to characterize the clinical PK of T-DM1 in HER2 positive breast cancer patients [13].

With the advent of site-specific conjugation technologies to regulate the level of heterogeneity and hydrophobicity within ADC formulation, the PK models to characterize deconjugation of ADC has also evolved. Development of one such model to characterize the distinct deconjugation processes of site-specific conjugates has been presented by Sukumaran et al. using MMAE-based Thiomab-drug Conjugates (TDCs) [32]. These conjugates are formed by engineering a cysteine residue on light and heavy chain. Figure 3c shows the model schematics, where complex deconjugation of higher to lower DAR ADC species is characterized. Each DAR species was individually purified and administered to feed into the final model structure, where it was assumed that every DAR species distribute via a 2-compartment model. The modeling work helped the authors elucidate that deconjugation rate of the drug was much faster (~4 times) from the heavy chain compared to the light chain. Additionally, they also incorporated DAR dependent clearance and potency for the TDCs within their model, highlighting a more mechanistic way of developing PK-PD relationships for ADCs [32].

Tumor Pharmacokinetics Models for ADCs

Although understanding and mathematically characterizing the plasma PK for ADCs is vital, it should not be the only deciding factor in selecting the lead candidates for the next phase of development. Plasma concentrations of majority of mAb-based therapeutics are not in rapid equilibrium with tissue concentrations. Moreover, additional complexity arises with ADCs, since the cytotoxic drug generally retains within the tumor due to strong intracellular binding to its pharmacological target (e.g. DNA, tubulin). Thus, the observed rate and extent of plasma exposure for different molecular species of ADCs can be very different than the one in the tumors. Consequently, a more systems based approach should be favored over empirical PK models for characterizing and predicting tumor PK of ADC, as this approach can integrate the physiological parameters underlying the system with the dispositional behavior of an ADC.

One such model has been developed by us and widely applied now for several ADCs with varying cytotoxic payloads and linker chemistries. Figure 4a shows the schematics for this model, where ADC disposition in the systemic circulation is represented using an integrated 2-compartment model shown in Fig. 3a. Due to high interstitial pressure and lack of any functional lymphatic system, the exchange of ADC/drug from systemic circulation to tumor microenvironment is predominantly characterized via diffusion, where the permeability or diffusivity exchange parameters are calculated *a priori* based on molecular weight of ADC/drug. At lower tumor sizes/volumes, the surface exchange (exchange from periphery of tumor) predominates, whereas at higher tumor sizes, the vascular exchange predominates. Once exchanged into the tumor extracellular matrix, both ADC/drug interacts with tumor cells in a similar manner as explained in the cellular disposition model (Fig. 1b) earlier. We have demonstrated the utility of this model by *a priori* predicting the experimentally obtained tumor exposures of different analytes of ADCs based on the plasma PK in xenograft mouse models. A priori predictions like this not just reduces the overall magnitude of tumor disposition studies required, but also provides a more mechanistic PK-PD approach which can be pivotal while translating it to higher species, especially where tumor PK is unavailable [12, 18, 20]. One can also incorporate an additional layer of complexity within these models by accounting for multiple populations of tumor cells (e.g. antigen-high and low expressing cells) to mimic the realistic scenarios observed with solid-tumor heterogeneity in the clinic. Parameters associated with the disposition of ADC and its analytes in each tumor cell-type can be obtained using the in vitro cell PK model explained earlier (Fig. 1b). This tumor PK model with various cell populations offer a more mechanistic framework for characterizing heterogeneous ADC disposition, ADC bystander effect, and immune-oncology effects of ADCs (e.g. immunogenic cell death – ICD). These models can also be used to determine the most important parameters (via global sensitivity analysis) and prominent pathways (via pathway analysis) responsible for tumor exposure of ADC, which can in turn help with the development of better ADCs [18].

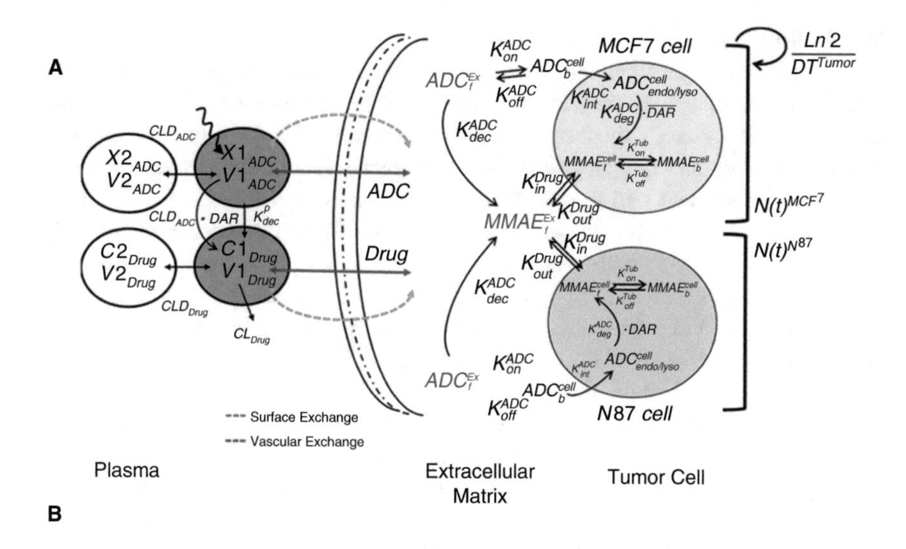

B

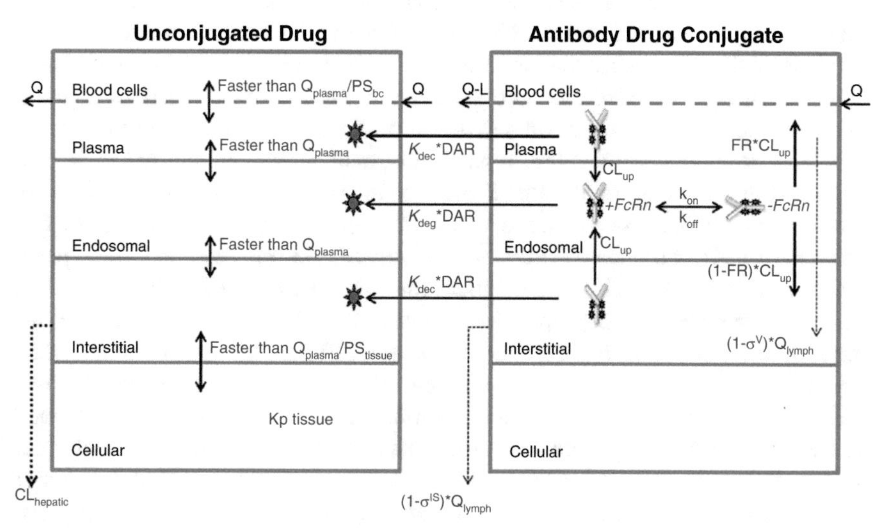

Fig. 4 In vivo system pharmacokinetic models for ADCs. (**a**) Mechanistic tumor disposition model for ADCs that is capable of incorporating multiple cell populations within the solid tumor. (**b**) Tissue-level diagram of the platform PBPK model for ADCs. The model accounts for simultaneous disposition of both ADC and the released drug. Each tissue compartment is subdivided into blood cell, vascular, endothelial, interstitial, and cellular spaces [21, 22]

Whole-Body Disposition Models for ADCs
Development of physiologically-based pharmacokinetic (PBPK) models has several additional advantages in comparison to mammillary models in establishing accurate exposure-efficacy and exposure-toxicity relationships. The plasma concentrations of the ADC and unconjugated drug may not always reflect their tissue concentrations, and hence one can lead to counterintuitive conclusions when correlating plasma exposure with efficacy and toxicity of ADC. Thus, more comprehensive PK models, which can integrate system-specific parameters (e.g. blood/lymph flows, tissue volumes) as well as drug-specific processes (e.g. protein binding, tissue binding, antigen and FcRn interaction), are much more reliable in characterizing and predicting tissue exposures of different ADC related analytes.

At the preclinical stage, the ADC PBPK models can be employed to assess the impact of differential expression of target antigen in tumor versus normal tissues on the therapeutic index of ADC. Such early-phase investigations can provide key insights towards target selection and can inform the development of lead ADC molecules. Once validated, such models can *a priori* recognize toxicity-prone tissues as well as predict exposures at the site-of-action. Because PBPK models are also systems PK models, the clinical PK predictions made by these models are more dependable than allometric scaling techniques or mammillary compartmental models. PBPK models can also be employed to identify drug-drug interactions and simulate therapeutic scenarios where ADCs are co-administered with other treatments.

While development of PBPK models for small molecules and mAbs is well described in the literature, the PBPK models for ADCs have been developed very recently. Mainly because one needs to simultaneously account for whole-body disposition of mAb and released drug, both of which have very distinct ADME properties. The first report on a PBPK model for ADCs was presented by Zhao et al. [33], who characterized the disposition of anti-CD70 ADC SGN-75 and its released metabolite cys-mcMMAF in plasma, tumor, and different tissues of a tumor bearing mice. Disposition of ADC was described using an antibody PBPK model where different tissues were arranged in an anatomical manner and connected via blood and lymph flows. Each tissue was further sub-divided into two parts to account for the disposition of mAb/ADC and the released drug cys-mcMMAF. In order to characterize the data, the authors estimated tissue partition coefficients of cys-mcMMAF, and also the vascular and lymphatic reflection coefficients of mAbs in each tissue. Additionally, total antigen (CD70) and tubulin density were also estimated along with clearances of mAb/ADC and the released drug. Although informative and first of its kind, there were several limitations of this analysis leading to poor characterization of datasets and lesser translatable potential. Later, a minimal PBPK model for ADCs was published by Chen et al. [34] to assess clinical drug-drug interaction potential for vc-MMAE based ADCs. The model was built to incorporate formation clearance of MMAE from ADC as well as its hepatic clearance from the liver compartment. The model was validated using two different ADCs, anti-CD22-vc-MMAE and brentuximab-vedotin, and was able to predict the changes in the AUC and Cmax ratios of released MMAE in the presence or absence of Rifampin, Midazolam and Ketoconazole. More importantly, the modeling analysis suggested that vc-MMAE based ADCs had a limited potential for causing significant DDIs. Although the minimal PBPK model was successful in addressing the questions at hand, the dispositional behavior of ADC and its related analytes was not explicitly characterized.

Cilliers et al. have recently presented another version of ADC PBPK model to characterize whole-body and intra-tumor PK of ADC using T-DM1 as a model compound [35]. The authors combined the PBPK model for mAbs [36] with a mechanistic Krogh cylinder tumor model to predict average concentrations of ADC in each tissue and heterogeneity of ADC distribution in tumor. Their modeling analysis and experimental investigations revealed that at the clinically approved dose of T-DM1 (3.6 mg/kg), its distribution is limited to perivascular regions of tumor tissue. In addition, the authors proposed that co-administration of ADC with naked antibody can result in a more homogeneous tumor disposition of ADC, while still maintaining similar average ADC concentrations within in tumor. While very elegant and useful, this model was used to characterize the PK of only the antibody component of the ADC, and it was validated using only single time-point tissue concentration measurements.

Recently, we have presented a more comprehensive and translational PBPK model for ADC to characterize whole-body disposition of ADC and its components, using T-DM1 as a model compound [21] (Fig. 4b). The model was developed in a sequential manner, where initially the biodistribution of DM1 was characterized using a small molecule PBPK model. Later, the small molecule PBPK model was integrated with our previously developed platform PBPK model of mAb, via deconjugation and degradation processes, to characterize the whole-body PK of ADCs. The model was able to effectively predict whole-body PK of T-DM1 in rats, and was also able to *a priori* predict the clinical PK for different analytes of T-DM1 reasonably well [21].

Pharmacokinetic-Pharmacodynamic Models for ADCs

Development of a reliable PK-PD relationship at an early preclinical stage is very valuable for further ADC development. Since the majority of ADCs are developed for oncology indications, ADC induced tumor regression in mouse xenografts, patient-derived xenografts, or orthotropic mouse models is usually investigated. Thus, development of PK-PD models for ADCs generally involve characterization of tumor growth inhibition (TGI) datasets, and estimation of efficacy parameters (e.g. K_{max} and KC_{50}). These efficacy parameters can help triage lead ADC candidates based on their preclinical performance and can also govern the prediction of clinical efficacy.

One of the earliest PK-PD analysis for ADC was performed by Jumbe et al. [37] for T-DM1 in trastuzumab-resistant mouse xenografts. Plasma PK of T-DM1 from multiple datasets in tumor bearing and tumor non-bearing mice was characterized using a 2-compartment model, and the plasma ADC concentrations from the central compartment were used as a forcing function to drive ADC tumor killing. The tumor growth in different xenografts was characterized using a unique set of equations that assumed spherical tumor shape. ADC exposure was assumed to initiate shuttling of tumor cells from growing to non-growing phases, which eventually led to cell death. The authors also introduced a novel secondary parameter, coined as 'Tumor Static Concentration (TSC)', which integrated information pertaining to both growth and killing components of PK-PD model. As described earlier for the in vitro setting, TSC is the theoretical concentration of ADC at which the growth and killing rates nullify each other and there is a static tumor volume over the period of time. Authors highlighted the translational value of this parameter by suggesting that for an efficacious dosing regimen both peak and trough concentrations of ADC should be above the in vivo TSC value [37].

A more comprehensive modeling analysis was later presented by Haddish-Berhane et al. [23] who explored the translational potential of 'TSC' for *a priori* predicting clinically efficacious dose of ADC. They use a hybrid tumor-kill cell distribution model (Fig. 5a) with a modified growth and kill functions [23]. Tumor growth rate was described as a function of tumor volume, initially starting with a faster 'exponential' phase, followed by a slower 'linear' phase, and eventually leading to saturation in growth rate once the tumor achieves the maximum carrying capacity. ADC induced tumor regression was presented using a non-linear killing function (with $\boldsymbol{K_{max}}$ and $\boldsymbol{KC_{50}}$). The model was employed to characterize the TGI datasets from multiple mouse models after administration of two different ADCs, T-DM1 and A1mcMMAF. The in vivo TSC values calculated from xenograft PK-PD model were then utilized to *a priori* predict clinically efficacious doses of ADC, using allometrically scaled human PK of ADCs. The developed strategy was validated with T-DM1, where the predicted doses based on preclinically obtained TSC values were very close to the clinically approved dosing regimen of 3.6 mg/kg Q3W (every 3 weeks) [23]. As described earlier, the 'TSC' values obtained from both *in vitro* and *in vivo* PK-PD analysis can also be utilized to develop IVIVC for ADC efficacy.

Empirical PK-PD relationships, such as the ones described above, fail to account for complex PK associated with ADCs as well as differences in the preclinical and clinical tumors. As a result, many mechanistic aspects are neglected while making PK and efficacy predictions using these models. Within the past few years, we have extensively worked on development of a general translational strategy, which integrates the information from different phases of ADC development to successfully predict clinical PK and efficacy. This strategy has been now validated for successful clinical translation of brentuximab-vedotin (Seattle genetics®), T-DM1 (Genentech®), and inotuzumab-Ozogamicin (Pfizer®) [3, 12, 15], in a retrospective manner. The strategy, which is shown in Fig. 5b, involves development of a mechanistic tumor distribution model (as described earlier, Fig. 4a) that incorporates all the system-specific values associated with ADC disposition in a single cell to *a priori* predict tumor payload concentrations. Tumor exposure of released payload/drug is then used as a driving function for characterizing the TGI data in different xenograft mouse models to estimate payload/drug induced efficacy parameters (i.e. $\boldsymbol{K_{max}}$ and $\boldsymbol{KC_{50}}$). Clinical translation of the preclinical tumor PK-PD model is then achieved by updating plasma PK of ADC and released drug, tumor growth rates, and tumor antigen expression levels to clinically relevant values reported in the literature. This translational strategy can help in predicting clinical endpoints such as

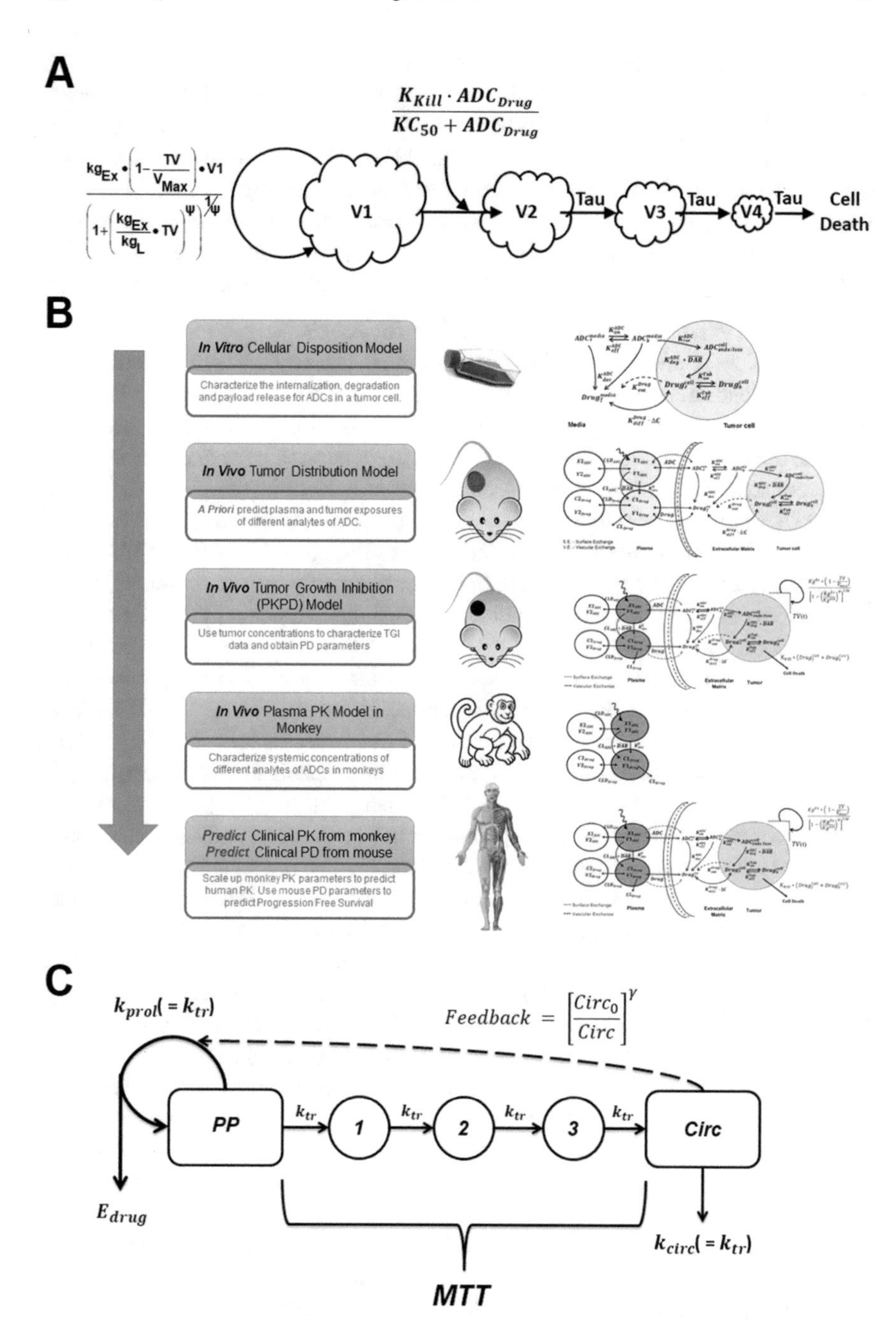

Fig. 5 In vivo PK-PD/TD models for ADC. (**a**) A semi-mechanistic tumor growth inhibition model that accounts for bi-phasic tumor growth, nonlinear cell killing, and cell-distribution mediated delay [23]. (**b**) A general PK-PD M&S driven strategy for clinical translation of ADC efficacy using the multiscale mechanistic model [3]. (**c**) A semi-mechanistic PK-TD model that is generally used to characterize ADC mediated toxicities (e.g. thrombocytopenia and neutropenia) [24]

progression-free survival (PFS) and objective response rates (ORRs) for ADCs. The translated models can also be employed to predict different clinical outcomes for ADCs under different dosing regimens and for different patient populations. For example, it has been shown that the translated PK-PD model developed for T-DM1 was able to predict the differences in the response to ADC by HER2-low (1+) and HER2-high (3+) patients reasonably well. The model simulations also suggested that the fractionated dosing regimen (e.g. once every week) may be more beneficial compared to the current clinical dosing regimen (once every 3 weeks) of T-DM1 [3].

Pharmacokinetics-Toxicodynamics Models for ADCs

A successful ADC molecule in the clinic is not necessarily the most potent one but the one that exhibits superior therapeutic index (TI). Thus, understanding the toxicity of ADCs is equally important. There can be multiple mechanisms associated with the observed toxicities for ADCs. Target expression in normal cells can lead to localized toxicity in different organs, and premature deconjugation of drug/payload from ADCs can lead to widespread systemic toxicities. The main toxicities associated with most commonly used payloads in the clinic (i.e. MMAE, MMAF, DM1, DM4, and Calicheamicin) include peripheral neuropathy, ocular toxicities, gastrointestinal/hepatic toxicities, neutropenia, and thrombocytopenia [38]. As mentioned earlier, development of whole-body PBPK models can be very helpful in predicting ADC exposure in target versus normal tissues, identifying toxicity-prone tissues, and developing reliable PK-TD relationships. However, all the PK-TD models developed for ADCs so far involve the use of semi-mechanistic PK-TD model to characterize blood related toxicities (e.g. thrombocytopenia and neutropenia).

A general TD model proposed by Friberg et al. [24] to characterize chemotherapeutic-induced myelosuppression has been extensively used to characterize the toxicities associated with ADC molecules. The model (Fig. 5c) consists of a growing pool of progenitor/stem cells (***PP***) that goes through a maturation step, via a series of transit compartments ($\boldsymbol{K_{tr}}$), to become circulating cells (***Circ***). In the absence of ADC, the progenitor cells (***PP***) are controlled by the growth rate ($\boldsymbol{K_{prol}}$) and the feedback mechanism from the circulating cells ($(\boldsymbol{Circ_0/Circ})^{\gamma}$). The plasma PK of ADC is then used to drive the reduction in cell proliferation rate via linear or non-linear functions [24]. Preclinical application of this model was first demonstrated by Tatipalli et al. [25], who evaluated the differences in ADC induced myelosuppression in monkeys for 10 different vc-MMAE based ADCs, which differed only in their specificity towards the therapeutic target. Plasma PK of different ADCs was characterized using a 2-compartment model, and ADC concentrations from the central compartment were utilized to drive the myelosuppression using a linear function (i.e. $\boldsymbol{E_{ADC} = C_{ADC} \cdot Slope}$). Authors later compared the estimated slope value, essentially indicative of potency of each ADC molecule, and reported that there was ~10-fold difference across different ADC molecules despite having the same linker-payload [25]. A more recent characterization of the ADC induced-myelosuppression was presented by Ait-Oudhia et al. [26] in xenograft mouse models for two clinically approved ADCs, T-DM1 and brentuximab-vedotin (SGN-35). Plasma PK of both ADCs was described using an integrated 2-compartment model (similar to PK model described in Fig. 3a). Their modeling analysis revealed that toxicity effects for T-DM1 (an example of non-cleavable linker based ADC) were driven by plasma concentration of conjugate, whereas the toxicity effects for brentuximab-vedotin (an example of cleavable linker based ADC) were driven by plasma concentration of payload (MMAE) [26].

Clinical Development

Application of PK-PD M&S for streamlining the clinical development process of drugs is widely recognized. In phase-1 clinical trials, the main focus is on determining the maximum tolerated dose (MTD) and establishing a safe dosing regimen for the subsequent clinical trial (phase 2 and phase 3). In the phase-2 and 3 trials, the focus is on establishing an effective exposure-response relationship for the drug across diverse patient population. There is a huge value in development of population based PK-PD models, which not only help with the estimation of the mean structural parameter, but can also help in estimation of inter-subject variability associated with each parameter. The source of the inter-subject variability can also be explained with the help of comprehensive covariate-analysis that helps in identifying statistically significant covariates within a population (e.g. age, body-weight, renal clearance etc.). The population PK-PD approach also encourages integration of multiple sparse datasets from different patient populations to come up with unified dose-exposure and exposure-response relationships. Within this section, we have discussed the most prominent modeling examples for ADCs where M&S was employed for making decisions in the clinical setting [39].

Pharmacokinetics Models for ADCs

There are multiple factors that contribute to the development of fit-for-purpose plasma PK models for ADCs in the clinical setting. This includes the availability of different analytical measurements (such as total antibody, free drug, total drug, and conjugated antibody), richness/abundance of PK samples, overall sample/population size, information available for the patient demographics (such as body-weight, age etc.), and the range of doses evaluated. The majority of the clinical PK analysis for ADCs in the literature is confined to smcc-DM1 and vc-MMAE based ADCs. One of the earliest examples includes the population PK analysis of T-DM1 in HER2-positive metastatic patients presented by Gupta et al. [40]. Authors incorporated datasets from three different clinical trials (phase-1 and phase-2) where conjugated antibody (i.e. T-DM1) was the primary analyte investigated at the dosing regimen of 3.6 mg/kg Q3W (every 3 weeks). Disposition of T-DM1 was characterized using a 2-compartment model with linear elimination from the central compartment. Authors identified that body-weight, albumin levels, tumor burden, and aspartate aminotransferase levels were the statistically significant covariates; among which body-weight was the major descriptor of the observed variability in clearance and central volume of distribution. These findings led authors to conclude that a BW-based dosing regimen of 3.6 mg/kg Q3W for T-DM1 may not need further adjustments to reach the desired exposure levels in different patients in the clinic [40].

A more comprehensive PK analysis for T-DM1 was presented by Lu et al. [41], who developed an integrated population PK model to characterize the disposition of two different analytes, total trastuzumab (TTmAb) and T-DM1 (conjugated antibody). Authors incorporated datasets from multiple studies (Phase-1 and 2) where different dose-levels (0.3–4.8 mg/kg) were investigated in a Q1W (once every week) and Q3W regimens. The model structure involved a common central compartment volume for TTmAb and T-DM1. Three different clearance mechanisms were incorporated, where clearances of TTmAb and T-DM1 from the central compartment was characterized using a linear catabolic process, and deconjugation of T-DM1 to TTmAb in the central compartment was characterized using a first order process. Additionally, both conjugated (T-DM1) and total antibody (TTmAb) were assumed to distribute to the peripheral tissue compartment with their own different distributional clearances and volumes. The model was able to characterize the TTmAb and T-DM1 profiles in diverse set of patient population reasonably well, with good precision for the estimated PK parameters. Authors also highlighted the importance of the deconjugation process of T-DM1 in the clinic, which leads to faster clearance of T-DM1 in plasma compared to TTmAb [41]. A semi-mechanistic PK model with complex catenary deconjugation processes has also been used by Chudasama et al. to characterize clinical PK of T-DM1 [13]. The model included disposition of four different conjugated antibody (T-DM1) and one naked antibody (trastuzumab) species via a 2-compartmental model with nonlinear Michaelis-Menten type elimination process from the central compartment. In addition, the model also included a 1st order deconjugation rate to characterize transformation of higher DAR species to lower DAR species. The model was able to characterize several PK datasets (both Phase-1 and Phase-2) generated with doses ranging from 0.3–4.8 mg/kg reasonably well. While the PK of T-DM1 is assumed to be linear at the clinically approved dose of 3.6 mg/kg, the wide range of doses allowed the authors to identify the non-linear elimination process of T-DM1 in the clinic.

Similar PK models have been also constructed for vc-MMAE based ADCs. An integrated 2-compartement model was constructed by Lu et al. [42] to characterize the disposition of vc-MMAE based ADCs using total antibody (TmAb) and antibody-conjugated MMAE (acMMAE) as two different analytes. Both analytes were characterized using a 2-compartment model with a linear elimination from the central compartment. An additional deconjugation clearance was incorporated to characterize the PK of acMMAE. Simultaneous fitting of clinical data for both the analytes enabled the authors to estimate the parameters associated with antibody disposition (clearances and volume of disposition) and MMAE deconjugation from the ADC. Importantly, the modeling analysis enabled the authors to remove the requirement of total antibody (TmAb) measurements from the subsequent late-stage clinical trials without compromising overall PK characterization of the ADCs [42]. A similar platform PK model was also presented by Kagedal et al. [43] to support the development of vc-MMAE based ADCs. The model was developed based on the clinical PK data of acMMAE from 8 different vc-MMAE based ADCs. Disposition of acMMAE was characterized using a two-compartment model with linear time-dependent clearance. Modeling analysis revealed that the time-dependent clearance only comes into play during the 1st dosing cycle, and had no effect later on. Additionally, authors identified body-weight and sex as the major descriptors of variability in clearance and volume of distribution of ADC. Their analysis also revealed that the estimated PK parameters were very consistent across 8 different vc-MMAE based ADCs that were targeted against different antigens in the clinic. The authors claim that the developed platform model can *a priori* predict clinical behavior of other vc-MMAE based ADCs in the future [43].

Pharmacokinetics-Pharmacodynamic Models for ADCs
Development of robust exposure-efficacy relationships in the clinical settings becomes challenging, especially for oncology therapeutics, because of the limited continuous tumor measurement data. Luu et al. [44] have presented an exposure-response relationship for clinically approved inotuzumab-ozogamicin (CMC-544) using a population PK-PD model. The plasma PK for CMC-544 was characterized using a 2-compartment model, and the total calicheamicin (total drug/payload) concentrations were used to drive the inhibition of exponentially growing tumor volumes. The tumor volumes were calculated using the tumor diameter measurements obtained via imaging in the clinic. The validated model was then able to inform about the duration required to get 10% shrinkage in tumor volume (~35 days). The modeling also gave an insight about the duration of time after the end of the therapy when the drug effects are still sustained at the clinically approved dose of 1.8 mg/m^2 Q4WX4. Another PK-PD analysis for ADC in the clinical setting was presented by Li et al. [45] for T-DM1 in HER2 positive metastatic breast cancer patients, which were previously treated with trastuzumab and a taxane. Authors utilized a previously validated PK model for T-DM1 to calculate the C_{min} and $AUC^{0\text{-}21d}$ (Area under the curve from time zero to 21 days) values during each cycle (3.6 mg/kg Q3W), and correlated the model predicted C_{min} and $AUC^{0\text{-}21d}$ values with PD endpoints like PFS and Overall Survival (OS). Importantly, the authors concluded that the model predicted C_{min} values demonstrated the strongest correlation with the efficacy of ADC [45].

A more mechanistic approach can also be taken by first translating a preclinical tumor disposition model to the clinic and then using the tumor exposures to drive the PD endpoints in the clinic. Using multiple case-studies with three different clinically approved ADCs (i.e. brentuximab-vedotin, T-DM1 and inotuzumab-ozogamicin) we have demonstrated the translational capabilities of the preclinical models for predicting the clinical efficacy of ADCs in different patient populations. Although, the utility of these models has been published using retrospective scenarios so far, one can envision incorporation of such mechanistic models for predicting clinically unknown scenarios (e.g. the effect of alternative dosing regimens) in a prospective manner going forward [3, 12].

Pharmacokinetics-Toxicodynamics Models for ADCs
Both exposure-efficacy and exposure-toxicity models should be utilized simultaneously in the clinic to determine an efficacious and well tolerated dose in clinic.

As discussed in the preclinical section, in the clinical situations as well mostly the blood related toxicities (e.g. thrombocytopenia and neutropenia) of ADCs have been mathematically characterized using the variations of the myelosuppression model (Fig. 5c).

Mugundu et al. [46] have developed a model to characterize the exposure-toxicity relationship of inotuzumab-ozogamicin (CMC-544, a calicheamicin based ADC), where total drug concentrations were utilized to suppress the proliferation of progenitor cells using a non-linear function. Using the population PK-PD analysis, authors identified baseline platelet count as a significant covariate for CMC-544 induced thrombocytopenia [46]. A similar approach was undertaken by Bender et al. [27] to characterize T-DM1 induced thrombocytopenia in HER2-positive metastatic breast cancer patients. They utilized the conjugated antibody (T-DM1) exposure (obtained using a 2-compartment model) in the plasma to drive the depletion of progenitor cells. However, they made two additional modifications to the Friberg et al. [24] model (Fig. 5c) to account for the clinical observations where the platelet nadirs were generally lower after the first dose. For the first modification, two separate efficacy parameters were incorporated to characterize the effects after first and subsequent doses. For the second modification, two different populations of progenitor cells were assumed, where one pool of progenitor cell was non-depletable and the other population was assumed to deplete with the effect of drug [27]. Data from two different phase 2 clinical studies was incorporated for the development of this model. Using the final model the authors concluded that the downward drifting of platelet-time profiles observed after T-DM1 treatment will be stabilized by the 8th treatment cycle. Additionally, the model also supported the clinical observation that the dosing regimen of 3.6 mg/kg Q3W will be well tolerated by the patients [27].

More recently the application of PK-TD modeling for vc-MMAE based ADC induced toxicities was presented by Li et al. [47]. Based on the diverse set of vc-MMAE based ADCs studied in the clinic, authors concluded that peripheral neuropathy (PN) and neutropenia were the most commonly observed toxicities. The authors utilized acMMAE (conjugated drug) PK simulated using a 2-compartmental model to drive both the PN and neutropenia toxicities. The Friberg et al. model [24] was adapted to drive ADC induced depletion of progenitor cells. The authors performed a model-based comparison of the toxicity parameters between monkey and humans for acMMAE induced neutropenia across different vc-MMAE ADCs, and concluded that they were very similar (within two-fold) for every molecule. More importantly, the modeling analysis revealed that occurrence of PN was both acMMAE exposure and treatment time dependent, and therefore restricting the ADC treatment for up to 8 cycles will avoid occurrence of peripheral neuropathy significantly. The authors also envisioned that their PK-TD M&S based strategy can be very helpful for *a priori* predicting the toxicity of vc-MMAE based ADCs in the clinic [47].

Summary

In this book chapter we have discussed an array of PK-PD models and model-based strategies that could be employed to impact the decision making process during ADC development. There is a range of PK and PK-PD/TD models available, ranging from complex systems models to simplified fit-for-purpose models, selection of which depends upon the specific questions to be addressed and the availability of resources at hand. In order for these models to be truly effective during the ADC development process, they need to be incorporated in the developmental process at an early stage. In addition, PK-PD modelers' perspective should be kept in mind while deciding preclinical and clinical studies. A robust mathematical characterization of existing data will not only provide the scientists an in-depth understanding of the mechanism-of-action of ADCs, but will also guide future studies and help in making go/no-go decisions.

Acknowledgements This work was supported by NIH grant GM114179 to D.K.S., and the Centre for Protein Therapeutics at the State University of New York at Buffalo. Authors would also like to thank Dr. Amrita V. Kamath (Genentech®, Inc) for her helpful discussion while conception of this book chapter.

References

1. Kimko H, Pinheiro J (2015) Model-based clinical drug development in the past, present and future: a commentary. Br J Clin Pharmacol 79(1):108–116
2. Seruga B, Ocana A, Amir E, Tannock IF (2015) Failures in phase III: causes and consequences. Clin Cancer Res 21(20):4552–4560
3. Singh AP, Shah DK (2017) Application of a PK-PD modeling and simulation-based strategy for clinical translation of antibody-drug conjugates: a case study with Trastuzumab Emtansine (T-DM1). AAPS J 19(4):1054–1070
4. Kamath AV, Iyer S (2015) Preclinical pharmacokinetic considerations for the development of antibody drug conjugates. Pharm Res 32(11):3470–3479
5. Lin K, Tibbitts J (2012) Pharmacokinetic considerations for antibody drug conjugates. Pharm Res 29(9):2354–2366
6. Sapra P, Betts A, Boni J (2013) Preclinical and clinical pharmacokinetic/pharmacodynamic considerations for antibody-drug conjugates. Expert Rev Clin Pharmacol 6(5):541–555
7. Behrens CR, Liu B (2014) Methods for site-specific drug conjugation to antibodies. MAbs 6(1):46–53
8. Singh AP, Shin YG, Shah DK (2015) Application of pharmacokinetic-pharmacodynamic modeling and simulation for antibody-drug conjugate development. Pharm Res 32(11):3508–3525
9. Singh AP, Shah DK (2017) Measurement and mathematical characterization of cell-level pharmacokinetics of antibody-drug conjugates: a case study with Trastuzumab-vc-MMAE. Drug Metab Dispos 45(11):1120–1132
10. Khot A, Sharma S, Shah DK (2015) Integration of bioanalytical measurements using PK-PD modeling and simulation: implications for antibody-drug conjugate development. Bioanalysis 7(13):1633–1648
11. Shah DK, Barletta F, Betts A, Hansel S (2013) Key bioanalytical measurements for antibody-drug conjugate development: PK/PD modelers' perspective. Bioanalysis 5(9):989–992

12. Shah DK, Haddish-Berhane N, Betts A (2012) Bench to bedside translation of antibody drug conjugates using a multiscale mechanistic PK/PD model: a case study with brentuximab-vedotin. J Pharmacokinet Pharmacodyn 39(6):643–659
13. Chudasama VL, Schaedeli Stark F, Harrold JM, Tibbitts J, Girish SR, Gupta M et al (2012) Semi-mechanistic population pharmacokinetic model of multivalent trastuzumab emtansine in patients with metastatic breast cancer. Clin Pharmacol Ther 92(4):520–527
14. Lu D, Jin JY, Girish S, Agarwal P, Li D, Prabhu S et al (2015) Semi-mechanistic multiple-analyte pharmacokinetic model for an antibody-drug-conjugate in cynomolgus monkeys. Pharm Res 32(6):1907–1919
15. Betts AM, Haddish-Berhane N, Tolsma J, Jasper P, King LE, Sun Y et al (2016) Preclinical to clinical translation of antibody-drug conjugates using PK/PD modeling: a retrospective analysis of inotuzumab ozogamicin. AAPS J 18(5):1101–1116
16. Workgroup EM, Marshall SF, Burghaus R, Cosson V, Cheung SY, Chenel M et al (2016) Good practices in model-informed drug discovery and development: practice, application, and documentation. CPT Pharmacometrics Syst Pharmacol 5(3):93–122
17. Baumann A (2008) Preclinical development of therapeutic biologics. Exp Opin Drug Discov 3(3):289–297
18. Singh AP, Maass KF, Betts AM, Wittrup KD, Kulkarni C, King LE et al (2016) Evolution of antibody-drug conjugate tumor disposition model to predict preclinical tumor pharmacokinetics of trastuzumab-emtansine (T-DM1). AAPS J 18(4):861–875
19. Singh AP, Sharma S, Shah DK (2016) Quantitative characterization of in vitro bystander effect of antibody-drug conjugates. J Pharmacokinet Pharmacodyn 43(6):567–582
20. Shah DK, King LE, Han X, Wentland JA, Zhang Y, Lucas J et al (2014) A priori prediction of tumor payload concentrations: preclinical case study with an auristatin-based anti-5T4 antibody-drug conjugate. AAPS J 16(3):452–463
21. Khot A, Tibbitts J, Rock D, Shah DK (2017) Development of a translational physiologically based pharmacokinetic model for antibody-drug conjugates: a case study with T-DM1. AAPS J 19(6):1715–1734. doi: 10.1208/s12248-017-0131-3
22. Shah DK, Betts AM (2012) Towards a platform PBPK model to characterize the plasma and tissue disposition of monoclonal antibodies in preclinical species and human. J Pharmacokinet Pharmacodyn 39(1):67–86
23. Haddish-Berhane N, Shah DK, Ma D, Leal M, Gerber HP, Sapra P et al (2013) On translation of antibody drug conjugates efficacy from mouse experimental tumors to the clinic: a PK/PD approach. J Pharmacokinet Pharmacodyn 40(5):557–571
24. Friberg LE, Henningsson A, Maas H, Nguyen L, Karlsson MO (2002) Model of chemotherapy-induced myelosuppression with parameter consistency across drugs. J Clin Oncol 20(24):4713–4721
25. Tatipalli MDH (2012) Semi-physiological population PK/PD model of ADC neutropenia. University of Florida, Gainesville
26. Ait-Oudhia S, Zhang W, Mager DEA (2017) Mechanism-based PK/PD model for hematological toxicities induced by antibody-drug conjugates. AAPS J 19(5):1436–1448. doi: 10.1208/s12248-017-0113-5
27. Bender BC, Schaedeli-Stark F, Koch R, Joshi A, Chu YW, Rugo H et al (2012) A population pharmacokinetic/pharmacodynamic model of thrombocytopenia characterizing the effect of trastuzumab emtansine (T-DM1) on platelet counts in patients with HER2-positive metastatic breast cancer. Cancer Chemother Pharmacol 70(4):591–601
28. Sadekar S, Figueroa I, Tabrizi M (2015) Antibody drug conjugates: application of quantitative pharmacology in modality design and target selection. AAPS J 17(4):828–836
29. Maass KF, Kulkarni C, Betts AM, Wittrup KD (2016) Determination of cellular processing rates for a trastuzumab-maytansinoid antibody-drug conjugate (ADC) highlights key parameters for ADC design. AAPS J 18(3):635–646
30. Maass KF, Kulkarni C, Quadir MA, Hammond PT, Betts AM, Wittrup KDA (2015) Flow cytometric clonogenic assay reveals the single-cell potency of doxorubicin. J Pharm Sci 104(12):4409–4416

31. Bender B, Leipold DD, Xu K, Shen BQ, Tibbitts J, Friberg LEA (2014) mechanistic pharmacokinetic model elucidating the disposition of trastuzumab emtansine (T-DM1), an antibody-drug conjugate (ADC) for treatment of metastatic breast cancer. AAPS J 16(5):994–1008
32. Sukumaran S, Gadkar K, Zhang C, Bhakta S, Liu L, Xu K et al (2015) Mechanism-based pharmacokinetic/pharmacodynamic model for THIOMAB drug conjugates. Pharm Res 32(6):1884–1893
33. Zhao B ZS, Alley SC (2011) Physiologically-based pharmacokinetic modeling of an anti-CD70 auristatin antibody-drug conjugate in tumor-bearing mice. In: American conference on pharmacometrics (ACoP), San Diego
34. Chen Y, Samineni D, Mukadam S, Wong H, Shen BQ, Lu D et al (2015) Physiologically based pharmacokinetic modeling as a tool to predict drug interactions for antibody-drug conjugates. Clin Pharmacokinet 54(1):81–93
35. Cilliers C, Guo H, Liao J, Christodolu N, Thurber GM (2016) Multiscale modeling of antibody-drug conjugates: connecting tissue and cellular distribution to whole animal pharmacokinetics and potential implications for efficacy. AAPS J 18(5):1117–1130
36. Ferl GZ, AM W, JJ DS 3rd (2005) A predictive model of therapeutic monoclonal antibody dynamics and regulation by the neonatal Fc receptor (FcRn). Ann Biomed Eng 33(11):1640–1652
37. Jumbe NL, Xin Y, Leipold DD, Crocker L, Dugger D, Mai E et al (2010) Modeling the efficacy of trastuzumab-DM1, an antibody drug conjugate, in mice. J Pharmacokinet Pharmacodyn 37(3):221–242
38. Donaghy H (2016) Effects of antibody, drug and linker on the preclinical and clinical toxicities of antibody-drug conjugates. MAbs 8(4):659–671
39. Bender BC, Schindler E, Friberg LE (2015) Population pharmacokinetic-pharmacodynamic modelling in oncology: a tool for predicting clinical response. Br J Clin Pharmacol 79(1):56–71
40. Gupta M, Lorusso PM, Wang B, Yi JH, Burris HA 3rd, Beeram M et al (2012) Clinical implications of pathophysiological and demographic covariates on the population pharmacokinetics of trastuzumab emtansine, a HER2-targeted antibody-drug conjugate, in patients with HER2-positive metastatic breast cancer. J Clin Pharmacol 52(5):691–703
41. Lu D, Joshi A, Wang B, Olsen S, Yi JH, Krop IE et al (2013) An integrated multiple-analyte pharmacokinetic model to characterize trastuzumab emtansine (T-DM1) clearance pathways and to evaluate reduced pharmacokinetic sampling in patients with HER2-positive metastatic breast cancer. Clin Pharmacokinet 52(8):657–672
42. Lu D, Gibiansky L, Agarwal P, Dere RC, Li C, Chu YW et al (2016) Integrated two-analyte population pharmacokinetic model for antibody-drug conjugates in patients: implications for reducing pharmacokinetic sampling. CPT Pharmacometrics Syst Pharmacol 5(12):665–673
43. Kagedal M, Gibiansky L, Xu J, Wang X, Samineni D, Chen SC et al (2017) Platform model describing pharmacokinetic properties of vc-MMAE antibody-drug conjugates. J Pharmacokinet Pharmacodyn 44(6):537–548. doi: 10.1007/s10928-017-9544-y
44. Luu KVE, Volkert A, Ogura M, Goy G, Boni J (2012) Antitumor response to inotuzumab ozogamicin (INO) in patients with refractory or relapsed indolent B-cell non-Hodgkin' s l ymphomas (NHL): pharmacokinetic-pharmacodynamic (PK-PD) modeling and interim results from a phase II study. In: AACR 103rd annual meeting, Chicago
45. Li C, Wang B, Chen SC, Wada R, Lu D, Wang X et al (2017) Exposure-response analyses of trastuzumab emtansine in patients with HER2-positive advanced breast cancer previously treated with trastuzumab and a taxane. Cancer Chemother Pharmacol 80(6):1079–1090. doi: 10.1007/s00280-017-3440-4
46. Mugundu GVE, Boni J (2012) Use of pharmacokineticpharmacodynamic modeling to characterize platelet response following inotuzumab ozogamicin treatment in patients with follicular or diffuse large B-cell non-Hodgkin's lymphoma. In: AACR 103rd annual meeting, Chicago
47. Li CLD, Samineni D, Kaagedal M, Chen C, Jin J, Girish S (eds) (2017) PK/PD modeling strategy to support the development of antibody drug conjugates. In: AAPS national biotechnology conference, San Diego

Regulatory Considerations and Companion Diagnostics

Elizabeth VanAlphen and Omar Perez

Abstract The combination of a small molecule and a biologic in an ADC has consequences for regulatory requirements and guidances with respect to nonclinical evaluation as well as clinical development. The complexity of ADCs with regards to manufacturing and analytics presents additional challenges from the regulatory perspective. The clinical development of most ADCs involves patient selection; companion diagnostic products are regulated as a medical device in the US and in most ex-US markets and require a development plan that is integrated with the clinical development strategy from the earliest stages.

Keywords Regulatory · FDA · Companion diagnostic · Precision medicine · Patient selection · GLP · GMP · Manufacturing

Introduction: Common Regulatory Elements for ADCs

Antibody drug conjugates (ADCs) represent a science driven experimental medicine approach that utilize the overexpression of specific tumor biomarkers to target cytotoxic agents to a tumor environment; this targeting strategy lends itself to a personalized medicine approach to treat cancer or other serious conditions. The composition of an ADC itself is a highly selective monoclonal antibody chemically conjugated to a small molecule drug. The antibody component is the delivery vehicle, while the attached small molecule drug is the cytotoxic agent. This composition results in a combination of two separate classes of products regulated by the United States Food & Drug Administration (FDA): a biologic and a drug. The Patient Protection and Affordable Care Act, which included The Biologics Price Competition

E. VanAlphen (✉)
Pfizer Inc., Worldwide Safety and Regulatory, Groton, CT, USA
e-mail: Elizabeth.VanAlphen@Pfizer.com

O. Perez
Pfizer Inc., Diagnostics, South San Francisco, CA, USA
e-mail: omar.perez@pfizer.com

M. Damelin (ed.), *Innovations for Next-Generation Antibody-Drug Conjugates*, Cancer Drug Discovery and Development,
https://doi.org/10.1007/978-3-319-78154-9_5

and Innovation Act of 2009, was signed into law on March 23, 2010 and amended the longstanding Public Health Service Act of 1944 regulating biologics. Consequently in May 2015, FDA released the Draft Guidance for Industry regarding "Implementation of the Biologics Price Competition and Innovation Act of 2009" which declared that as a therapeutic class, ADCs are to be regulated as biologics. Nonetheless regardless of regulatory therapeutic class, a sponsor of an investigational ADC must carry out appropriate chemistry, manufacturing and controls (CMC) assessments for the antibody, the small molecule, and the final conjugated ADC molecule as well as the standard nonclinical toxicology evaluations in order to open an Investigational New Drug (IND) application with FDA and initiate first in human clinical studies. Meanwhile, the composition of an ADC presents unique pharmaceutical manufacturing challenges because the small molecule components are typically potent cytotoxic agents such as classical chemotherapy drugs, microtubule inhibitors, and DNA-damaging drugs, which also require appropriate measures to prevent potential cross-contamination in multiproduct manufacturing facilities and potential exposure to involved personnel. Furthermore, ADCs targeting expression of a tumor specific antigen may also call for the co-development of an in vitro diagnostic test to identify patients whom would benefit most with treatment of the ADC but also for which would require compliance with device regulations resulting in additional regulatory considerations.

In the U.S., currently the FDA has approved four ADC therapeutic drugs to the market. The first early generation ADC, gemtuzumab ozogamicin (targeting CD33), to be marketed in the US received an accelerated approval in 2000 for treatment of acute myelogenous leukemia. However, this drug was voluntarily withdrawn from the market in 2010 after the required post-approval phase III study did not confirm the clinical benefit when compared to chemotherapy treatment alone. This first generation ADC did not previously receive marketing approval in the EU [1]. Although more recent trials with new dosing regimens have shown good results suggesting benefit and therefore have warranted reassessment and reapplication in both the US and EU markets. As a result, FDA approval for new dosing regimens was ultimately granted in 2017 and the EU market application was in review at the time [2]. Two other early generation ADCs, brentuximab vedotin (targeting CD30) and ado-trastuzumab emtansine (targeting HER2), both for oncology indications were FDA approved for marketing in 2011 and in 2013 respectively [3, 4]. Finally also granted in 2017, inotuzumab ozogamicin (targeting CD22), is the fourth ADC to have achieved approval from U.S. regulators contributing to the changing ADC regulatory landscape [5].

Nonclinical Evaluation: General Considerations

To this date, no specific regulatory guidance to industry on ADC development has been published. Aligned with International Council on Harmonisation (ICH) S9: Nonclinical Evaluation for Anticancer Pharmaceuticals and (ICH) S6(R1):

Preclinical Safety Evaluation of Biotechnology-Derived Pharmaceuticals guidelines, FDA has generally followed an adaptive approach using existing guidelines for small molecule drugs and monoclonal antibodies. However, this guidance is very limited to small subsections within ICH S6 (R1) and ICH S9. The ICH has announced a "question and answer" subsection discussing ADCs, planned for ICH S9 inclusion, but has only published a draft version in 2016 requesting public comment [6]. Therefore, there is no set "blueprint" to follow for the design of nonclinical safety assessments of ADCs allowing for some flexibility to teams in designing these studies.

Factors for ADC success depend on optimization of each component: linker, small molecule drug, and monoclonal target antibody. The unique biochemical properties of these components can significantly affect the safety profile of the final conjugated molecule in comparison to the individual components alone and certainly as the next-generation ADCs continue to evolve. As an example, the recent efforts in more stable next-generation ADC design attempt to avoid systemic toxicities such as premature release of drug in the circulation and attempt to improve the therapeutic index of these molecules. Furthermore, the target antigen chosen will optimally have high expression levels in tumors and little or no expression in normal tissues in order to achieve an acceptable therapeutic index and reduce observed toxicity; ADCs with the same cytotoxic small molecule drug can also have different toxicity profiles dependent on the tumor antigen target. With that said, it can be difficult to predict potential for toxicity based on these expression patterns alone. Presently, the relationship between the linker choice, tumor antigen target, efficacy and safety is not well understood and challenging to model in preclinical settings. For all these reasons, appropriate toxicology evaluations are expected of all novel ADC regulatory filings and are also necessary prior to human clinical trials.

Primary Goals of Nonclinical Safety Evaluation

ADC nonclinical studies should be consistent with ICH and animal research guidelines. Prior to initiation of any clinical study, characterization of pharmacology, mechanism of action, anti-tumor activity in addition to the nonclinical safety assessment are expected in accordance with ICH S9 guidelines. An investigational ADC in development can also have a unique pharmacokinetic profile with significantly changed half-life, clearance, elimination, and biodistribution when compared to the unconjugated components alone. For example, elimination of an ADC involves properties of both large and small molecules. Therefore, assessing these characteristics is also a primary goal of nonclinical evaluations. The specifications for ADC stability have not been established through any relevant regulatory guidelines, but the goal of these studies is to provide data that is representative of the potential stability when dosed in humans. According to the ICH S6(R1) guideline, metabolic stability can be measured *in vitro*, by incubation of the ADC in human and animal plasma, but also during the conduct of rodent in vivo studies for the conjugated and unconjugated molecule [7].

As ADCs consist of a monoclonal antibody, small molecule, and linker, each individual component may contribute a measure of toxicity, and the ADC molecule as a whole may have its own toxicity. This complexity of ADC's requires a case-by-case scientifically-based approach and strategy for design and conduct of the nonclinical safety evaluations. For example in the case of ADCs, an aspect to consider is the presence of the highly potent small molecule which can produce significant toxicities unrelated to target binding. In this case, a study in rodent that does not express the intended target although will not inform target-dependent toxicity may provide relevant information regarding anticipated off-target toxicities. Furthermore, a brief discussion in ICH S6(R1) notes the importance of an additional rodent study specifically with novel unconjugated cytotoxic small molecules never studied before. For the conduct of nonclinical toxicity studies, principles for species selection are outlined in ICH S6(R1) to guide researchers. While the required regulatory toxicology studies are typically conducted in two relevant species, rodent and non-rodent for investigational small molecule drugs, exceptions do exist for the complete ADC molecule for example due to the lack of target cross-reactivity in rodent. The ability to identify two species that are both pharmacologically and toxicologically relevant may not always be possible, as many monoclonal antibodies will only bind to the target antigen in non-human primates. Therefore in those circumstances, research teams may choose to conduct the safety evaluation of the complete ADC molecule limited to a single non-rodent species which is typically non-human primates due to high homology with the human target. Required studies in rodent may be conducted with the small molecule and/or linker-small molecule component alone as an alternate option for research teams to consider. Studies conducted in non-relevant species may be considered misleading and are discouraged in the guidelines [8].

Consequently, the biological activity profiles of each ADC component should be considered when selecting the relevant and appropriate species and choosing which individual ADC components to assess. For small molecule components which are not novel and for which there is a sufficient body of scientific information available, ICH S6(R1) states in this situation a separate evaluation of the unconjugated small molecule is not warranted. Meanwhile per ICH S9 recommendations, the safety of the unconjugated components of the molecule can have a more "limited" evaluation. Additional toxicity studies associated with the free linker component alone may not be necessary because studies with the conjugated ADC or linker-small molecule component are expected to identify potential toxicities associated with the linker. For instance, a FDA review of ADC INDs showed that toxicities of the small molecule compared to the linker-small molecule were comparable [9]. A table outlining the generally accepted minimum data package of nonclinical safety studies is illustrated in Table 1 for both IND applications and ultimately marketing biologic license application (BLA) submissions. ADCs are not expected to access DNA because of their large molecular size but the cytotoxic drug and linker can be of potential genotoxic concern, therefore if nonclinical testing is warranted it should

Table 1 Nonclinical safety studies of ADC and its small molecule component

Study	Molecule	IND	BLA
GLP toxicology in relevant species (including safety pharmacology endpoints)	ADC	☒	☒
GLP toxicology study in rat[a]	Small molecule	☒	
In vitro plasma stability	ADC	☒	
Tissue cross-reactivity (human and tox species)	ADC	☒	
Genotoxicity[a]	Small molecule		☒
Embryofetal development	ADC		☒

[a]separate evaluation not warranted if the small molecule has been previously tested and sufficient body of scientific information is available

be conducted as ADC development proceeds. According to ICH S9 for advanced cancer indications, an embryofetal development toxicity assessment of potential risks for the developing embryo or fetus in patients who are or who might become pregnant is generally expected at the time of a marketing application (BLA).

FIH Dose Selection for ADCs

As previously discussed, FDA has not published guidance for ADCs including methodology for first in human (FIH) clinical trial dose selection. Thus, there remains a lack of best practices for both designing animal toxicity studies and calculating FIH starting dose to support ADC clinical trials. As a result, research teams have historically chosen various designs for toxicology studies and approaches to select the FIH dose such as traditional approaches used for small molecules or biological products in oncology and scaling either to body weight or body surface area. In the current ICH S9 guidelines for the nonclinical evaluation for anticancer pharmaceuticals, a common approach to select the (FIH) dose is to use 1/10th the severely toxic dose to 10% (STD_{10}) of the animals identified in a rodent good laboratory practice (GLP) study [7]. However due to the cross-reactivity requirements noted, ADC nonclinical programs are more likely to be conducted in non-human primates with 3 or more dose levels of the ADC to support the dose selection for clinical trials. In fact, the FDA recently disclosed in a review of 20 IND applications many ADC IND sponsors have generally chosen to use 3 or more dose levels of the ADC in a GLP toxicology study conducted in cynomolgus monkeys [9]. The review also revealed that some sponsors of ADC INDs elected to study effects of the small molecule alone in an additional rodent study [9]. But, FDA noted because the conjugated small molecule drives the human toxicity this makes a study with the free antibody less informative for FIH dose decisions generally. As a result, the FDA recommended that ADC FIH clinical dose setting not be based on studies with doses of the free antibody alone [9]. FDA's ADC IND review concluded that a non-human primate toxicology study with the clinical candidate has provided sufficient information regarding organ toxicities as the dose limiting toxicities were most often related to the small molecule independent of the target binding. Moreover, while the definition of HNSTD can be subjective in animal toxicology studies because there is no set criteria to define severity of toxicities in animals, the published FDA review found an acceptable balance of safety and efficient dose-escalation for a phase 1 trial resulted from a FIH dose that is 1/6th the highest non-severely toxic dose (HNSTD) in cynomolgus monkeys or 1/10th the STD_{10} in rodents scaled according to body surface area (BSA) rather than body weight (BW) [9]. To define the HNSTD, when an unacceptable toxicity was observed in the toxicology study in monkeys then a dose below it was defined as the HNSTD. In order to define STD_{10} in the rodent toxicology studies, when a dose exceeded mortality, the next lower dose was defined as the STD_{10}. Furthermore, dose selection based on 1/6th the HNSTD, 1/10th HNSTD, and 1/10th STD algorithms using body weight for animal-to-human dose conversions were considered unsafe in this FDA review. The published FDA review also found that ADCs sharing the same cytotoxic small molecule drug, linker, and drug:antibody ratio (DAR), should also use prior clinical data to help inform the design of a phase 1 clinical trial, such that if nonclinical studies support a higher starting dose than would be expected from clinical experience with other ADCs meeting the above criteria, a lower starting dose should be proposed. Overall, it is most important that ADC IND sponsors choose a starting dose that has potential for antitumor activity but provides an acceptable toxicity profile because FIH clinical studies are typically conducted in patients with advanced cancer.

Expedited Pathways and Mechanisms in US

In situations of serious or life-threatening diseases with limited therapeutic options, FDA can expedite patients' access to important treatments for serious conditions, such as cancer. The FDA first formally articulated expediting the availability of promising new therapies in regulations codified at part 312, subpartE in 1988 as it was specifically recognized that patients and physicians are generally willing to accept greater risks and side effects from treatment of life-threatening and severely debilitating diseases than they would for other diseases. The four principal US regulatory programs that support these principles are fast track designation, breakthrough therapy designation, accelerated approval, and priority review designation. The features of these four programs are outlined in Table 2. For drugs to qualify for regulatory expedited pathways, the drug must be intended to treat a serious condition and the scientific data (nonclinical or clinical) demonstrates the potential to address an unmet medical need; a drug may qualify for more than one program [10]. These programs were instituted to ensure therapies are approved and available to patients as soon as it can be concluded that the therapies' benefits justify their risks and have been becoming more standard in oncology drug development. For some drug development programs, demonstrating an effect on survival or morbidity

Table 2 Principal FDA regulatory programs as of 2017

	Fast track	Breakthrough therapy	Accelerated approval	Priority review
Nature of program	Designation	Designation	Approval Pathway	Designation
Qualifying criteria	Drug intended to treat a serious condition	Drug intended to treat serious condition	Drug treats serious condition	Application for a drug that treats a serious condition
	Nonclinical or clinical data show unmet medical need potential	Preliminary clinical evidence that may demonstrate substantial improvement on clinically significant endpoint(s) over available therapies	Generally meaningful advantage over available therapies	If approved would provide significant improvement in safety or efficacy
			Demonstrates an effect on a surrogate endpoint that is reasonably likely to predict clinical benefit or on a clinical endpoint that can be measured earlier than irreversible morbidity or mortality (IMM)	
Features	Actions to expedite development and review	Actions to expedite development and review	Approval based on effect on a surrogate or intermediate clinical endpoint reasonably likely to predict clinical benefit	Shorter review clock for marketing application: 6 months compared to 10 month standard review
	NDA/BLA rolling review	Intensive guidance on efficient drug development		
		Organizational commitment involving senior staff		
		Rolling review		

(continued)

Table 2 (continued)

	Fast track	Breakthrough therapy	Accelerated approval	Priority review
When to submit request	With IND or after	After IND opened	Discussion with review division during development: To acquire support for planned endpoints as basis for approval as well as discuss plans for confirmatory trials	With BLA or NDA
	No later than pre-BLA/ pre-NDA meeting	No later than End of Phase 2 meeting		
Timeline for FDA response	Within 60 calendar days of receipt of request	Within 60 calendar days of receipt of request	Not specified	Within 60 calendar days of receipt of BLA/ NDA
Additional considerations	Designation may be rescinded if it no longer meets the qualifying criteria	Designation may be rescinded if it no longer meets the qualifying criteria	Confirmatory trials to verify and describe the anticipated effect on IMM or other clinical benefit	Designation assigned at time of BLA or NDA filing
			Subject to expedited marketing withdrawal	

requires lengthy and large trials because of the duration of the typical disease course. Therefore, accelerated approval of important drugs has been exercised in these settings. Both previously approved ADCs, gemtuzumab ozogamicin in 2000 and brentuximab vedotin in 2011, were granted an accelerated approval base on phase 2 trials in the US [2, 3]; brentuximab vedotin converted the US accelerated approval to regular approval after successful completion of a required phase 3 confirmatory trial in 2015 [3]. Additionally, a priority review was granted in 2013 for ado-trastuzumab emtansine [4].

Patient Selection for Targeted Therapy Clinical Trials

Targeted agents often require a patient selection strategy that may involve the development of a diagnostic product to specifically identify the intended population or the patients more likely to respond to treatment. The FDA defines a companion diagnostic (CDx) as an in vitro diagnostic product that is used for the safe and effective administration of a therapeutic agent. In most circumstances, the FDA considers a companion diagnostic as a Class III (high-risk device) requiring premarket approval. CDx products are regulated as a medical device in the US and in most ex-US markets and require a development plan that is integrated with the clinical development strategy. Targeted agents that are efficacious in only a biomarker selected population, need to evaluate if a companion diagnostic development is required for successful drug registration and subsequent commercialization. Oncology has been the leading therapeutic area where the CDx paradigm has emerged; however the advancement of precision medicine in all therapeutic fields is demonstrating that companion or complementary diagnostics can be useful aids in maximizing patient benefit. A complementary diagnostic is a Class III medical device that may aid in the benefit risk decision making about the therapeutic product, however is not required for the safe and effective use of the therapeutic product. Complementary diagnostics have been discussed elsewhere [11].

Patient selection strategies are generally rooted in the biology of the disease within the context of the mechanism of action of the drug. The development path of two ADCs provide contrasting examples of this point. Adcetris (brentuximab vedotin) is an ADC that comprises an anti-CD30 monoclonal antibody attached by a protease-cleavable linker to a microtubule disrupting agent, monomethyl auristatin E (MMAE). The ADC is internalized into CD30-expressing tumor cells. The approvals of Adcetris in 2011 were based on data from two open-label, single-arm clinical trials: a pivotal trial in Hodgkin lymphoma patients who relapsed after autologous stem cell transplant (ASCT) and a pivotal trial in relapsed systemic anaplastic large cell lymphoma (ALCL) patients. As CD30 is a marker for the disease diagnosis, a separate companion diagnostic was not necessary [3]. However for drug Kadcyla (trastuzumab emtansine,T-DM1), an ADC that incorporates the HER2-targeted antitumor properties of Herceptin (trastuzumab) with the cytotoxic activity of the microtubule-inhibitory agent DM1 (derivative of maytansine), the co-development of a companion diagnostic was pursued based on the expectation that T-DM1 would be most effective in the subset of breast cancers with high expression of HER2. Anti-HER2 agents including Herceptin inhibit or block the oncogenic signaling properties of HER2. As such, the drug agent requires a test to detect which patients are HER2 positive, as HER2 negative patients do not benefit from the treatment. The requirement of the HER2 test to be eligible for Herceptin treatment was one of the first examples of a CDx launched at the time when the concept of a CDx was in its infancy. Subsequently, the labels of the approved HER2 CDx tests were expanded to also include T-DM1 in the test label. Several other targeted agents have been developed that require a diagnostic test in order to accurately determine which patients should be considered for treatment with the targeted therapeutic agent. ADCs developed in the future will also need to evaluate if a companion diagnostic would be required to identify the appropriate population for treatment.

Development strategies for the diagnostic test are recommended to be factored in early within the clinical development plans, and are of particular importance in accelerated drug development strategies that do not always take into account the diagnostic test development cycles. Identification of the specific marker or sets of markers, technology platform, assay development and validation for clinical use are the initial steps in consideration for a CDx development. As the development plans mature, regulatory and commercialization considerations are factored into the planning and often involve partnership with IVD manufacturers to undertake the design control governed CDx process in support of the pharma companies drug development plans.

There is a variety of external guidance documents including, industry standards (Clinical & Laboratory Standards Institute: CLSI Guidelines; Clinical Laboratory Evaluation Program, New York State Department of Health; International Council on Harmonisation) and FDA issued guidances on analytical validation of assays as well as co-development principles. Several guidances have been drafted and issued to highlight the considerations for a CDx development. On July 31, 2014 the FDA issued "Guidance for Industry: In Vitro Companion Diagnostic Devices," to help companies identify the need for companion diagnostics at an earlier stage in the drug development process and to plan for co-development of the drug and companion diagnostic test. However, the guidance did not outline how to best approach the co-development or recommended strategies. Consequently, the FDA recognized there was a need to describe the processes both device and pharmaceutical companies should take during the co-development process. On July 15, 2016, FDA released the draft guidance, "Principles for Codevelopment of an In Vitro Companion Diagnostic Device with a Therapeutic Product." This guidance document was intended to be a practical guide to assist therapeutic product sponsors and IVD sponsors in developing a therapeutic product and an accompanying IVD companion diagnostic.

Every drug program is unique and should evaluate what a co-development plan would entail, if the strategy should be regional or global, and incorporate considerations for the expected contemporaneous filing and approval of both the CDx and the (Rx) drug. Thus, the guidance recommends that sponsors should seek input from both the drug division, CDER, and the device division, CDRH, through frequent communication or meetings. In principle, the stages of a CDx development can be broken down into a similar phase 1, phase 2, phase 3 paradigm that exists for drug development largely representing assay development, assay validation and assay verification.

The challenge for the CDx, is that the rigor of a design controlled process and the validation and verification of the GMP manufacturing often do not align with the accelerated development scenarios that are becoming standard in oncology. It is often the case that oncology development strategies go from a phase 1 to either an accelerated phase 2 model or sometimes directly into a phase 3, compressing the development time for the device. This presents significant challenges for diagnostic tests that empirically require determining the optimal threshold on a continuum to define a positive and negative determination. This adds incredible pressure for the diagnostic manufacturer as the equivalent breakthrough designation status and conditional approval scenarios that exist for drugs do not translate over into the regulated device space. However, recently there has been an expedited premarket approval (PMA) program introduced by FDA that is a mechanism that can be considered. In addition, drug sponsors need to carefully evaluate how much resources need to be expended on a CDx development in advance of knowing if the drug product will successfully provide a proof of concept. The balancing act of two product developments is unique for each drug (Rx)/CDx pair; however some key points can be applied.

The FDA has issued guidance which summarizes the regulations around the CDx development and with the suggestion to engage the agency early in the planning process through the device pre-submission and drug pre-IND process. Prior to being utilized in a prospective trial, a CDx requires an Investigational Device Exemption (IDE) filing with the CDRH division in order to be classified as an Investigative Use Only device (IUO) if the trial data is to be used for registration purposes. This is analogous to an IND filing for the drug product within the CDER division and required in order to be able to submit the premarket authorization (PMA) for the CDx product. In this process, there are typically a series of pre-submission meetings outlining and discussing the device principles, the analytical validation plans, any specific thresholds for determining positive versus negative, and how they were developed and specifically how it will be used within the clinical trial. Sponsors are encouraged to engage early, particularly with high complexity tests to ensure there is alignment on the development and validation plans. This is of high importance with newer technologies that have not been established through the regulatory process and also for follow on products that may leverage a pre-existing companion diagnostic test for the same target. Sponsors are also encouraged to discuss the diagnostic strategy in non-registration studies if they are to be used to support a future registration as it is important to ensure that the same patient populations will be selected from one study to another.

One component that requires alignment for the CDx development is the design of the clinical trial itself. Oftentimes, in biomarker positive only trials where patients are being selected for a given marker and the biomarker negative patient population is being excluded from treatment, the safe and effective assessment of the device has missing data. In an ideal world, a clinical trial designed to evaluate both the biomarker positive and biomarker negative population with a companion diagnostic and treatment outcome would provide both the screening information as well as the efficacy assessment to adequately assess if the threshold setting for the device was accurately determined. This model tends to be large in design and is often not straightforward in oncology studies. For example, with respect to epidermal growth factor receptor (EGFR) tyrosine kinase inhibitor (TKI) drugs, one can argue that it would be unethical to treat an EGFR mutation negative patient with a new EGFR TKI given the precedent and understanding of EGFR TKI response only in the EGFR mutated population. In an example where it is a first in class molecule and there is no history or precedent for response in the biomarker negative population, there may be a request on behalf of regulators to generate this information in a post marketing scenario. These considerations and design principles require engagement with the regulatory agency early so that it is clearly understood how the trial is designed, what data outputs will be available and importantly which ones will not be, and proposals be agreed upon for mitigating around expected analyses.

In several cases, it may not be possible to ensure a CDx test is ready at the time of the trial start. In such cases it is recommended that a well validated clinical trial assay (CTA) be utilized while the plans for a formal CDx become finalized. In these situations a bridging study is required to bridge the CTA generated data to the final CDx. This often requires analytical performance assessment as well as re-testing the clinical specimens with the final CDx. The timing of this process can introduce unexpected challenges that would require proactive mitigation plans. In many cases samples or material may not be available for re-testing, stability requirements for a given analyte may have been exceeded by the time it's recognized a CDx is required, or patient samples may not be properly consented for a diagnostic test development. A summary of some of these challenges is presented in the following guidance: *Statistical consideration and challenges in bridging study of personalized medicine*, including several approaches to consider when "missing data" is present in biomarker positive only trial designs [12]. The advancement of precision medicine is helping identify the molecular mechanisms of many diseases. In combination with targeted therapy development, identifying the right drug for the right patients requires the development of diagnostic products. Given the parallel developments that must occur for both the drug as well as the future companion diagnostic, active engagement with health authorities is recommended to align on the strategy for a given program.

Summary and Conclusions

There is no single all-encompassing nonclinical strategy, no general rule as to what level of efficacy is required, or what level of toxicity is acceptable to determine regulatory success. With possible indications for next-generation ADCs as single agent monotherapy, in palliative settings or in combination with other agents, the main criteria that will determine regulatory success will be a significant advantage in at least one clinically meaningful parameter such as in tumor response efficacy, survival, or in the ADC's toxicity profile in relation to currently available therapy alternatives to positively influence the benefit: risk profile. Each nonclinical development plan for ADCs should begin with the selection of assays and studies evaluated on a scientifically-based approach that are required to be conducted consistent with ICH and animal research guidelines and according to existing published regulatory guidances. However, because detailed strategies for ADC nonclinical development are not currently specified in existing regulatory guidelines, development plans should be scientifically based and determined on a case by case basis and will likely be unique to each ADC. In situations qualifying for accelerated regulatory pathways, the need for a companion diagnostic test should be identified in the earliest phases of development of a therapeutic ADC molecule so that ideally both are developed and launched on the market at the same time. As noted, various approaches may be acceptable to obtain the data needed to support contemporaneous marketing authorization of a therapeutic ADC and an accompanying *in vitro* CDx but should be discussed with regulatory authorities early in development. While not in scope for this chapter, additional assays for the qualification of the ADC after manufacturing to characterize ADC concentration, cytotoxic drug: antibody ratio (DAR), percent of unconjugated cytotoxic drug, purity and bioassay information will be required to assess the preparation of dose formulations and the stability of the ADC under the conditions of use prior to and during the conduct of clinical trials as well. And with the anticipated innovations for novel ADCs, the proposed approaches in this chapter should be considered in the design of drug development plans of next-generation ADCs in order to support their safe clinical use and potential for positive clinical outcomes, but also to ultimately support the potential for achieving regulatory approval.

References

1. Rowe JM, Lowenberg B (2013) Gemtuzumab ozogamicin in acute myeloid leukemia: a remarkable saga about an active drug. Blood 121(24):4838–4841
2. FDA Approved Drug Products (2017) MYLOTARG 2017 BLA. Accessdata.fda.gov. U.S. Food and Drug Administration, N.p, n.d Web. 15
3. FDA Approved Drug Products (2017) ADCETRIS 2011 BLA. Accessdata.fda.gov. N.p., n.d. Web. 31
4. FDA Approved Drug Products (2017) KADCYLA (ado-trastuzumab emtansine, T-DM1) 2013 BLA. Accessdata.fda.gov. N.p., n.d. Web. 31
5. FDA Approved Drug Products (2017) BESPONSA 2017 BLA. Accessdata.fda.gov. U.S. Food and Drug Administration, N.p, n.d. Web 15 Dec 2017
6. S9 Implementation Working Group ICH S9 Guideline (2016) Nonclinical Evaluation for Anticancer Pharmaceuticals Questions and Answers
7. ICH Harmonised Tripartite Guideline nonclinical evaluation for anticancer pharmaceuticals S9 (2009)
8. ICH Harmonised Tripartite Guideline Preclinical Safety Evaluation of Biotechnology-Derived Pharmaceuticals S6(R1) (2011)
9. Saber H, Leighton JK (2015) An FDA oncology analysis of antibody-drug conjugates. Regul Toxicol Pharmacol 71(3):444–452
10. Food and Drug Administration Center for Drug Evaluation and Research, Center for Biologics Evaluation and Research (2014) Guidance for industry: expedited programs for serious conditions – drugs and biologics. FDA, Maryland
11. Beaver JA, Tzou A, Blumenthal GM, McKee AE, Kim G, Pazdur R, Philip R (2017) An FDA perspective on the regulatory implications of complex signatures to predict response to targeted therapies. Clin Cancer Res 23(6):1368–1372
12. Li M (2014) Statistical consideration and challenges in bridging study of personalized medicine. J Biopharm Stat 25(3):397–407

Outlook on Next Generation Technologies and Strategy Considerations for ADC Process Development and Manufacturing

Olivier Marcq

Abstract In the chapter, we review new conjugation technologies from the standpoints of process development and manufacturability and identify potential process hotspots. We briefly review recent progress in conventional conjugation methods and assess, for instance, how new linkers impact process. We also consider antibody modeling and its untapped potential to help design ADCs. We address outsourcing options and trends and provide an overview of single use technologies. Finally, strategies for efficient early process development to ensure CMC consistency across clinical phases and manufacturing scales and ensure readiness for accelerated regulatory approval paths are discussed.

Keywords ADC · Process development · Analytical development · Scale-up · Manufacturing · GMP · Drug substance · Drug product · Bulk drug substance · DS · DP · BDS · Conjugation technologies · Site specific · Bridging · Thiobridge · Conventional cysteine · Engineered cysteine · Lysine · Serine · Unnatural amino acid · Non-natural amino acid · Maleimide · Valine-citruline · Maleimidocaproyl · Thiosuccinimide · Haloacetamide · Click chemistry · Azide · Cyclooctyne · Glycan · Enzyme · Enzymatic ligation · Transglutaminase · Seleno mAb · AmbrX · Eucode · Xpress · THIOMAB · Glycoconnect · Fleximer · Hydraspace · Auristatin · Ozogamicin · Talirine · Maystantin · Quaternary amine · Glucuronide · Linker · Payload · Aggregate · Aggregation · Stability · Hydrophobicity · DAR · Drug antibody ratio · Modeling · Antibody · Probody · Extracellular · Bispecific · TFF · HIC · Chromatography · Tangential flow filtration · Regulatory approval · CMC · Accelerated approval · Single use · Outsourcing · CMO · CQA · Critical quality attribute · Toxicity · Cytotoxicity · MTD · MED · Therapeutic index · PK · PD

Content herein does not necessarily reflect the positions of Astellas and its affiliate Agensys.

O. Marcq (✉)
Agensys, an affiliate of Astellas Pharma, Santa Monica, CA, USA

SutroVax, Foster City, CA, USA
e-mail: omarcq@sutrovax.com

M. Damelin (ed.), *Innovations for Next-Generation Antibody-Drug Conjugates*, Cancer Drug Discovery and Development,
https://doi.org/10.1007/978-3-319-78154-9_6

Abbreviations

ADC Antibody Drug Conjugate
ADC Antibody Drug Conjugate
BDS Bulk Drug Subtance
BDS Bulk Drug Subtance
BLA Biologics License Application
BLA Biologics License Application
Cit Citruline
CMO Contract Manufacturing Organization
CQA Critical Quality Attribute
Cys Cysteine
DAR Drug Antibody Ratio
DL Drug Linker
DoE Design of Experiments
DP Drug Product
DS Drug Substance
DSI Drug Substance Intermediate
FIP First In Patient
HIPS Hydrazino-Pictet-Spengler
MED Minimum Effective Dose
MFG Manufacturing
MTD Maximum Tolerated Dose
NNAA Non-Natural Amino Acid
PBD Pyrrolobenzodiazepine
PEG Polyethylene Glycol
PK Pharmacokinetics
POC Proof Of Concept
PPE Personal Protection Equipment
QA Quality Attribute
QbD Quality by Design
SME Subject Matter Expert
SPAAC Strain promoted azide–alkyne cycloaddition
SUT Single Use Technology
TFF Tangential Flow Filtration
TI Therapeutic Index
UAA Un-natural Amino Acid
UF/DF Ultrafiltration/Diafiltration

Introduction

ADCs entered the commercial arena and first became a therapeutic option available to cancer patients with MYLOTARG® (gemtuzumab ozogamicin) in 2000. The field has since grown steadily with around 60 candidates at different stages of clinical development and several additional approvals (ADCETRIS® (brentuximab vedotin), KADCYLA® (ado-trastuzumab emtansine), BESPONSA® (inotuzumab ozogamicin) and re-approval of MYLOTARG®). The field has also grown in complexity with an ever expanding array of payloads and conjugations technologies [1] and advances in non-oncology applications [2, 3]. With time, understanding of ADCs pharmacokinetic (PK) properties and Therapeutic Index (TI) has improved and so have characterization methods [4, 5]. With site specific conjugation technologies seemingly offering the best avenue to therapeutic agents with better safety profile and simpler analytical profiles *via* lower heterogeneity, so called Next Generation ADCs have become the focus of intense research and represent a growing proportion of on-going pre-clinical and clinical studies. In parallel, introduction of accelerated regulatory approval paths (e.g. Breakthrough Therapy designation) and increased competition have often resulted in accelerated development timelines.

In this context, it is useful to complement other sections of this volume with process development considerations that often come in focus when commercial stage is in sight.[1] Therefore, we first set out to take a candid look at the developability of next generation technologies. We identified potential process hotspots or pitfalls that could present risks from a CMC standpoint. We briefly review recent progress in conventional conjugation methods and assess, for instance, how introduction of new linkers impacts process. We also take a look at mAb modelling and its untapped potential to help design ADCs.

In a second part, we discuss development and manufacturing strategies including single use technologies and outsourcing strategies. We finally advocate early investment in process development to deliver robust processes, alleviate risks to deviations in the critical quality attributes during clinical development and support accelerated development and accelerated approval opportunities.

Conjugation Technologies Process Development and Manufacturing

In this section we attempt to provide a process development and manufacturing outlook on the varied and expanding array of conjugation technologies being developed by the many inventive research organizations in the pharmaceutical industry or academia. Understanding of how the make-up of drug substance impacts PK and safety, the ability of a process to control composition during manufacturing and across manufacturing scales is important. Building and expanding on a few excellent reviews [1, 6, 7], we go over a number of representative conjugation technologies (a

[1] While we tried to support comments and positions with literature or conference reports, publications on ADC process development are scarce and some considerations are based on the author's experience and assessment.

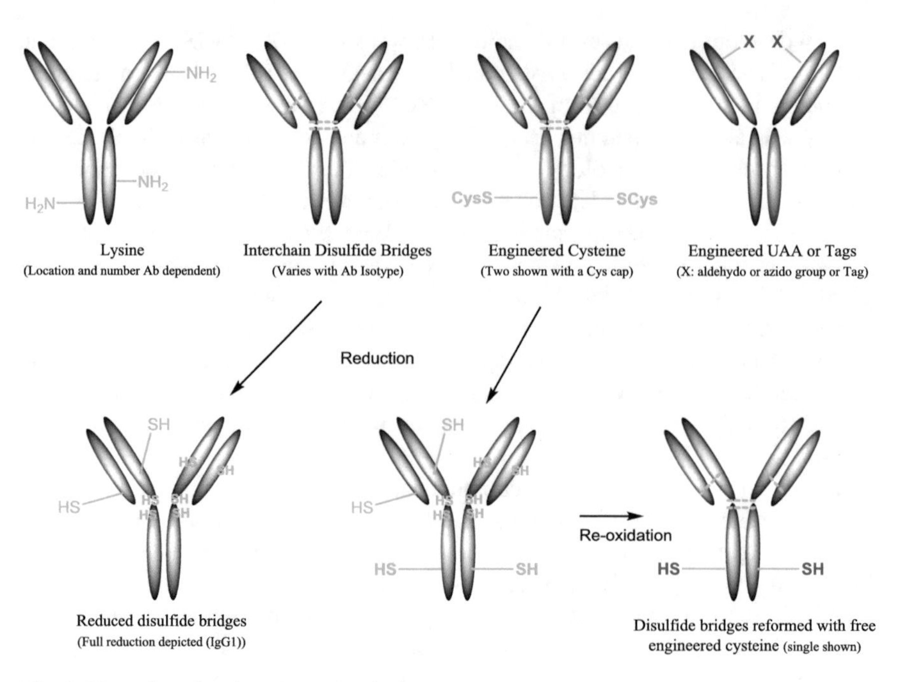

Fig. 1 Examples of conjugation technologies

few of them are depicted on Figs. 1 and 3) with a process development view point to highlight the corresponding processes salient points (Tables 1 and 2).

Manufacturing Challenges Presented by New Technologies

With the advent of site specific technologies allowing better control of DAR distribution, a deviation in DAR (e.g. higher DAR) is far less likely but if it does occur, it is likely to result in adverse safety event. Despite better control of DAR, site specific technologies are no less challenging from a manufacturing and process control standpoint than their non-site specific predecessors.

Overview of Site Specific Technologies

Research in site specific conjugation technologies was initially driven by a desire to better control DAR and improve DS characterization by decreasing heterogeneity but it quickly became evident that the selection of the conjugation site impacted pharmacokinetics and therapeutic index [56]. A number of studies focusing on different technologies highlight the importance of conjugation site selection on PK and TI [41, 43, 48, 56–59]. It is therefore likely that site specific ADCs will continue to

Table 1 Conventional and site specific technologies: native antibodies

Target site	Technology (Designation, Owner or published reference	DAR target	Control of DAR around target	Process assessment
Native Antibody				
A – Native Lysine [8, 9]	Often referred to as "conventional chemistry"	Depends on mAb sequence and conjugation conditions	Strong dependence on process controls such as pH, concentration and Temperature	Certain lysine residues can be preferentially conjugated [10] but the observation cannot be generalized [11]. This technology yields complex mixture even with a well-controlled process.
B – Native Cysteine [12]	Often referred to as "conventional chemistry".	Typical target: DAR 4.0 featuring a distribution of DAR species 0, 2, 4, 6, 8 with IgG1 or higher with IgG2 [13].	Primarily dependent on reduction step and strongly dependent on conjugation conditions. However control of DAR range should not be a challenge. Typical range of ± 0.5 easily maintained even with process variations.	With hydrophobic drugs, conditions during conjugation and quench can lead to aggregation affecting yield, DAR and soluble aggregates [14]. Stability of the DS and DP depends on DAR [15] as well as on DL hydrophobicity [16]. Process parameters can provide control over positional isomers [17]. Presence of Trisulfide affects the reduction step [18] as well as the properties of the conjugate [19] and mAb production needs to control for trisulfide formation. The conformational and colloidal destabilization induced by conjugation on IgG1 is discussed briefly in section "The Antibody Component: Can We Design mAbs with ADC Manufacturing in Mind?".
C – Re-bridging	Thiobridge by PolyTherics [20] Next Generation Maleimides (NGM) of University College London [21] SNAP technology by Igenica [22] McSAF SA and University of Tours (see WO2015004400)	Typical target: DAR 4.0 with DAR species 4 as the main product. DAR 2 can be produced with controlled reduction.	Failure to control re-bridging can lead to significant DAR variations.	Disulfide scrambling is a potential concern. Formation of HL intra-chain isoform instead of the desired HHLL inter-chain isoform is possible. Monitoring during process optimization and scale up is a must.

(continued)

Table 1 (continued)

Target site	Technology (Designation, Owner or published reference	DAR target	Control of DAR around target	Process assessment
D – Native Glycan	[23–25]	DAR 2	Significant amount of DAR1 to be expected	Control of the oxidation is difficult [8] and is often partial. Variations in the glycan composition of the native mAb will affect the conjugation. Advisable to monitor for amino acids oxidation.
	Fucose oxidation (Philogen) [26]	DAR 2	Significant amount of DAR1 to be expected	
E – Remodeled Glycan	GlycoConnect – Synaffix [27]	DAR 2	Expecting DAR ~ 1.9. No species with loading >2 expected.	The process comprises two stages, including enzymatic remodeling (trimming and tagging with azide), followed by ligation of the payload based on SPCA. Efficient conjugation step (>90%).
	[28]	DAR 2	No species with loading >2 expected.	The process comprises two stages, including enzymatic remodeling (trimming and C2-*keto*-Galactose attachment), followed by ligation of the payload via oximation.
	[29]	DAR 2		No cytotoxic ADC application yet. The process comprises two stages, including enzymatic remodeling (trimming and Azido-N-acetylgalactosamine attachment).
	U of Georgia [30]	DAR 2		1. Galactosyltransferase, Sialyltransferase – introduction of an azido group
	Genzyme/Sanofi Sialic acid on N297 [31]	DAR 2	1.3–1.9 reported	1. Sialyltransferase 2. Oxidation
	[32]	DAR 2	Unknown	1. Neuraminidase + Galactose oxidase 2. Reductive amination

Hippach M, Schwartz I, Pei J, Huynh J, Kawai Y, Zhu M, (2017 – Unpublished Data) Fluctuations in Dissolved Oxygen Concentration During a CHO Cell Culture Process Affects Monoclonal Antibody Productivity and the Sulfhydryl-drug Conjugation Process.

Table 2 Site specific technologies – engineered antibodies

Engineered antibodies (sequence alteration or extension)				
Target site	Technology	DAR target	Control of DAR around target	Process assessment
A -Cysteine	Engineered Cysteine (capped Cysteine)	Typically DAR 2 or DAR 4	Decent DAR control. Incomplete Re-oxidation can lead to higher DAR.	Full reduction can lead to aggregation and scrambling. Controllable to an extent through process control (e.g. stabilizers) with major dependency on mAb sequence. Selective reduction of capped engineered site might be achievable [33].
	Variation Cys Insertion (Medimmune) [34]			
	Actibody (Lc)-Q124C [35, 36]	DAR 2	Reliance on Q124C on expressed antibody being uncapped.	Attractive technology avoiding reduction and re-oxidation steps. Likely mAb to mAb variation either in the degree of capping or the conjugatability owing expected variation in the environment around the site based on sequence.
B – Serine	Medimmune [37] Immunogen (Seri Mabs) [38]		Conjugation efficacy and DAR control similar to AmbrX aldehyde based conjugation.	Mild oxidation followed by oxime ligation. Possible mAb degradation during oxidation.
C – Enzyme targeted	Transglutaminase [39] Refined technology by full deglycosylation [40, 41] Q-tag Engineering (Pfizer) [42, 43]	DAR 2 or 4	Likely to feature more DAR 1 than engineered Cysteine technology. Up to DAR 4 achievable in theory either at Q295,Q297 (ETH Zurich/ Innate Pharma)[a] or at various sites on heavy and light chains (Pfizer) but 3.8 is practically expected.	Unless solid supported enzyme are used, chromatographic removal of enzyme necessary with impact on yield and/or aggregate formation. Conversion dependent on tag location and amino acid sequence in the vicinity. Bacterial transglutaminase now expressed in E. Coli. Assay needed to assess Tag integrity. Unless solid supported enzyme are used, chromatographic removal of the enzyme is necessary.
	S. aureus sortase A-NBE therapeutics(SMAC-Technology ™) [44] Duke University (NC, USA) [45]	sortase A recognition motif LPETG on C-terminal of H and or L chains allows for DAR 2 or 4.	Improved mutants should allow for high transpeptidation and average DAR close to targets but under non optimized conditions DAR 3.2–3.6 are reported and up to 3.9 depending on the linker [46]	Sortase not highly efficient. Large amounts of SrtA or long reaction time required. Unless solid supported enzyme are used, chromatographic removal of enzyme necessary. Advantageous use of the Strep II-tag present in unconjugated sites has been reported by NBE Therapeutics for high DAR species enrichment [46]

(continued)

Table 2 (continued)

Engineered antibodies (sequence alteration or extension)				
Target site	Technology	DAR target	Control of DAR around target	Process assessment
D – Enzymatically generated conjugation site	Mushroom tyrosinase oxidation of a genetically encoded tyrosine Y-tag [47]	DAR 2 with low dispersity		MAb to mAb variation possible depending on environment around the tag insertion site. Hard to address through conjugation process. Unless solid supported enzyme are used, chromatographic removal of enzyme necessary.
	Enzyme formylglycine generation: SmartTag, Catalent [48, 49]	DAR 2 or 4	Lowest level of low DAR species when C-terminus targeted.	Efficient, non-reversible aldehyde targeted conjugation (HIPS). No catalyst required. Best efficiency (>90%) achieved with C-terminus or C_{H1}.
E – Unnatural Amino acids (also referred to as non natural amino acids)	Eucode [50] – AmbrX p-acetylphenylalanine and p-azidomethylphenylalanine	Typically DAR 2	Very narrow distribution can be achieved. DAR >1.8. No high DAR species.	As for other UAA technologies, antibody cell culture is the most challenging (titer ~ 1 g/L). Optimizing ligation catalyst to accelerate and maximize oxime formation is a worthy discovery or continuous process development endeavor. Potential IP opportunity.
	Xpress CF+ – Sutro [51]	Up to DAR 8	Ability to control distribution should be similar to other UAA technologies.	Only a preliminary report is available but the cell free technology should allow for great flexibility in the selection of insertion sites. Antibody titers are likely to be very low initially.
	Azide – Medimmune N6-((2-azidoethoxy) carbonyl)-l-lysine expression [52]	Target DAR 2 or DAR 4	Very narrow distribution can be achieved. DAR >1.8. No high DAR species.	Titer ~2 g/L
	Seleno mAbs [53]			Titer varies depending on the number of insertion sites [54]
F – Metabolic variants Glycans				
	Seattle Genetics [55]			

[a]A depiction of utilization of native Q295 after deglycosilation at N297 is shown on Fig. 3. Engineering of the antibody via N297Q mutation allows to achieve DAR4 with this technology. Pfizer Q-Tag technology requires Q-Tag engineering and can achieve various DAR levels without deglycosylation

represent a growing portion of the entities entering the clinic and therefore be subject to process development and GMP manufacturing activities.

Site selection is also critical from a manufacturing standpoint where parameters such as antibody structure integrity and conjugatability are typically considered. In-process issues remain hard to predict and relationship between antibody sequence/conjugation site and ADC aggregation are not yet understood to the point where full prediction through modeling is possible. However as more and more data is generated efforts to understand these relationships are being pursued and will be discussed in section "The Antibody Component: Can We Design mAbs with ADC Manufacturing in Mind?".

While site specific technologies solve some of the problems associated with conventional methods, chiefly heterogeneity, efficacy and safety, clinical data regarding these new technologies is currently very limited. Site specific technologies represent a fast growing field but they still represent less than 15–20% of global ADC clinical trials. In addition all of them are still in Phase I with the exception of Vadastuximab talirine. Innovators choices are guided by a combination of parameters including target, available payloads, literature, safety, PK and efficacy data as well as access to technology (internally or through licensing). After considering the elements above in the discovery phase, process considerations are often secondary but given the option it is worth assessing potential issues and limitations associated with each technology in the context of portfolio acceleration or product sensitivity to aggregation, hydrophobicity, DAR (high loaded species) or low MTD.

In the following sections, we give a short overview of the implication of site selection as well as an overview of typical process unit operations associated with common site specific technologies and a review of recent development in conventional conjugation methods with an update on process solutions to maleimide instability and alternatives to maleimido-caproyl linker.

Site Specific Technologies from a Process Standpoint

Whatever the technology, the ADC manufacturing process involves antibody activation, conjugation, purification (process impurities and residual drug linker removal) and formulation. While the conjugation step is simple, activation can involve multiple process units. For conventional lysine and cysteine technologies, the activation step is typically limited to pH adjustment and mAb reduction. Engineered cysteine technologies require an additional purification step after mAb reduction and before the necessary re-oxidation step. Glycan targeted technologies require a glycan tailoring step followed by purification and, depending on the chemistry, an activation step (e.g. oxidation). Enzymatic conjugation may require deglycosylation if the location of the target site requires it. Technologies relying on unnatural amino acid and aldehyde tag incorporation typically do not require activation. The activation step can be further complicated if a two-step conjugation is selected (conjugation of an anchor to the antibody followed by drug linker conjugation) or if an intermediate chromatography is required (e.g. enzyme removal, aggregate removal). Similarly the purification step can be limited to a simple UF/DF for buffer exchange or include a chromatography step. The chromatography step can reliably be used at scale for aggregate removal for instance [14]. Though scale or scalability are not specified, a report [60] considers the use of chromatography for DAR distribution control.

Figure 2 below provides a comparison between expected process steps for different ADC technologies. It highlights the impact of technology choices on process complexity. A small number of steps does not necessarily correlate with better CQAs or control of the CQAs. Simply the process optimization can be expected to be shorter with fewer steps.

Typical Process Flowchart For Conventional and Next Generation ADC Processes

	Convention Lysine or Cysteine	Cysteine Bridging	Engineered Cys / Selenocysteine	Enzymatic Conjugation	Glycan	UAA/aldehydo tag
Post-Translational Modification				Deglycosylation	GlycanTailoring	
mAb pH Adjustment / Dilution	pH Adjustment / Dilution	pH Adjustment / Dilution	pH Adjustment / Dilution	TFF (with or without chromatography)	pH Adjustment / Dilution	pH Adjustment / Dilution
Activation	Reduction	Reduction	Reduction	Conjugation anchor enzymatic attachment(*)	Activation(e.g. oxidation)	
Purification / Buffer Exchange			TFF (with or without chromatography)	Chromatography/ TFF		
mAb Treatment			Re-Oxidation			
Purification			TFF (with or without chromatography)			
Conjugation	Conjugation/ Quench	Conjugation/ Quench	Conjugation/ Quench	DLConjugation (*)	Conjugation (Reductive amination,Click chemistry)	Conjugation
Selective Purification	Chromatography	Chromatography	Chromatography	Chromatography(*)	Chromatography	Chromatography
Impurity Removal / Buffer Exchange	TFF	TFF	TFF	TFF	TFF	TFF

Fig. 2 Typical process unit operations for conventional and site specific technologies

Engineered Cysteine Technologies

The current lead site specific strategy is the engineered cysteine technology [61, 62] optimized to its first scalable version as THIOMAB by Genentech [56].

Reduction to ensure deprotection of the engineered Cysteine thiols requires a subsequent oxidation step to reform the interchain disulfide bridges (Fig. 1). These steps can theoretically lead to significant challenges such as over or under oxidation, aggregation during reduction, yield loss during post-reduction chromatographic step, scrambling of the interchain disulfides during re-oxidation, and possible formation of higher loaded species than the theoretical target due to incomplete re-oxidation and potential mAb degradation during conjugation. Formation of DAR 3 and DAR 4 species is possible but controllable assuming the re-oxidation step is reasonably optimized. If the engineered Cysteine site has been selected with solvent exposure and conjugatability in mind, the process with efficient reduction should lead to low levels of DAR 0 and DAR 1 species.

Selective reduction would help to significantly simplify the overall process and eliminate or limit interchain scrambling and formation of higher DAR species but information shared in publications on process development are scarce at this point and presentation at conferences only report on the default reduction approach. A recently published patent from Pfizer claims selective uncapping of engineered sites [33]. If the method is generalizable, conjugation processes involving engineered cysteine would compete with conjugation resorting to UAA in terms of ease of manufacturing.

From an ADC manufacturing standpoint, THIOMAB and related technologies currently require more complex conjugation processes than un-natural amino acid (UAA) based technologies but conjugates can be manufactured at several hundred grams with good consistency.[2] From an antibody production standpoint, production of Cys engineered IgG antibodies is now mainstream with yields in range with other therapeutic antibodies and good process control can reliably deliver constant quality attributes across scale.

A recent report [63] highlights the potential for innovation in cell culture processes to deliver antibodies with un-capped unpaired engineered surface cysteine or functionalized engineered surface cysteine. Such antibodies would simplify the manufacturing process by eliminating the reduction and re-oxidation steps.

Unnatural Amino Acids (UAA)

Several technologies are given in Table 2 Row E. AmbrX's technology can be considered as the first UAA technology designed for ADCs [50]. Currently low antibody titers are a drawback of UAA technologies but improvements are possible.[3]

[2] Marcq O, Tawfiq Z, Parker R, Tomas F, Zhu M (2017 - Unpublished Data).

[3] Hippach M, Kyung S Y, Kikuchi T, Kawai Y, Huynh J, Gredder J, Zhu M (2017 – Unpublished Data). Enhancing Production of an Engineered Antibody Containing Non-native Amino Acid for Site-Specific Conjugation: Considerations for Early and Late Stage Development.

A narrow loaded species distribution of the conjugate is observed with these technologies making them attractive site specific technology options. In our experience, specific technologies combine improved PK profile [58] and reliable manufacturability at more than 100g scale.[4] An anti-FLT3 ADC [64] is currently in Phase 1 clinical trial (NCT02864290). With regards to the antibody, availability of cell free expression technology should allow for increased flexibility in the selection of the conjugation sites [51].

Glycan Targeted Technologies

Glycan targeted conjugation is an attractive approach as it relies on the antibody's natural glycosylation sites for conjugation and therefore requires no sequence engineering. A few methods use native glycans for conjugation after mild oxidation while most methods resort to a remodeling of the glycans. See Table 1 Row E. The former methods have lower efficiency with presence of low DAR species and the risk of oxidation of amino acids on the antibody scaffold. The latter methods require specialized enzymes and usually two steps to achieve the desired glycan structure. This requires two or three extra process steps including a purification step and, at commercial stage, GMP grade enzymes. Furthermore, each step carries the risk of product changes resulting in specificity, efficiency or material loss.

Glycan Targeted Technologies: CMC Strategy

It is not yet public knowledge as to how companies utilizing one of these glycan targeted methods will handle the glycan remodeled intermediate. There would be advantages in rolling the glycan modification step in the antibody intermediate production and release a conjugation ready antibody. From a manufacturing strategy standpoint this presents both advantages and drawbacks. Operations associated with the mAb can be handled in a regular antibody GMP production facility thus decreasing the number of process steps associated with the DS requiring OEB4/5 facilities. However the steps associated with glycan remodeling are not typical for most antibody manufacturing facilities and would probably be better accomplished by technical teams used to conduct ADC related operations. Whatever strategy is selected for early stage development and GMP manufacturing, it will need to be thought thoroughly for commercial operations. Depending on the supply chain, the manufacturing site and process validation timelines there might be advantages going one way or the other.

In the specific case of Innate Pharma's Gln295 targeted transglutaminase site specific conjugation, full deglycosylation is needed and it makes sense for the antibody intermediate to be the deglycosylated antibody. This is automatically achieved by their reliance on Asn297 mutation. An approach that Lhospice et al. [41] have used to generate the cAC10Q antibody with 4 conjugation sites (N297Q and native Q295).

[4] Marcq O, Schwartz I, Tawfiq Z, Tomas F, Zhu M (2016 – Unpublished Data).

Enzymatic Conjugation

As shown in Tables 1 and 2, a number of enzymatic conjugation technologies are being studied either based on native antibodies via glycan remodeling (Table 1 – Row E and Fig. 3) or engineered antibodies via introduction of enzyme targeted tags (Table 2 – Rows C and D).

Enzyme activity, site accessibility and therefore antibody sequence and linker payload structure are all parameters that will affect the reliability and ultimately the relevance enzymatic conjugation technologies for ADC manufacturing. Enzymatic conjugation methods are either restricted to a limited number of sites by choice (e.g.

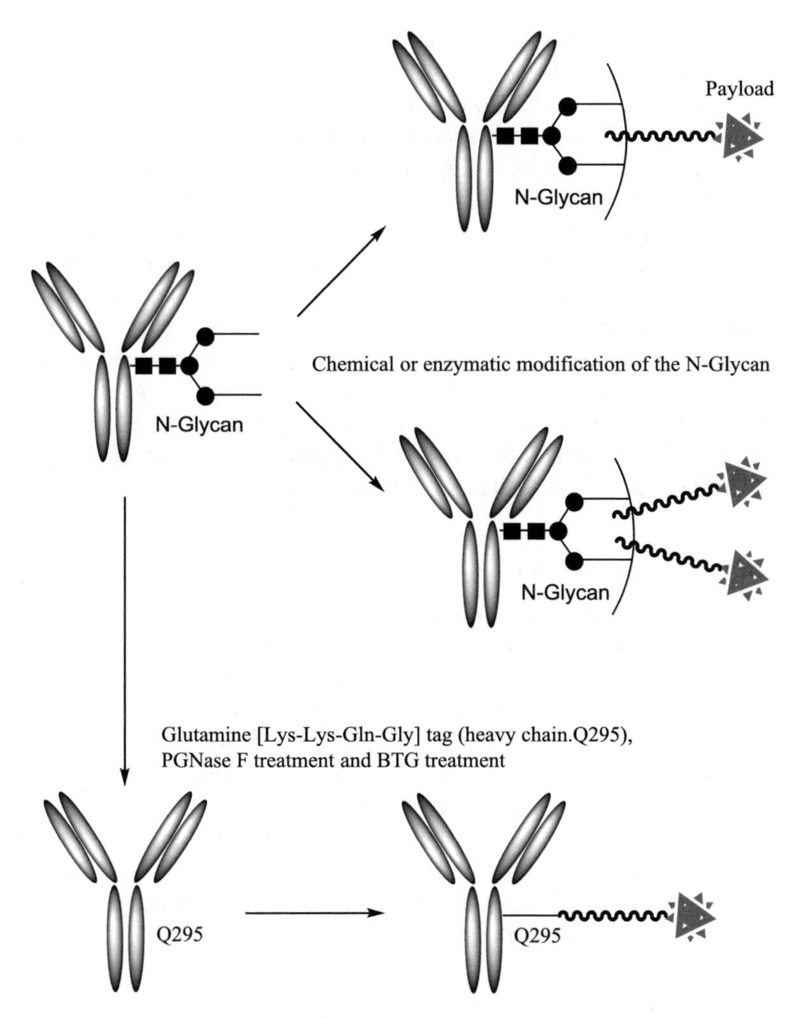

Fig. 3 Schematic illustration of conjugation technologies relying on native glycan (Asn297) modification or removal

based on *in vivo* data), conjugation efficacy limitations depending on site or Tag expression restrictions while others seem to offer a broader array of sites. An interesting example is the reported flexibility Pfizer's bacterial transglutaminase offers in terms of Q-tag localization compared to microbial transglutaminase applied to our knowledge to N297 or Q295 after Q mutation.

Transglutaminase, sortase and few other methods offer the possibility to enzymatically attach the linker payload directly while other methods are geared toward enzymatically introducing a new conjugatable moiety. That is the case with Catalent's SmartTag technology that evolved from Bertozzi's lab. The formylglycine generating enzyme results in the incorporation of an aldehyde tag that serves as a handle to a very efficient HIPS ligation.

From a process standpoint, enzymatic conjugation requires an enzyme removal step. That can be achieved via chromatography unless a solid supported enzyme process is developed. The latter is likely to be time consuming but worth pursuing if a definite commitment to the enzymatic platform is warranted. Without being a general rule, enzymatic conjugation is likely to deliver higher percentage of DAR 1 species compared to chemical conjugation methods unless the conjugation site is optimized. Methods involving initial enzymatic attachment of a small linker prior as an anchor for a subsequent drug linker attachment will be easier to generalize and could lead to more homogeneous mixtures agnostic of the antibody sequence and payload. Using an excess of such small linker would have minimal impact on the operation costs and would allow optimization of the expensive drug linker to avoid over addition in the subsequent chemical step. This approach, favored for instance by SynAffix [27] in the last step of their glycan targeted chemoenzymatic conjugation (an azidoglycosyl tag is appended by glycosyltransfer), is also reported by Dennler et al. [40] as part of their two steps approach (An azido amine spacer is attached to the antibody by a microbial transglutaminase).

CMC Strategies: Enzymes as Raw Materials

Sourcing high quality and consistent supply of the respective enzymes will be necessary for clinical manufacturing. Early investment in identifying quality attributes for the enzyme as raw materials ensuring consistent activity is highly advisable.

If enzyme based conjugations are to reach commercial scale, GMP manufacturing of corresponding enzymes will need to be scalable and adaptable to existing manufacturing facilities. To that end, recent reports by two Pfizer teams indicate that efforts are already underway to achieve this. Rickert et al. [65] reported the production of transglutaminase in E. coli, the platform of choice for GMP therapeutic proteins while Chen et al. reported the design of high efficiency sortase variants [66]. It is reasonable to assume that other companies pursuing enzymatic ligation for ADC manufacturing are pursuing similar efforts.

Conventional Cysteine Chemistry: Updates and Process Considerations

ADC based on conventional Lysine or Cysteine chemistries still represent the vast majority of drugs currently under clinical evaluation. Recently two conventional ADCs (Gentuzumab ozogamicin and Inotuzumab ozogamicin) were approved or re-approved whereas the Phase III trial of the most advanced site specific ADC, Vadastuximab Talirine (SGN-CD33A), had to be discontinued.[5] Additionally, a recent paper demonstrated, in animals, that careful design of the linker can result in safe and efficacious DAR 8 ADC generated by conventional Cysteine chemistry [67]. Conventional methods may remain very relevant for a while until more site specific based ADCs enter the late stage clinical arena.

General process considerations on conventional Cysteine chemistry are given in Table 1.

Strategies to Address Thiol/Maleimide Instability

The structures of all ADCs currently in pre-clinical or early clinical development are not known but most ADCs rely on cysteine conjugation. Whether relying on glutathione induced cleavage (di-sulfide linkage) or lysosomal proteases induced cleavage (valine-citruline "vc" dipeptide linker) drug linker attached to Cysteine residues are anchored via a Michael addition between the cysteine thiol and the maleimidocaproyl-like moiety (mc or mcc for maleimidomethyl cyclohexane-1-carboxylate) to generate a thiosuccinimide link (see Fig. 4). Thiosuccinimide moieties are susceptible to retro-Michael reaction [68].

The latter is not a process related issue *per se* but a significant drawback with regards to plasma stability. Process solutions were reported [69] that require treatment at pH greater than 9 for extended period of time and relatively high temperature that could lead to degradation with certain antibodies. Various linker modifications efficiently favoring self-hydrolysis and thus avoiding post conjugation treatments that can be detrimental to the antibody have been reported [70, 71]. A stabilized hydrolyzed linker is shown on Fig. 4.

Plasma instability due to glutathione or albumine by thiol exchange (represented by XS-H in Fig. 4) or direct retro-Michael reactions are also elegantly and efficiently avoided by careful conjugation site selection as demonstrated by Shen et al. [72]. It was found that a positively charged environment induced self-hydrolysis hence stabilizing the linker.

New thiol specific linkers are also described in Table 3. Experience at several hundred gram scale under GMP of thioether ADCs with haloacetamides indicate that these thiol reactive moieties are amenable to scale-up.[6]

[5] As of June 19, 2017, based on public information releases from Seattle Genetics.

[6] Marcq O, Tawfiq Z, Parker R, Tomas F, Zhu M (2017 - Unpublished Data)

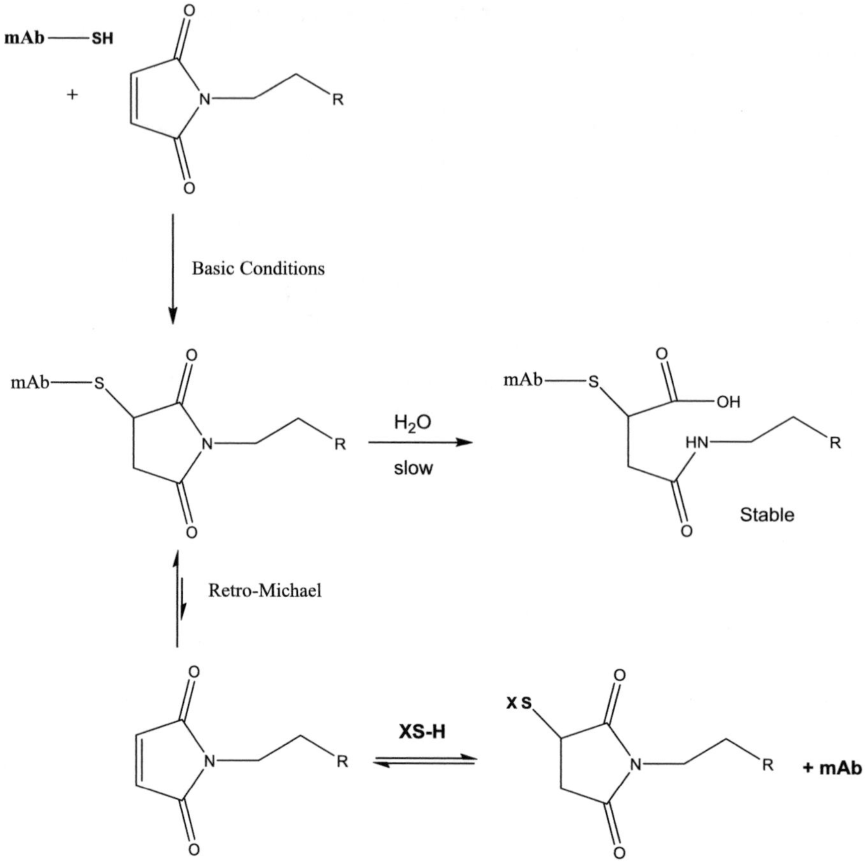

Fig. 4 Retro-Michael and hydrolysis reactions affecting a thio-succinimide linkages

Table 3 Selected examples of alternatives to maleimide linker

Alternatives to mc	Comments
Haloacetamides [73]	Good reactivity and selectivity
Keto Sulfones [74]	Ketone reduction necessary but mild conditions make the approach interesting
Methylsulfonylphenyloxadiazole [75]	Good reactivity and selectivity. New diazole moiety introduced potentially requiring immunogenicity assessment.
Carbonylacrylic reagents [76]	pH 8.0 in Tris but prohibitively high number of DL equivalent

Multi Payloads and High Loaded ADCs from a Process Standpoint

The ADC field (conventional Lysine and conventional Cysteine) initially moved away from high DAR because a DAR of 4 [77] was empirically demonstrated as optimal *in vitro* with non-site specific conjugation methods. The trend was further supported by findings that high loaded species had faster *in vivo* clearance and/or were responsible for off-target toxicity [78]. With the advent of site specific technologies and progress in the understanding of cellular processing, it became clear that high DAR was not necessarily detrimental provided that the conjugation site on the antibody was optimized [59]. In addition, the idea of modulating trafficking and internalization by addition of an extra function to the antibody (bispecific antibody or lysosomal protein targeting peptide) was investigated.

In parallel, the research on payload went in two opposite directions. One seeking ever more toxic payloads and another considering less toxic payloads used in a much higher stoichiometry. The latter prompted the need for high loaded ADCs. Some examples are given below and briefly described from a drug substance process standpoint. The synthesis of linkers or drug linkers as drug substance intermediates (DSI) is not discussed in this chapter.

Different approaches exist to reduce the dependence of average DAR on the number of conjugation sites (Table 4). One can either rely on orthogonal conjugation methods to introduce sequentially different warheads or resort to a carrier allowing for multiple payloads. From a process standpoint the preferred option is site specific conjugation of a linker bearing two payloads in order to take advantage of conjugation site specificity and the use of a purified drug substance intermediate. If drug linker intermediates bearing two payloads are not used, achieving dual drug loading requires resorting to orthogonal conjugation on the antibody or orthogonal conjugation of two different payloads on a linker after its conjugation to the antibody. A priori, the latter is the least preferred from a manufacturing standpoint as it requires exquisite conjugation efficacy and selectivity at each step in order to avoid very complex mixtures. With regards to screening linker and payload combinations, the latter method is the most flexible and will likely be favored by discovery groups.

Approach A (Table 4) is an example of methodology designed for payload combination screening. The successive deprotections are elegantly designed. However if the linker conjugation following the antibody reduction is not complete, one of the payloads will conjugate directly to the antibody since all payloads in this approach target Cysteine.

Approach C relies on the same azide click chemistry to orthogonally attach payloads. If motifs associated with cyclooctyne are found to be immunogenic, this approach may not be suitable for ADCs.

Approach E delivers DAR 4 ADC using glycan targeted conjugation. The tagged glycoform bear two reactive azido moieties. Selective introduction of two different payloads is not achievable with the current method.

Approach G: Control of loading dependent on linker conjugation and linker loading. Aggregation is theoretically possible with hydrophobic payloads but unlikely thanks to the hydrophilic carbohydrate derived linker. Characterization of linker payload will have to include degree of conjugation and, potentially, polydispersity if the linker is not of defined length.

For a review of strategies for dual modification of biomolecules see Maruani et al. [79] (Table 4).

Table 4 Technologies to achieve dual or high loading

Approach	Targeted Site	Linker	1st payload	2nd payload	
Dual Loaded ADCs					
A	Cysteine	Dual Cysteine multiplexing linker with a maleimide moiety for conjugation to the antibody	Attached by deprotection of S-Isopropyl disulfide group on the linker	Attached by deprotection of Acetamidomethylcsyteine moiety on the linker	[80]
B	Cysteine	2-Azidoacrylate mono payload linker	Already on the linker	Alkyne-azide cycloaddition	[81]
C	Cysteine	Orthogonal Click dibromopyridazinedione bridge	Alkyne	Strained alkyne	[82]
D	Thio-selenomabs	The method relies on orthogonal conjugation on two engineered cysteine sites on the mAb and one C-terminal selenocsyteine			[83]
E	Glycan site specific	HydraSpace connects to the azido tagged mAb preferably via bicyclo[6.1.0]nonyne Cu-Free cycloaddition.	Not disclosed		Glyconnect overview [27]
F		Tagged glycoform (two azido groups per glycation site)	Dual loading achieved per conjugation site on the mAb		[84]
High Loaded					
G	Cysteine	Fleximer (Poly-1-hydroxymethylethylene hydroxymethyl-formal) from Mersana	Selective payload attachment technique not disclosed.		[85]

New Linkers from a Process Standpoint

The search for new payloads with different mode of actions, the drawbacks of initial maleimide linkers and the understanding that payload attachment site could impact the drug linker stability in plasma or its release after internalization prompted the search for new linkers offering new chemical attachment options. The need to reduce drug linker hydrophobicity has also influenced new linker selection.

Listed below are second generation linkers (Table 5). Hydraspace (SynAffix) and Fleximer (Mersana) are recently reported proprietary hydrophilic linkers. Sulfonates have the potential to increase hydrophilicity of lysine targeted heterobifunctional cross-linkers. Glucuronide are components of the linker and not involved in the anchoring to the antibody. They represent an interesting alternative to the Val-Cit motif as a target for lysosomal release of the payload. Quaternary amine linkers should enable the use of new drugs/payloads by offering new attachment options. Similarly pyrophosphate diesters are ideally suited for payload attachment via hydroxyl moieties. All the linkers listed below decrease hydrophobicity and should help alleviate aggregation phenomena encountered with hydrophobic payloads and possibly help simplifying processes through elimination of certain chromatographic steps.

While payloads are not discussed in this chapter, overall conjugate hydrophobicity can also be addressed by using hydrophilic payload variants as an alternative or in complement to hydrophilic linkers. A hydrophilic and potent Auristatin analog was reported recently [91].

Table 5 Examples of new linkers

New linkers	Information	Advantage	Reference
Quaternary amines	New anchoring chemistries. Should allow new payloads to be used	Increases DL hydrophilicity	[86] [87]
Glucuronide	Hydrophilic alternative to Val-Cit. Cleavage by lysosomal enzyme β-glucuronidase	Increases DL hydrophilicity	[67] [88]
Sulfonate	Studied as a variant for heterobifunctional cross-linkers	Increases DL hydrophilicity	[89]
Pyrophosphate Diesters	Selected for payload (Dexamethasone) attachment via its C-21 hydroxyl	Increases DL hydrophilicity	[90]
HydraSpace	Sulfamide based linker	Hydrophilic linker	Synaffix – US 9,636,421 B2
Fleximer	Poly-acetyl (DAR > 10)	Hydrophilic linker	Mersana [85]

The Antibody Component: Can We Design mAbs with ADC Manufacturing in Mind?

Significant progress has been made in understanding and controlling antibody therapeutics properties such as aggregation and thermal stability by correlating behavior and structure/sequence [92–96].

It is now common practice to optimize sequences at early stage of development based on computational modeling and experimental work around formulation composition. Antibody Drug Conjugates would benefit from antibody optimization for easier and more efficient conjugation and more stable ADCs via rational design (Table 6).

By studying different mAbs with the same linker payload under thermal stress conditions, Beckley et al. [97] demonstrated the impact of sequence on aggregation propensity of DS and the involvement of CH2 domain secondary and tertiary conformational changes in the destabilization of the conjugate. Aggregation and fragmentation of high DAR species (MMAE conjugates) was observed by Adem et al. in presence of high ionic strength buffer. Pan et al. reported that the CH2 region and the region between CH2 and CH2-CH3 domains undergo limited destabilization in MMAE or MMAF conjugate mixtures in their HDX-MS studies. Conformational destabilization is also reported with Menstansine conjugates [5]. A DAR dependence with an increased destabilization of not only secondary and tertiary structures [98] but also of quaternary structure [16] was demonstrated. These latter findings results from a complementary use of physical and molecular modeling assessments on two different mAbs conjugated with different Auristatin payloads with our report studying different DAR species separated via preparative hydrophobic interaction chromatography [16]. Beyond the disulfide bridges cleavage resulting in local increase in solvent exposure and hydrophobicity, the payload was also confirmed by modeling, to have an impact on the ADC's overall hydrophobicity [16, 99] in agreement with earlier reports based on physicochemical assessments [15].

Table 6 Opportunities for ADC molecular modelling

Behavior/property of interest	Modelling focus
DS Aggregation	Relationship between sequence, conjugation technology and aggregation Relationship between mAb sequence, payload and aggregation propensity during DS manufacturing process and in the Bulk Drug Substance.
Stability during conjugation Process	MAb sequence optimization to favor stability during reduction/ Re-oxidation steps (Engineered Cysteine technology)
Conjugatability	mAb Sequence optimization to increase site accessibility and/or selectivity Drug Linker structure optimization to avoid charge repulsion and increase reactivity with target sites on the antibody.

Applying molecular modeling to characterization of conjugate species can therefore provide insight into the impact of conjugation on the conformational and colloidal factors that underpin physical stability. This is relevant not only to the conjugate during conventional cysteine conjugation process but also to formulated conjugates (BDS or DP) based on any conjugation technology. Conformational factors could become less of concern in next generation site specific ADCs, either by virtue of lower average DAR or by virtue location of conjugation site in the antibody's structure. Colloidal factors are likely to still remain a concern especially with highly hydrophobic payloads such as certain PBDs. Additionally, site specific mutations and/or introduction of unnatural amino acids could significantly lower conformational stability of the mAb warranting mAb sequence assessment alongside mutation site selection.[7]

Work by Voynov et al. [100] which focused on selecting cysteine introduction sites to prevent IgG1 oligomerization, illustrates the potential value of modelling of site specific ADCs requiring site selection for introduction of cysteines or other amino acids or tags. Tumey et al. [101] recently applied the same logic to cysteine engineered antibodies. In their review on antibody design [102], Tiller and Tessier dedicate a section on methods for optimizing folding stability. A similar thinking could help design sequences making antibodies more favorable to proper refolding during re-oxidation step (e.g. engineered cysteine) following full reduction hence limiting risks of aggregation. A practical advantage of reducing antibody aggregation during conjugation reaction is that it obviates the need for costly chromatographic purification of the ADC. Additionally, reduced aggregation can also translate into improve product yields.

Prediction of biophysical behavior based on antibody sequences is an iterative process between modelling and experimental data. Modeling an ADC accounting for payload and solvent is obviously a daunting task but one that is no longer beyond most institutions' computing capacity. The accumulation of data as molecules are being screened and candidates progress through development should enable directed data mining supporting optimization of subsequent constructs, payloads or conjugation sites to address specific concerns such as aggregation, conjugatability, stability during manufacturing process, stability of the Drug Product.

New Antibody Formats

Drug conjugates expand beyond IgG formats and a few new formats that have entered the preclinical and clinical arena. We therefore attempt an early process assessment of a limited number of formats, namely probodies [103], extracellular drug conjugates [104] and bispecific antibodies as they remain close to IgGs discussed throughout this chapter.

[7] Sandeep Kumar, Pfizer (2017 – Personal Communication).

Probodies

From a manufacturing standpoint, we think probodies will present similar challenges as bispecific ADCs or dual payload ADCs. Indeed, the naked probody itself might present heterogeneity due to requirement of a masking peptide and linker. The heterogeneity associated with the conjugation of the linker-payload to the probody will potentially make for a complex mixture that will be difficult to characterize and control. There is a potential for such technology to need two chromatographic purifications. However, when using site specific conjugation approaches that provide good conjugation specificity and efficiency, a single chromatographic clean-up will likely be sufficient. Interestingly, variations in DAR are less of a concern with probody ADCs even though probodies are aimed at targets expressed in healthy tissues as well as tumors (a good example is Cytomix's CD166 program targeting CD6). Indeed the probody component (masked binding site) of such ADC can be expected far more critical to safety than drug loading. This should be the focus of early process development and also lead to a specific CQA related to binding site masking.

Extracellular ADCs or EDCs

Introduced by Centrose these ADCs are binding surface antigens and releasing payloads aimed at surface targets. Aside from their synthesis using longer chain linkers these conjugates should not present unexpected challenges from a manufacturing standpoint.

Bispecific Antibody Drug Conjugates

Bispecific antibody therapeutics is a very active field but one that Brinkmann et al. [105] describes as a "zoo" to highlight the diversity and vibrancy of research efforts fueled by competitive and IP landscape and critically by the need to adapt the format to the target or avoid stability or immunogenicity issues of specific constructs [102]. The fact that Blinatumomab, a T-cell recruiting BITE targeting CD19 and CD3 is commercial proves that developability of bispecific antibody is achievable. Clearly, manufacturing of bispecific construct is not trivial and for most formats is still far from being amenable to platform approaches we are accustomed with regular monoclonal therapeutics [106].

With regards to targeting small molecule drugs to specific cells, two approaches are being pursued. The first relies on using one of the targeting moieties of the antibody to the functionalize surface of nanoparticles and the other relies on covalent attachment of drug or drug carrier to a bispecific antibody.

Examples of the former are EDV technology (EnGenIC), anti-digoxigenin tetravalent bispecific antibody [107] or some of the constructs based on Immunomedics Dock-and-Lock technology [108].

Several bispecific antibodies bearing covalently attached drugs have also entered the clinic. MEDI4276 [109]; OXS1550/DT2219ARL (Oxis) and AMG570 a bispecific antibody peptide conjugate for the treatment of Lupus. MEDI4276 [109] appears to feature 2 engineered Cysteine conjugation sites (S239C and S442C) giving an average DAR of 3.6 [110] indicating a distribution of loaded species. From a process or analytical development and CMC standpoints, two conjugation sites would be preferable. Note that the reliance on Tubulysin, avoiding p-glycoprotein pump efflux, rather than more toxic payloads such as Spirogen's PBDs may require a higher DAR. GenmAb is pursuing DuoBody-ADC conjugates including an anti Her2xCD63 Lysine conjugate [111] with a Duostatin-3 payload [112] and achieves a DAR of 1. Regeneron compared DM1 lysine conjugated anti-HER2 antibody and anti-Her2xProlactin bispecific antibody and achieves a DAR of 3.3 [113]. Pfizer has used a bispecific approach to improve anti-tumor activity of a non-cleavable MMAD anti-Trop2 ADC by targeting one arm against Trop2 for tumor selectivity and one arm against a protein traveling directly to the lysosome to shift intracellular trafficking of the ADC [114].

We can expect quality attributes and properties associated with the antibody format to have significant impact on the corresponding drug conjugate CQAs and properties. The conjugate manufacturing process of bispecific conjugates will present challenges that will intimately depend on the antibody stability but also the drug linker. Particular attention should be paid to isoelectric point of the bispecific construct both to ensure ease of purification after conjugation and resistance to aggregation during the process where pH transitions are inevitable. In order to add as little complexity as possible to the purification steps and analytical profiles of these bispecific conjugates, the antibody intermediate will have to be thoroughly purified and the design should focus on site specific conjugation approaches with ideally two optimized conjugation sites to limit heterogeneity.

Strategies for ADC Process Development and Manufacturing

As illustrated is section "Conjugation Technologies Process Development and Manufacturing", mAb isotype, conjugation technology or linker payload can lead to simple or complex BDS processes. While the search for a novel and universal platform has seen the rise of many successful platform centric start-ups, most companies are still dealing with 1st or 2nd generation platforms and assessing multiple 3rd generation i.e. site specific technologies [1]. As a result, process development groups and manufacturing facilities are still currently dealing with multiple processes and will be for the foreseeable future. As for antibodies, the antibody conjugate developability should be included in the candidate selection process.

In this section we discuss the key features of an ADC manufacturing facility, some examples of CMO offerings in the field of ADCs, the pros and cons of production and development outsourcing as well as the trend in single use technologies. We also propose some considerations of the impact of process development on portfolio acceleration and strategies to achieve rapid development of robust processes, quality manufacturing and timeline optimization. We also highlight the importance of investing in early process development by discussing the impact of early phase process choices on target BDS and DP quality attributes.

ADC Manufacturing

Unique Requirements of ADC Biologics Manufacturing

The hybrid nature of ADCs is reflected in the type of operations that need to be conducted during manufacturing and how these operations are conducted [115, 116]. Overall, process unit operations are very similar to antibody downstream purification polishing steps (TFF, chromatography, dilution, formulation, …). The drug linker conjugation however requires the use of a reactor with cooling/heating, mixing and material/solution addition requirements closer to small molecule chemistry. Additionally, each conjugation technology introduces a certain level of complexity (See Fig. 2). The cytotoxic character of the drug linker imposes a unique set of protection and containment protocols and practices (in alignment with ICH Q9 guidelines) that significantly increase the complexity of processes [115, 117]. The drug linker powder itself needs to be handled in a glove box while operators need to receive special training for handling the drug linker powder, operating the glove box and need to wear dedicated PPE during the entire set of operations. Depending on the toxicity of the drug linker and conjugate, the entire process may require to be handled in isolators. This is however rare and adapted PPE and operation in properly designed controlled access GMP suite is enough to handle dissolved drug linker and conjugation steps in otherwise normal biologics GMP manufacturing conditions. The cytotoxic nature of ADCs also influences plant design with focus on cross contamination, safety and containment. Air handling has to be specially designed, flow of raw materials and waste optimized to ensure proper tracking of cytotoxic materials and waste. Safe handling of cytotoxic material, completion of process steps involving both small molecule and antibody components and the hybrid ADC require specially trained and skilled GMP operators.

Single Use for ADC Manufacturing

Single use technologies for ADC manufacturing have gained traction over the last decade with an increasing array of options adopted from protein and antibody manufacturing.

While fully single use manufacturing for ADCs are still a rarity, the trend is toward more single use components and several plants are now designed for full single use operations. Single use technology is an ideal fit for modular manufacturing and multiproduct facilities.

SUT components that are becoming common place are UF/DF disposable path compatible with automated skids but also smaller scale pumps.

The offering for disposable glove boxes and biosafety hoods is improving in quality and allowing for both cytotoxic powder weighing and DS bulk fill to be completed in collapsible film containment enclosures. The newest GMP suite at Piramal in the UK features no fixed equipment and can rely on SUT to complete ADC manufacturing.

Disposable reactors are still a topic of debate due to concerns with extractables and leachables or risk of leak or rupture of the bags through mechanical tear or structural weakening through exposure to organic solvents.

Notable examples of early adoption of SUT for ADC manufacturing are the Lonza facility in Visp [118, 119] where a mostly disposable approach is implemented for non-commercial manufacturing and the Pfizer Pearl River facility where both clinical and commercial manufacturing relies heavily on SUT [120]. A recent communication by Bayer discussed the design, in collaboration with Sartorius, of a single use manufacturing approach of ADCs within their mammalian cell culture pilot facility [121].

Aside from the variety and quality of SUT options on the market, several factors will lead to SUT becoming mainstream for ADC manufacturing:

- Reliance on outsourcing by sponsor organization and the investment in SUTs at CMOs
- The diversity of payloads and their different mode of action requiring strict segregation either through efficient cleaning procedures or use of disposable components
- The increased size of portfolio in most developers in the ADC field leading to high production turnover rate at sponsors or at their partnered CMOs.

Table 7 provides examples of areas where SUTs are available.

Outsourced Manufacturing

Expanding CDMO and CMO Offering

The outsourcing market is ready for a strong expansion fueled by the increasing number of companies working in the ADC field and the ever expanding clinical portfolios from which a significant number of late stage clinical trials and commercial products are bound to come. Additionally, most small innovative biotechs developing payloads, drug linker, conjugation technologies or identifying new biological targets are unlikely to have a dedicated process development group skilled across all aspects of ADC development and are more likely to outsource or partner to access GMP manufacturing capacities. This brings an influx of process development needs and a significant volume of early stage small scale manufacturing requests. Cases like Wyeth (now Pfizer) building a facility to produce calicheamicin payload and drug linker as well as the GMP BDS production and DP fill finish

Table 7 SUT examples and implementation trends

Equipment or Unit Operation	Glove box	UF/DF	Reactors	Tubing and filter assemblies	Bulk fill	Biosafety Cabinet
Examples of Single Use options	Disposable glove box	Example 1: Disposable TFF membranes	Disposable reactors	Example 1: Pre-welded filter assemblies with quick connects	BDS stored in bags	Disposable biosafety hoods
		Example 2: Disposable TFF cassette with integrated holder/ capsule [122]		Example 2: TFF flowpath with integrated connectors, sensors		
Adoption	Becoming default choice for new facilities	On the path to adoption		Increasingly mainstream	Mainstream for mAb	Becoming default choice for new facilities
Concerns			Reservations with regards to compatibility		Resistance to tear, storage, shiping	

facility or Agensys (now part of Astellas) building its own antibody and ADC manufacturing structures to cover Phase 1/2 needs are very valuable assets but also may become a thing of the past. Both Seattle Genetics and Genentech opted initially for outsourced commercial manufacturing and that is now the default path from early stage clinical manufacturing to commercial manufacturing. At this point, more than two-thirds of all ADC manufacturing is outsourced, though the proportion varies among companies and molecules. These considerations did not escape the CMO industry and the offering of cytotoxic capable facilities has increased significantly in the last few years along with start to finish offerings either by a single CMO or alliances (Table 8). From the sponsor side, outsourcing must be part of a corporate strategy and continuously managed and constantly reassessed (Table 8).

Outsourcing Manufacturing

ADC manufacturing is complex and requires specialized facilities able to handle biologics and cytotoxic small molecules with appropriate containment and cleaning/decontamination procedures [123–125]. The cytotoxic component adds a level

Table 8 Non-exhaustive list of CMOs and their offering.

CMO or alliance	Cytotoxic Drug Linker GMP manufacturing	mAb GMP manufacturing	Cytotoxic GMP DS manufacturing	Cytotoxic GMP DP manufacturing	Note
Althea		√	√	√[&]	[&] Fill finish: 2018
Baxter	(A)		(A)	√	(A) via SAFC
BSP	√		√	√	
Carbogen	√		√	√	
DPx Holdings		√		√	
Lonza	√	√	√		
Novasep	√	√	√*		* 2017
Pierre Fabre		√		√	
Piramal/ Fujifilm	√		√	√	
Proveo (IDT, CMC, Cerbios, Oncotec)	(B)	(B)	(B)	(B)	Unified offering via Proveo alliance (B)
SAFC	√		√	(C)	(C) via Baxter
WuXi	√	√	√		

Based on commercial and marketing information available to the author

of complexity in the design of GMP areas and extra cost in the build-up and operation. With only three commercial launches of ADCs, the field is open and extremely promising but also complex, highly competitive and risky. Companies that do have existing facilities will rely on outsourced manufacturing for extra capacity and smaller biotechnology companies without a commercial product will not spend significant capital money in building GMP facilities and rather resort to CMOs at least until their candidates reach clinical POC.

So while outsourcing manufacturing makes good sense and the offering is large, there are potential pitfalls [126]. Table 9 provides considerations on outsourcing.

Outsourced Development

Outsourcing manufacturing and outsourcing development pertain to very different strategies that need careful consideration and present risks if not managed properly. Early and late stage developments also need to be distinguished [126–128].

Table 9 Key considerations when considering manufacturing outsourcing

	General comments	Potential future developments
Scheduling	Negotiated with CMO.	Portfolio growth across the industry might lead to high demand and competition for slots. Advance purchase of slots might be necessary. Consider identifying strategic CMO partner to become an extension of sponsor's operations.
Capacity	Assess during CMO selection. CMO may impose sharing certain components (e.g. reactors) across customers. Batch scale, especially late stage and commercial may be limited by what the CMO as. Need to account for extra cost if new equipment is needed.	
Supply Chain	Remains the responsibility of the sponsor.	Relying on one end-to-end partner should simplify supply chain. Maintaining alternate suppliers advisable.
Flexibility	Significantly less flexible than internal manufacturing. Flexibility will depend on the CMOs level of occupancy.	
IP	Contract typically contain an IP clause the terms of which need careful review.	
Cross contamination/ Multiproduct Facilities	Dependent on CMO's cleaning procedure. Thorough review and vetting by internal QA needed.	
Quality Monitoring	Reliance on CMO's QA system. Regular audit on site necessary.	Question of who's QA system will apply to the various sites and partners of an end-to-end alliance. How harmonious and consistent will the Quality system be.
Issue escalation	A clear path and key decision makers must be identified	A site by site approach is advisable. Some alliances will offer unified systems with single point person.

Table 10 Outsourcing development

Drawbacks and pitfalls	Advantages
Outsourcing Early stage Development	
– Future dependence on CMO for know-how. – Slower buildup of internal expertise. – Work may take longer at a CMO. – Less flexibility in case of priority change. – The CMO may focus on facility fit (Potentially lesser focus on process understanding and process portability). – Possible issue with IP ownership of process. – Accountability and decision-making remain with the sponsor organization.	– Ideal when extra capacity needed. – Faster Tech Transfer if using the same CMO for MFG. – In case of issue during GMP operation, CMO quickly able to help. – Opportunities to benefit from CDMO's experienced team. – CMOs experience with commercial stage manufacturing know what works and understand ADC scalability issues. – CMO likely to suggest best practices.
Outsourcing Late Stage Development – BLA activities	
– Should be done at identified commercial launch site. – Loss of internal expertise growth opportunity. – Significant oversight by SMEs and project management still necessary. – Thorough strategy assessment needed to align outsourced activities with late stage/BLA filling strategy and timelines. – May not get the CMO's "A team".	– Enables internal focus on pipeline growth by outsourcing time consuming activities (e.g. process characterization, validation). – CMOs with experience with commercial stage manufacturing know what works and have been involved with at least part of process validation activities. – Possible synergies and time saving opportunities if CMO also handles antibody and drug linker aspects.

These views represent the author's position and not necessarily those of his past or current employers

The drawbacks and potential pitfalls of outsourcing early development [126] such as development toward manufacturing of toxicity batches or phase 1 clinical materials are listed in below (Table 10). Situations that should lead to selecting outsourced development and possible advantages are also listed. A new kind of hybrid offering by Lonza, coined IBEX, presents interesting opportunities for start-ups in need of both space and trained personnel, with a full spectrum of services, development lab space or GMP facility space renting or build-up and hiring of dedicated staff or reliance on the CMO's personnel.

Process Development Strategies

In this section, we aim at demonstrating the value of investing in early development by assessing the impact of process development on quality attributes and the importance of early investment in process development to enable portfolio acceleration.

DS Process Development in the Continuum of Clinical Development and Regulatory Filing

Regulatory agencies enounce clear requirements in terms of product DS and DP characterization, stability studies and analytical method qualifications. Early process development is implicitly mandated through requirements for comparability between Discovery toxicology material, regulatory toxicology material and clinical materials. Commercial process characterization and validation are mandatory for BLA filing. Early process development however is not the object of specific guidelines or opinions. Quality-by-Design (QbD) approaches are encouraged, yet, QbD filings have been rejected [129] and process parameters such as PARs and NORs selected based on small scale DoEs without at-scale process validation would most likely be rejected by regulatory agencies. It remains that QbD approaches are a core component of any process development aiming at delivering robust and scalable processes. Antibodies, component of ADC molecules, have well established development stages and drug linker, the other component of the ADC molecule, have very clear regulatory requirements by virtue of being small molecules. Similarly DP formulation development often followed a linear staged development derived from protein and antibody therapeutics with the added level of complexity inherent to ADCs [130]. The hybrid nature of ADCs, the limited number of commercial products and the ever expanding variety of conjugation technologies, payloads and linkers and the lack of quality attributes universally associated with clinical efficacy are responsible for the absence of regulatory guidelines or opinions or even ADC community documented practices for ADC drug substance process development.

The expectation is that the drug substance process will change as manufacturing scale increases and antibody and drug linker processes mature. Strict observance of GMP practices, appropriate analytical development, formulation and stability studies, clinical trial protocol review and approval process are sufficient to initiate clinical trials in a safe manner for patients. Early process development is nonetheless critical as highlighted in Table 11.

Table 11 Impact of early process development on DS quality profile, on clinical manufacturing and on portfolio acceleration

Quality	Early process dictates the quality attributes of reference materials against which all clinical materials will be compared through comparability studies
	Robust early process development ensures consistency of the clinical materials with maintenance of quality within specifications from run to run.
Clinical Manufacturing	The scalability of early DS process impacts the scale of clinical manufacturing and manufacturing timelines
Portfolio Acceleration	In case of accelerated approval for instance, a robust early clinical manufacturing process and a strong development data package can be the basis for a commercial process with minor adjustments.

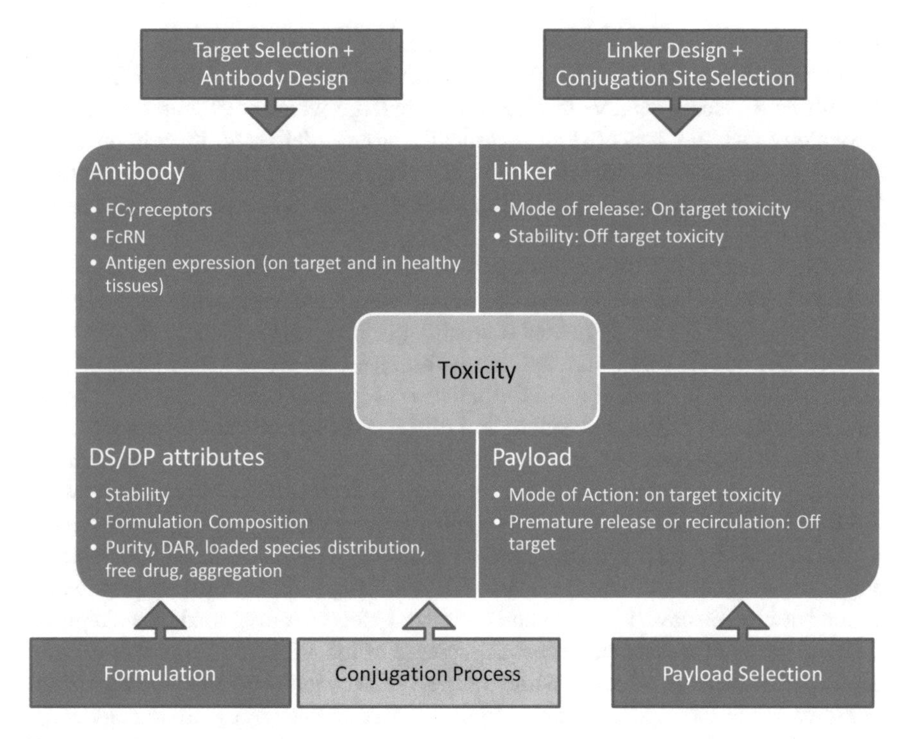

Fig. 5 ADC components and design steps impacting toxicity. (Center panels adapted from Roberts et al. [131])

Impact of Process on Quality Attributes: Example of Cytotoxicity

Figure 5 illustrates what parameters impact the toxicity of an ADC. The inner compartments present the contribution of the different component of the ADC molecule and the outer arrows illustrate what element and stage of the candidate selection process has the most impact. Antibody selection, linker selection and payload have, by design, determining impacts on the candidate toxicity.

The DS and DP attributes and associated toxicity are controlled by the selection of the conjugation technology primarily but ultimately DS manufacturing process and the DP formulation and manufacturing process control the actual toxicity of the clinical materials. In this context the process should deliver the intended target molecule and efficiently control impurities, free drugs and levels of conjugated species other than the target molecule.

Via comparability and through specifications setting, early process choices can have long term impact on a product toxicity profile. As an example we discuss cytotoxicity. The complexity of the ADC molecules makes cytotoxicity assessment difficult from a biology standpoint during discovery stages but also in the context of *in vitro* assay used as a surrogate *in vivo* cytoxicity and used to characterize the molecule and assess its stability [132, 133]. Process controlled drug substance components such as high DAR species affect cytotoxicity *in vivo* and potentially *in vitro* depending on assay design and optimization stage [78]. Knowing that *in vitro* cytotoxicity is measured relative to a reference material which is often the regulatory toxicology material, it is obvious that quality profiles delivered by early processes dictate, in a more or less narrow fashion, but very direct way, future CQA specifications by defining a target and setting some key clinical manufacturing process features.

Finally, associated with effective cytotoxicity, it is common to see a shift in observed MTD between discovery stage toxicology studies and regulatory enabling toxicology. That is directly related to quality profile changes associated with mAb quality, DL quality and critically, drug substance process *via* generation of high DAR species for instance. Figure 6 expands on Fig. 5 by highlighting the relationship between DS CQAs and Safety and efficacy parameters on the one hand and what process steps can be foreseen as having the most impact on the other hand. A recent article using human FcRn binding assay confirms a direct correlation between DAR and FcRn binding [134] and therefore *in vivo* half-life, toxicity and efficacy.

Though MTDs are not discussed in the article by Prashad et al. [17], an interesting example of conventional cysteine IgG1 ADC drug substance quality profile evolution between discovery process and optimized process is discussed. In a simplistic fashion, we can for instance expect an increase of the MTD if a better control over high DAR species is achieved while a higher conversion (lower D0) could, on the contrary, lower the MTD. Considering the impact of Regulatory Toxicology MTD

Safety Efficacy Parameters	Impactful ADC CQA	Relevant mAb QAs	Relevant DL DSI QAs	Most Impactful Process Step or Parameter	
				ConventionalCys	Site Specific Eng Cys
Potency PK Safety	Average DAR		Purity (conjugatable impurities)	• Reduction • Aggregate Removal	• Reduction • Re-oxidation
	Loaded Species Distribution		Purity (conjugatable impurities)	• Reduction • Aggregate Removal	• Reduction • Re-oxidation
PK Potency Immunogenicity	Aggregates	Aggregates		• Conjugation Conditions • Filtration • Chromatography	• Reduction • Re-oxidation
PK Potency Safety	Charge Variants	Charge Variants	Purity (conjugatable impurities)	• Reduction • Process pH extremes	• Reduction • Re-oxidation • Process pH extremes
Safety	Free Drug and associated impurities		Purity	• Final TFF	• Final TFF

Fig. 6 Drug substance, mAb, drug linker quality attributes and process steps impacting safety and efficacy parameters

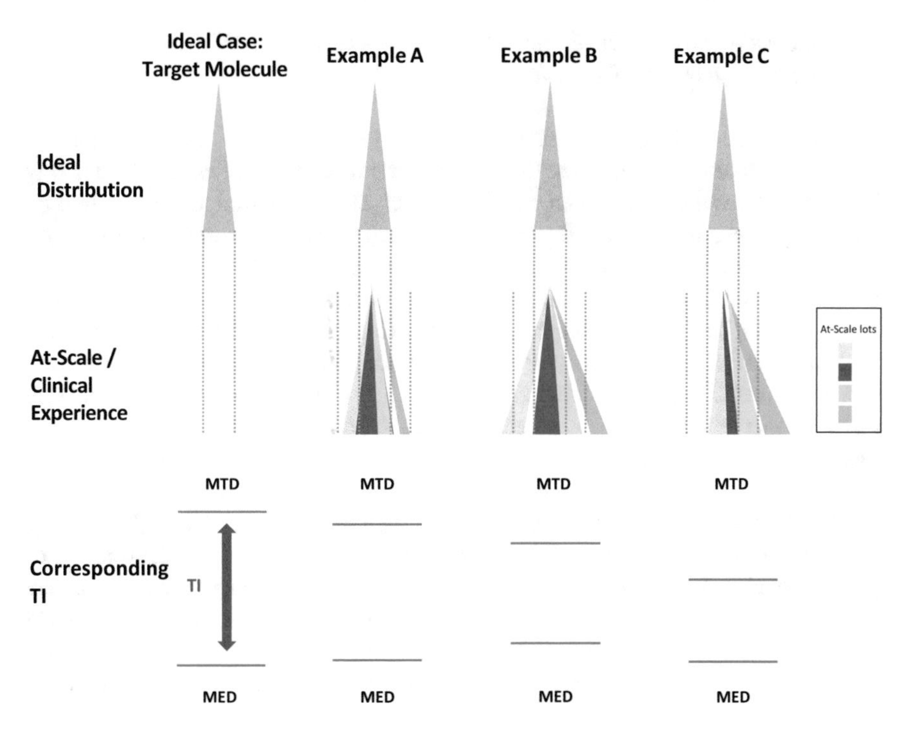

Fig. 7 Relationship between theoretical therapeutic index and quality attribute profile based on at-scale or clinical experience

on subsequent dose escalation design [131, 135], optimization and consistency of the BDS quality profile through early process development should be regarded as important [127].

Figure 7 illustrates the difference of TI that can be expected when the process delivers a composition that differs (e.g. loading species distribution or monomer content) from the ideal molecule quality attribute (e.g. 4-loaded species from a conventional Cysteine process or a DS with 100% monomer). The top row represents an ideal narrow distribution for a given quality attribute. The first column depicts the MED and MTD for such a narrow distribution close to the target molecule. Assuming a DP combining four BDS is generated, examples A, B and C illustrate what the theoretical MED and MTD are depending on the level of control over the process. With a reproducible and well controlled process, clinical lots will be closely similar and the corresponding DP would have a theoretical MED and MTD close to the ideal target molecule (Example A). If at-scale experience results in a distribution wider (e.g. wide variation of average DAR) than initial specifications defined around the target molecule a lower MTD and higher MED will be recorded (Example B). If at-scale experience results in skewed distribution such as the one depicted in Example C, a lower MTD can be expected. While combining four BDS is uncommon, Fig. 7 illustrates the potential impact of lot to lot variation and process control can have on actual TI.

Approaches to Process Development: Meeting the Timelines While Keeping an Eye on the End Game

Companies seem to have different approaches to early process development and considerations on what should be the focus of early process optimization. Toxicology Material can for instance be generated using polyclonal material and platform conjugation process at less than 50 g scale or produced using optimized process monoclonal antibody at hundred g-scale or higher to generate Toxicology material at several hundred gram-scale. The level of process development for later stages also varies and can be limited until clinical Proof of Concept is achieved. The same logic applies to analytical development and Reference Material for assay qualification can be derived from the regulatory toxicology run, an engineering run or a clinical run for concomitant qualification and release. We consider early process development as paramount to be in control of the process and be able to increase scale as needed or pursue, with some level of comfort, accelerated approval paths or simply shorten the time between candidate selection and reach First In Patient (FIP).

To better discuss acceleration, it is important to highlight what the deliverables of process development groups are in terms of toxicology, analytical reference or clinical materials and how the corresponding timelines align with analytical, formulation and regulatory timelines. Figure 8 provides an example of ADC development timelines.

In addition to process development itself, process development groups are typically responsible for:

- Technology transfer from research
- Supply of development material to support animal studies, analytical development and formulation development. Often referred to as Team Supply (TS) as done in Fig. 8.

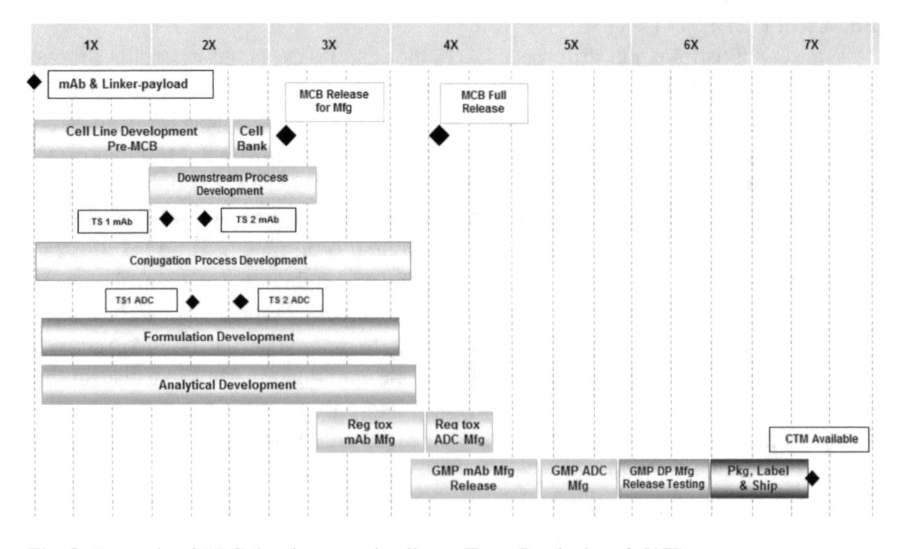

Fig. 8 Example of ADC development timelines. (From Prashad et al. [17])

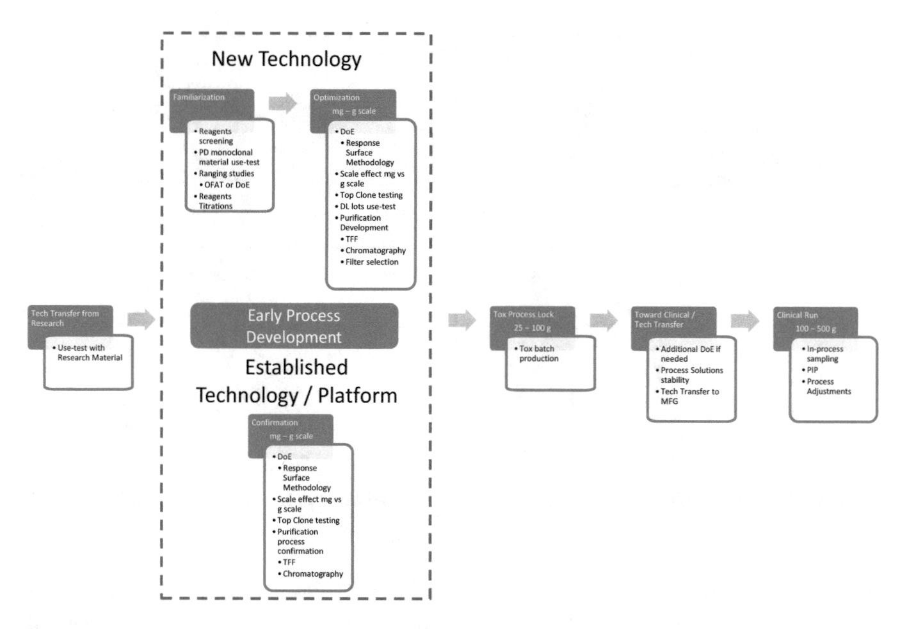

Fig. 9 Elements of early process development and sequence

- Use test of antibody development lots (conjugatability) to support top clone selection
- Technology transfer to manufacturing organization
- Production of regulatory enabling toxicology material
- Co-authoring of relevant IND sections

The figure below illustrates some of the activities and sequence of the process development work (Fig. 9).

Importantly, strategies for development work will evolve depending on the level of platform adoption for advancement of the technology [126, 127]. Technology selection significantly impacts process unit operations (Fig. 2).

Early Process development focuses on quality, consistency and scalability while cost of goods, raw materials specifications, commercial scale and process validation are typically the focus of Late Stage Development. Process Characterization as it applies to BLA considers commercial process and associated validated antibody and drug linker production, raw materials sourcing, facility fit, equipment validation and validated analytical methods [10]. However some minimum level of process characterization must be part of early stage work along with characterization of the drug substance. As we discuss in section "Shortening Process Development in the Context of Multiplying Technology Options: Investing in Analytical Characterization", advanced analytical development helps rational process design.

Figure 10 illustrates the value of QbD approaches in early stages of process development we advocate in Fig. 9. Section A illustrates the ideal outcome of a QbD

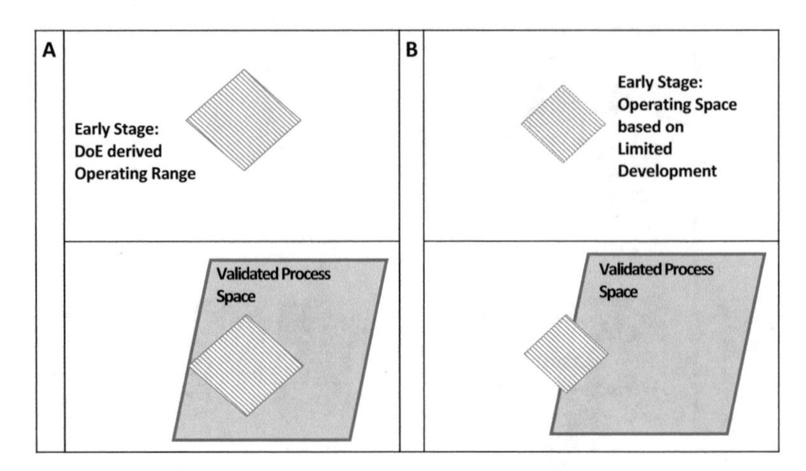

Fig. 10 Possible outcomes of QbD based early development (**A**) *vs* Limited Early Development (**B**)

approach leading to the operating space defined by limited DoE studies prior to early clinical phases. Typically this early operating space will be encompassed by the validated operating space for commercial manufacturing. The process should then be able to deliver CQA in range with clinical experience and facilitate comparability studies. Section B illustrates the possible outcome of limited process development, limited process understanding and the reliance on acceptable product quality as a demonstration of process robustness. It is likely that the validated space and the early operating space will not overlap. Alignment with clinical experience might require narrow operating ranges in that situation..

Limited early process development can lead to process variability with shifts in quality profile manifesting itself several years down the road [126, 127].

QbD is a reliable way to provide manufacturing organizations with comfortable operating range with an economy of development work [136]. Parameter ranging studies, buffer and reagent screening and M/OFAT (Multiple/One Factor At a Time) and DoE experiments at mg scale enable to build process understanding and identify critical parameters. Finally, confirmation of operating ranges established by DoE around target parameters confirmed at g-scale serves as a basis for Toxicology Lot production and subsequent clinical manufacturing. Chances of successful transition from process development lab scale to GMP manufacturing at several hundred grams are significantly increased by use of scale down versions of manufacturing equipment (e.g. TFF membranes, filter cartridges), utilization during process development of GMP reagents, minimal optimization of TFF operations focusing on impurity clearance and avoidance of aggregate formation. In process hold times and addition times need to be assessed and are of high importance at large scale.

If a chromatographic step is needed, aim for integration to the process as early as Toxicology batch production but only if the chromatographic purification is well defined. If the chromatographic step is likely to change, weigh CQA modifications i.e. quality profile changes brought by the chromatographic purification [14]. For instance, less HMW is always positive whereas a change of DAR is more difficult to handle from a comparability standpoint. Therefore a chromatographic step affecting DAR should probably be introduced early in process development. Specific details on process development are rarely published but a few reports featuring chromatographic purification discussions with a process development perspective have been presented [14, 17, 137, 138]. On a case by case basis depending on technologies, certain process unit operation will be obvious choices for thorough assessment early on. That is the case for the re-oxidation step involved in engineered cysteine conjugation as mentioned in Table 2. In our hands, early development OFAT studies followed by DoE on two closely related engineered cysteine mAbs led to early adjustments to their respective re-oxidation processes steps. This enabled better control over CQAs and successful toxicology batch and GMP ADC manufacturing at Agensys/Astellas.

In a very competitive landscape, while quality is always paramount, speed is also critical Acceleration often means shorter times between team supply lots (e.g. used for formulation development or analytical development) and toxicology run and avoidance of pilot scale runs prior to GMP engineering. This allows for accelerated development of analytical methods, qualification, DP engineering run and ultimately FIP. For this to be successful, development priority decisions need to be made in order not to jeopardize process robustness. Indeed, acceleration to the clinic is best achieved by being successful during clinical manufacturing.

Shortening Process Development in the Context of Multiplying Technology Options: The Tool Box Approach and Continuous Improvement

In the context of platform technology, well designed platform development approaches are highly efficient as illustrated for instance by Lacoste et al. [137]. Recently, companies have been exploring a broad array of technologies as they become available and process implications of the various conjugation technologies are discussed in section "Manufacturing Challenges Presented by New Technologies". Process Development groups are unlikely to contemplate single process flow diagrams across ADC candidates where the antibody and drug linkers would be the only variants over a long period of time.

When the focus is on quality and timelines, process development groups must develop a "tool box" approach [14] i.e. develop sets of process step units that they can select from based on the conjugation technology and still fit into a platform approach as much as possible. This allows the manufacturer to build process step knowledge, process step understanding and control across projects and simplifies recurring Technology Transfers to manufacturing organizations even as the ADC format or technology varies. Adopting a type of TFF membrane (material and pore size) across technologies is an obvious first step. Favoring buffer adjustment by buffer spike rather buffer exchange is attractive as it simplifies pH adjustment steps. With regards to formulation, a given technology applied to different mAbs is likely

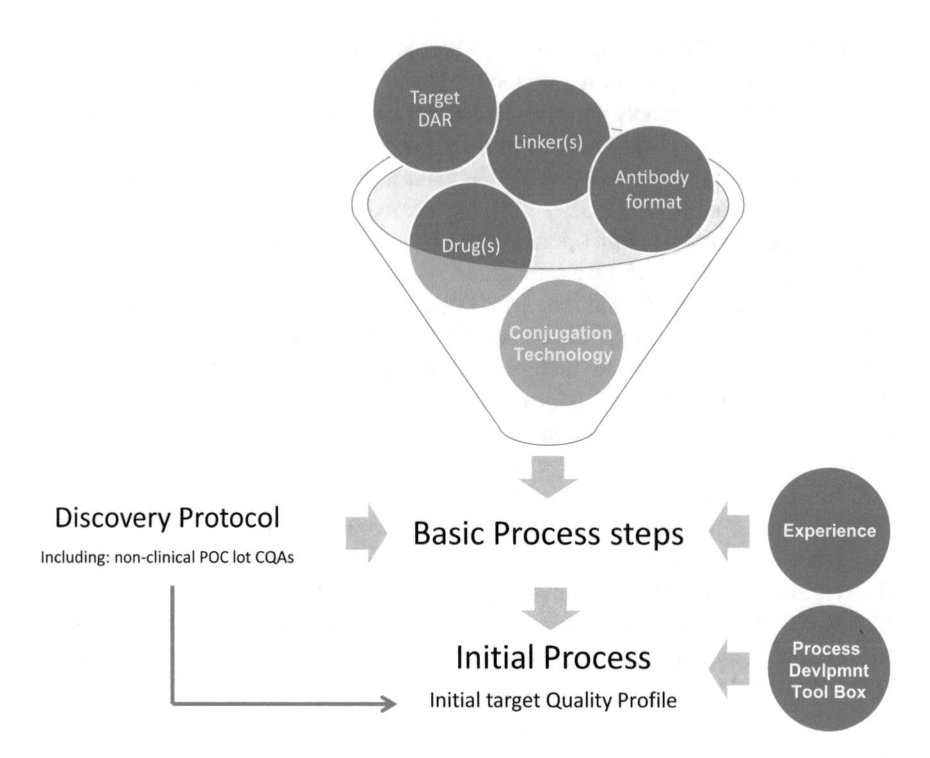

Fig. 11 Generation of an initial ADC conjugation process

to require a limited set of buffers and stabilizers with virtually a single, albeit critical, main variant: pH. As experience is gained, such knowledge becomes a component of institutional "experience" referred to in Fig. 11 and help selecting default buffers and speed up development times.

When it comes to chromatography to remove high DAR species or aggregates, the goal should be adoption of universal and scalable chromatographic equipment compatible with single use operation. The solid support is likely to vary depending on the purpose of the chromatography but also the mAb and/or the DL. Investing in pro-active resin screening to identify a limited set of universal resins is a worthy investment. Similarly, seeking new or better catalysts for oxime ligation [139, 140] required in certain UAA based conjugation technologies can prove valuable. SUTs are discussed earlier in this chapter and their early adoption is advisable to accelerate transfers to CMOs using SUTs.

Another component of quality process development in a context of portfolio acceleration is continuous improvement that relies on a formal risk assessment or an exercise inspired by risk assessment methods. The result is an early ranking of process steps in terms of criticality to quality or simply to robustness or transferability. In doing so, development activities can be prioritized and planned in parallel to more immediate deliverables or partially outsourced to a CRO or CDMO while process development teams remain focus on the next portfolio item.

Also pertaining to continuous improvement is technology platform optimization and understanding. Some examples are development of conditions favoring succinimide ring opening to prevent retro-Michael [69] or understanding of payload impact on conjugate hydrophobicity [16].

Finally, spending time on the very first process development step, namely the tech transfer from Research and providing feedback for future candidates is often hampered by time constrains but important over time to eliminate some of the shifts in quality attributes discussed in section "Impact of Process on Quality Attributes: Example of Cytotoxicity".

Figure 11 summarizes the elements that lead to the initial process flow diagram and process choices. Technology choices made by discovery, methods used by discovery to prepare their initial materials and process development tool box discussed above and institutional experience are critical. Institutional experience and institutional knowledge in general is hard to capture or track but should be kept in mind. Knowledge capture in development report is one obvious solution. Focusing on staff cross-training and retention is also important. As discussed in section "Outsourced Development", outsourcing development presents a risk in that regard unless the CMO institutional knowledge is made available.

Shortening Process Development in the Context of Multiplying Technology Options: Investing in Analytical Characterization

A platform approach is necessary not only for BDS and DP manufacture, but also in the context of portfolio acceleration and that applies to analytical assays as well. However, while a process robustness and consistency is assessed by analysis of the quality of the resulting DS via a range of analytical assays, assessment of the ability of an individual assay to truly depict the nature of its analyte requires development of orthogonal methods that a platform approach does not support. If the initial version of a process leads to high DAR species, it is possible that a platform HIC would not resolve all high loaded species. A platform SEC assay could show multimers, monomer and fragments but fail to resolve dimers. Early access by analytical groups to DS is critical to allow them to adapt assays to the new molecules. Also, focus should not solely be on fit for purpose methods and qualifiable methods as this may lead to a lack of knowledge of the molecule. Prashad et al. [17] discuss the characterization of two positional DAR 4 species isoforms in a conventional cysteine conjugate that gave the process development team the ability to monitor the species and to optimize the process and deliver primarily the more stable and putatively most efficacious isoform.

Early product analytical characterization i.e. structural features and detailed composition is very useful to process development group to understand at the molecular level the impact of process conditions. Constant progress in mass spectrometry techniques [141, 142] should allow almost routine extensive characterization of ADC molecules.

Another important component of process development and process understanding and control is access to in-process assays to help with process understanding and process control. While full development of in-process assay methods is unlikely during early development, securing collaboration with an analytical team dedicated to supporting process development is paramount. Early assessment of the suitability of release methods for analysis of in-process samples can be a component of late stage acceleration with direct impact on timelines for process characterization and validation.

We are not treating formulation development in this chapter but accelerated stability studies supported by formulation development and analytical groups are also critical to conjugation process decision and optimization.

Process Development and Accelerated Approval

Chizkov et al. [143] and Shea et al. [144] review trends in Breakthrough Therapy designation and oncology is the first or second leading therapeutic area for designation. There are other paths leading to accelerated approvals and whatever the path manufacturing readiness is critical to maximize chances of early licensure [145]. Antibody Drug conjugates are not covered in this document but the principals of this collective white paper apply to the antibody component and the drug linker component of the ADC. Several case studies are provided by Dye et al. [146]. For the ADC, the planning and strategy to identify development priorities are significantly more complex. Some elements of a conservative path to process characterization and validation under normal approval timelines are given in a late stage development case study on Inotuzumab Ozogamicin by Hu et al. [10]. A parallel characterization/validation of the ADC components is challenging but still conservative as it already relies on intense and efficient coordination of supply chain, manufacturing, process development, analytical development and quality review activities. Further acceleration requires negotiations with the regulatory agencies to delay certain activities post-licensures or potentially implementing more audacious multipurpose utilization of manufactured lots (validation lots, team supply, stability program, reference materials). As discussed in the previous sections, ability to actually accelerate late stage development is significantly increased if analytical methods, mAb, drug linker and drug substance processes have been designed for robustness, consistency and scalability. Any discussion with the regulatory agency around flexible filing process (delaying post-licensure certain activities), will hinge on solid QbD development data, well documented process development reports indicating not only that the process scaled up successfully during GMP manufacturing but also that process development data were able to predict it. Process development data become even more critical, both for companies to assess their readiness and for discussions with regulatory agencies, when breakthrough designation is granted based on phase 1 data.

With time and hopefully a larger number of approved antibody drug conjugates drugs, companies will start sharing examples of successful strategies in the field of

ADCs that will help others. It is also likely that regulatory agencies will continue the outreach efforts undertaken in the recent years, share their expectations and define these through better mutual understanding. White papers like the one by Dye et al. [146] and efforts by the EBE initiative on ADC [147] are to be encouraged.

References

1. Beck A, Goetsch L, Dumontet C, Corvaia N (2017) Strategies and challenges for the next generation of antibody-drug conjugates. Nat Rev Drug Discov 16(5):315–337
2. Lehar SM, Pillow T, Xu M, Staben L, Kajihara KK, Vandlen R, DePalatis L, Raab H, Hazenbos WL, Hiroshi Morisaki J, Kim J, Park S, Darwish M, Lee B-C, Hernandez H, Loyet KM, Lupardus P, Fong R, Yan D, Chalouni C, Luis E, Khalfin Y, Plise E, Cheong J, Lyssikatos JP, Strandh M, Koefoed K, Andersen PS, Flygare JA, Wah Tan M, Brown EJ, Mariathasan S (2015) Novel antibody–antibiotic conjugate eliminates intracellular S. aureus. Nature 527:323
3. Lim RK, Yu S, Cheng B, Li S, Kim N-J, Cao Y, Chi V, Kim JY, Chatterjee AK, Schultz PG, Tremblay MS, Kazane SA (2015) Targeted delivery of LXR agonist using a site-specific antibody–drug conjugate. Bioconjug Chem 26(11):2211–2222
4. Beck A, Wagner-Rousset E, Ayoub D, Van Dorsselaer A, Sanglier-Cianferani S (2013) Characterization of therapeutic antibodies and related products. Anal Chem 85(2):715–736
5. Wakankar A, Chen Y, Gokarn Y, Jacobson FS (2011) Analytical methods for physicochemical characterization of antibody drug conjugates. MAbs 3(2):161–172
6. Agarwal P, Bertozzi CR (2015) Site-specific antibody–drug conjugates: the nexus of bioorthogonal chemistry, protein engineering, and drug development. Bioconjug Chem 26(2):176–192
7. Deonarain MP, Yahioglu G, Stamati I, Marklew J (2015) Emerging formats for next-generation antibody drug conjugates. Expert Opin Drug Discovery 10(5):463–481
8. Hamann PR, Hinman LM, Hollander I, Beyer CF, Lindh D, Holcomb R, Hallett W, Tsou H-R, Upeslacis J, Shochat D, Mountain A, Flowers DA, Bernstein I (2002) Gemtuzumab ozogamicin, a potent and selective anti-CD33 antibody−calicheamicin conjugate for treatment of acute myeloid leukemia. Bioconjug Chem 13(1):47–58
9. Chari RVJ (2008) Targeted cancer therapy: conferring specificity to cytotoxic drugs. Acc Chem Res 41(1):98–107
10. Hu X, Bortell E, Kotch FW, Xu A, Arve B, Freese S (2017) Development of commercial-ready processes for antibody drug conjugates. Org Process Res Dev 21(4):601–610
11. Kim MT, Chen Y, Marhoul J, Jacobson F (2014) Statistical modeling of the drug load distribution on trastuzumab emtansine (Kadcyla), a lysine-linked antibody drug conjugate. Bioconjug Chem 25(7):1223
12. Lyon RP, Meyer D, Setter JR, Senter PD (2012) Conjugation of anticancer drugs through endogenous monoclonal antibody cysteine residues. Methods Enzymol 502:123
13. Wiggins B, Liu-Shin L, Yamaguchi H, Ratnaswamy G (2015) Characterization of cysteine-linked conjugation profiles of immunoglobulin g1 and immunoglobulin G2 antibody–drug conjugates. J Pharm Sci 104(4):1362–1372
14. Marcq O (2015) Impact on new linker payloads on drug substance quality attributes and process solutions. BPD Week, Huntington Beach, IBC Life Science
15. Adem YT, Schwarz KA, Duenas E, Patapoff TW, Galush WJ, Esue O (2014) Auristatin antibody drug conjugate physical instability and the role of drug payload. Bioconjug Chem 25(4):656–664
16. Guo J, Kumar S, Chipley M, Marcq O, Gupta D, Jin Z, Tomar DS, Swabowski C, Smith J, Starkey JA, Singh SK (2016) Characterization and higher-order structure assessment of an

interchain cysteine-based ADC: impact of drug loading and distribution on the mechanism of aggregation. Bioconjug Chem 27(3):604–615
17. Prashad AS, Nolting B, Patel V, Xu A, Arve B, Letendre L (2017) From R&D to clinical supplies. Org Process Res Dev 21(4):590–600
18. Cumnock K, Tully T, Cornell C, Hutchinson M, Gorrell J, Skidmore K, Chen Y, Jacobson F (2013) Trisulfide modification impacts the reduction step in antibody–drug conjugation process. Bioconjug Chem 24(7):1154–1160
19. Liu R, Chen X, Dushime J, Bogalhas M, Lazar AC, Ryll T, Wang L (2017) The impact of trisulfide modification of antibodies on the properties of antibody-drug conjugates manufactured using thiol chemistry. MAbs 9(3):490–497
20. Badescu G, Bryant P, Bird M, Henseleit K, Swierkosz J, Parekh V, Tommasi R, Pawlisz E, Jurlewicz K, Farys M, Camper N, Sheng X, Fisher M, Grygorash R, Kyle A, Abhilash A, Frigerio M, Edwards J, Godwin A (2014) Bridging disulfides for stable and defined antibody drug conjugates. Bioconjug Chem 25(6):1124
21. Morais M, Nunes JPM, Karu K, Forte N, Benni I, Smith MEB, Caddick S, Chudasama V, Baker JR (2017) Optimisation of the dibromomaleimide (DBM) platform for native antibody conjugation by accelerated post-conjugation hydrolysis. Org Biomol Chem 15(14):2947–2952
22. Behrens CR, Ha EH, Chinn LL, Bowers S, Probst G, Fitch-Bruhns M, Monteon J, Valdiosera A, Bermudez A, Liao-Chan S, Wong T, Melnick J, Theunissen J-W, Flory MR, Houser D, Venstrom K, Levashova Z, Sauer P, Migone T-S, van der Horst EH, Halcomb RL, Jackson DY (2015) Antibody–drug conjugates (ADCs) derived from interchain cysteine cross-linking demonstrate improved homogeneity and other pharmacological properties over conventional heterogeneous ADCs. Mol Pharm 12(11):3986–3998
23. Hamann PR (2005) Monoclonal antibody-drug conjugates. Expert Opin Ther Pat 15(9):1087
24. Hinman LM, Hamann PR, Wallace R, Menendez AT, Durr FE, Upeslacis J (1993) Preparation and characterization of monoclonal antibody conjugates of the calicheamicins: a novel and potent family of antitumor antibiotics. Cancer Res 53(14):3336–3342
25. Rodwell JD, McKearn TJ (1987) Antibody conjugates for the delivery of compounds to target sites. Patent Number US4671958 A
26. Zuberbuhler K, Casi G, Bernardes GJL, Neri D (2012) Fucose-specific conjugation of hydrazide derivatives to a vascular-targeting monoclonal antibody in IgG format. Chem Commun 48(56):7100–7102
27. van Geel R, Wijdeven MA, Heesbeen R, Verkade JMM, Wasiel AA, van Berkel SS, van Delft FL (2015) Chemoenzymatic conjugation of toxic payloads to the globally conserved N-glycan of native mAbs provides homogeneous and highly efficacious antibody–drug conjugates. Bioconjug Chem 26(11):2233–2242
28. Zhu Z, Ramakrishnan B, Li J, Wang Y, Feng Y, Prabakaran P, Colantonio S, Dyba MA, Qasba PK, Dimitrov DS (2014) Site-specific antibody-drug conjugation through an engineered glycotransferase and a chemically reactive sugar. MAbs 6(5):1190–1200
29. Zeglis BM, Davis CB, Aggeler R, Kang HC, Chen A, Agnew B, Lewis JS (2013) An enzyme-mediated methodology for the site-specific radiolabeling of antibodies based on catalyst-free click chemistry. Bioconjug Chem 24:1057
30. Li X, Fang T, Boons G-J (2014) Preparation of well-defined antibody–drug conjugates through glycan remodeling and strain-promoted azide–alkyne cycloadditions. Angew Chem Int Ed 53(28):7179–7182
31. Zhou Q, Stefano JE, Manning C, Kyazike J, Chen B, Gianolio DA, Park A, Busch M, Bird J, Zheng X, Simonds-Mannes H, Kim J, Gregory RC, Miller RJ, Brondyk WH, Dhal PK, Pan CQ (2014) Site-specific antibody–drug conjugation through glycoengineering. Bioconjug Chem 25(3):510–520
32. Stan AC, Radu DL, Casares S, Bona CA, Brumeanu T-D (1999) Antineoplastic efficacy of doxorubicin enzymatically assembled on galactose residues of a monoclonal antibody specific for the carcinoembryonic antigen. Cancer Res 59(1):115–121
33. Zhong X, Prashad AS, Kriz RW, He T, Somers W, Wang W, Letendre LJ (2017) Capped and uncapped antibody cysteines, and their use in antibody-drug conjugation. Patent Number WO2017025897 A2

34. Dimasi N, Fleming R, Zhong H, Bezabeh B, Kinneer K, Christie RJ, Fazenbaker C, Wu H, Gao C (2017) Efficient preparation of site-specific antibody–drug conjugates using cysteine insertion. Mol Pharm 14(5):1501–1516
35. Shinmi D, Nakano R, Mitamura K, Suzuki-Imaizumi M, Iwano J, Isoda Y, Enokizono J, Shiraishi Y, Arakawa E, Tomizuka K, Masuda K (2017) Novel anticarcinoembryonic antigen antibody–drug conjugate has antitumor activity in the existence of soluble antigen. Cancer Med 6(4):798–808
36. Shinmi D, Taguchi E, Iwano J, Yamaguchi T, Masuda K, Enokizono J, Shiraishi Y (2016) One step conjugation method for site-specific antibody-drug conjugates through reactive cysteine-engineered antibodies. Bioconjug Chem 27:1324
37. Thompson P, Bezabeh B, Fleming R, Pruitt M, Mao S, Strout P, Chen C, Cho S, Zhong H, Wu H, Gao C, Dimasi N (2015) Hydrolytically stable site-specific conjugation at the N-terminus of an engineered antibody. Bioconjug Chem 26(10):2085–2096
38. Harris L, Tavares D, Rui L, Maloney E, Wilhelm A, Costoplus J, Archer K, Bogalhas M, Harvey L, Wu R, Chen X, Xu X, Connaughton S, Wang L, Whiteman K, Ab O, Hong E, Widdison W, Shizuka M, Miller M, Pinkas J, Keating T, Chari R, Fishkin N (2015) Abstract 647: SeriMabs: N-terminal serine modification enables modular, site-specific payload incorporation into antibody-drug conjugates (ADCs). Cancer Res 75(15 Supplement):647–647
39. Jeger S, Zimmermann K, Blanc A, Grünberg J, Honer M, Hunziker P, Struthers H, Schibli R (2010) Site-specific and stoichiometric modification of antibodies by bacterial transglutaminase. Angew Chem Int Ed 49(51):9995–9997
40. Dennler P, Chiotellis A, Fischer E, Bregeon D, Belmant C, Gauthier L, Lhospice F, Romagne F, Schibli R (2014) Transglutaminase-based chemo-enzymatic conjugation approach yields homogeneous antibody-drug conjugates. Bioconjug Chem 25(3):569
41. Lhospice F, Brégeon D, Belmant C, Dennler P, Chiotellis A, Fischer E, Gauthier L, Boëdec A, Rispaud H, Savard-Chambard S, Represa A, Schneider N, Paturel C, Sapet M, Delcambre C, Ingoure S, Viaud N, Bonnafous C, Schibli R, Romagné F (2015) Site-specific conjugation of monomethyl auristatin E to anti-CD30 antibodies improves their pharmacokinetics and therapeutic index in rodent models. Mol Pharm 12(6):1863–1871
42. Strop P, Dorywalska MG, Rajpal A, Shelton D, Liu SH, Pons J, Dushin R (2012) Engineered polypeptide conjugates and methods for making thereof using transglutaminase. Patent Number 2,012,059,882
43. Strop P, Liu SH, Dorywalska M, Delaria K, Dushin RG, Tran TT, Ho WH, Farias S, Casas MG, Abdiche Y, Zhou D, Chandrasekaran R, Samain C, Loo C, Rossi A, Rickert M, Krimm S, Wong T, Chin SM, Yu J, Dilley J, Chaparro-Riggers J, Filzen GF, O'Donnell CJ, Wang F, Myers JS, Pons J, Shelton DL, Rajpal A (2013) Location matters: site of conjugation modulates stability and pharmacokinetics of antibody drug conjugates. Chem Biol 20(2):161
44. Beerli RR, Hell T, Merkel AS, Grawunder U (2015) Sortase enzyme-mediated generation of site-specifically conjugated antibody drug conjugates with high in vitro and in vivo potency. PLoS One 10(7):e0131177
45. Bellucci JJ, Bhattacharyya J, Chilkoti A (2015) A noncanonical function of sortase enables site-specific conjugation of small molecules to lysine residues in proteins. Angew Chem Int Ed 54(2):441–445
46. Stefan N, Gébleux R, Waldmeier L, Hell T, Escher M, Wolter FI, Grawunder U, Beerli RR (2017) Highly potent, anthracycline-based antibody drug conjugates generated by enzymatic, site-specific conjugation. Mol Cancer Ther 16(5):879–892
47. Bruins JJ, Westphal AH, Albada B, Wagner K, Bartels L, Spits H, van Berkel WJH, van Delft FL (2017) Inducible, site-specific protein labeling by tyrosine oxidation–strain-promoted (4 + 2) cycloaddition. Bioconjug Chem 28(4):1189–1193
48. Drake PM, Albers AE, Baker J, Banas S, Barfield RM, Bhat AS, de Hart GW, Garofalo AW, Holder P, Jones LC, Kudirka R, McFarland J, Zmolek W, Rabuka D (2014) Aldehyde tag coupled with HIPS chemistry enables the production of ADCs conjugated site-specifically to different antibody regions with distinct in vivo efficacy and PK outcomes. Bioconjug Chem 25(7):1331

49. Rabuka D, Rush JS, deHart GW, Wu P, Bertozzi CR (2012) Site-specific chemical protein conjugation using genetically encoded aldehyde tags. Nat Protoc 7(6):1052
50. Axup JY, Bajjuri KM, Ritland M, Hutchins BM, Kim CH, Kazane SA, Halder R, Forsyth JS, Santidrian AF, Stafin K, Lu Y, Tran H, Seller AJ, Biroc SL, Szydlik A, Pinkstaff JK, Tian F, Sinha SC, Felding-Habermann B, Smider VV, Schultz PG (2012) Synthesis of site-specific antibody-drug conjugates using unnatural amino acids. Proc Natl Acad Sci 109(40):16101–16106
51. Yin G, Stephenson HT, Yang J, Li X, Armstrong SM, Heibeck TH, Tran C, Masikat MR, Zhou S, Stafford RL, Yam AY, Lee J, Steiner AR, Gill A, Penta K, Pollitt S, Baliga R, Murray CJ, Thanos CD, McEvoy LM, Sato AK, Hallam TJ (2017) RF1 attenuation enables efficient non-natural amino acid incorporation for production of homogeneous antibody drug conjugates. Sci Rep 7(1):3026
52. VanBrunt MP, Shanebeck K, Caldwell Z, Johnson J, Thompson P, Martin T, Dong H, Li G, Xu H, D'Hooge F, Masterson L, Bariola P, Tiberghien A, Ezeadi E, Williams DG, Hartley JA, Howard PW, Grabstein KH, Bowen MA, Marelli M (2015) Genetically encoded azide containing amino acid in mammalian cells enables site-specific antibody-drug conjugates using click cycloaddition chemistry. Bioconjug Chem 26:2249
53. Li X, Nelson CG, Nair RR, Hazlehurst L, Moroni T, Martinez-Acedo P, Nanna AR, Hymel D, Burke TR, Rader C (2017) Stable and potent selenomab-drug conjugates. Cell Chem Biol 24(4):433–442. e436
54. Li X, Yang J, Rader C (2014) Antibody conjugation via one and two C-terminal selenocysteines. Methods 65(1):133–138
55. Okeley NM, Toki BE, Zhang X, Jeffrey SC, Burke PJ, Alley SC, Senter PD (2013) Metabolic engineering of monoclonal antibody carbohydrates for antibody–drug conjugation. Bioconjug Chem 24(10):1650–1655
56. Junutula JR, Raab H, Clark S, Bhakta S, Leipold DD, Weir S, Chen Y, Simpson M, Tsai SP, Dennis MS, Lu Y, Meng YG, Ng C, Yang J, Lee CC, Duenas E, Gorrell J, Katta V, Kim A, McDorman K, Flagella K, Venook R, Ross S, Spencer SD, Lee Wong W, Lowman HB, Vandlen R, Sliwkowski MX, Scheller RH, Polakis P, Mallet W (2008) Site-specific conjugation of a cytotoxic drug to an antibody improves the therapeutic index. Nat Biotech 26(8):925–932
57. Dorywalska M, Strop P, Melton-Witt JA, Hasa-Moreno A, Farias SE, Galindo Casas M, Delaria K, Lui V, Poulsen K, Loo C, Krimm S, Bolton G, Moine L, Dushin R, Tran TT, Liu SH, Rickert M, Foletti D, Shelton DL, Pons J, Rajpal A (2015) Effect of attachment site on stability of cleavable antibody drug conjugates. Bioconjug Chem 26(4):650–659
58. Jackson D, Atkinson J, Guevara CI, Zhang C, Kery V, Moon S-J, Virata C, Yang P, Lowe C, Pinkstaff J, Cho H, Knudsen N, Manibusan A, Tian F, Sun Y, Lu Y, Sellers A, Jia X-C, Joseph I, Anand B, Morrison K, Pereira DS, Stover D (2014) In vitro and in vivo evaluation of cysteine and site specific conjugated herceptin antibody-drug conjugates. PLoS One 9(1):e83865
59. Strop P, Delaria K, Foletti D, Witt JM, Hasa-Moreno A, Poulsen K, Casas MG, Dorywalska M, Farias S, Pios A, Lui V, Dushin R, Zhou D, Navaratnam T, Tran T-T, Sutton J, Lindquist KC, Han B, Liu S-H, Shelton DL, Pons J, Rajpal A (2015) Site-specific conjugation improves therapeutic index of antibody drug conjugates with high drug loading. Nat Biotech 33(7):694–696
60. Müller-Späth T, Ulmer N, Aumann L, Kennedy C, Bavand M (2015) Twin-column cation-exchange chromatography for the purification of biomolecules. BioPharm Int 28(4):32–36
61. Lyons A, King DJ, Owens RJ, Yarranton GT, Millican A, Whittle NR, Adair JR (1990) Site-specific attachment to recombinant antibodies via introduced surface cysteine residues. Protein Eng Des Sel 3:703
62. Stimmel JB, Merrill BM, Kuyper LF, Moxham CP, Hutchins JT, Fling ME, Kull FC (2000) Site-specific conjugation on serine right-arrow cysteine variant monoclonal antibodies. J Biol Chem 275:30445
63. Zhong X, He T, Prashad AS, Wang W, Cohen J, Ferguson D, Tam AS, Sousa E, Lin L, Tchistiakova L, Gatto S, D'Antona A, Luan Y-T, Ma W, Zollner R, Zhou J, Arve B, Somers

W, Kriz R (2017) Mechanistic understanding of the cysteine capping modifications of antibodies enables selective chemical engineering in live mammalian cells. J Biotechnol 248(Supplement C):48–58
64. Rudra-Ganguly N, Lowe C, Virata C, Leavitt M, Jin L, Mendelsohn B, Snyder J, Aviña H, Zhang C, Russell DL, Mattie M, Yang P, Randhawa B, Liu G, Malik F, Vest M, Abad JD, Kemball CC, Hubert R, Karki S, Anand B, An Z, Grant J, Dick JE, Doñate F, Morrison K, Challita-Eid P, Joseph IB, Pereira DS, Stover DR (2015) AGS62P1, a novel anti-FLT3 antibody drug conjugate, employing site specific conjugation, demonstrates preclinical anti-tumor efficacy in AML tumor and patient derived xenografts. Blood 126(23):3806–3806
65. Rickert M, Strop P, Lui V, Melton-Witt J, Farias SE, Foletti D, Shelton D, Pons J, Rajpal A (2016) Production of soluble and active microbial transglutaminase in Escherichia coli for site-specific antibody drug conjugation. Protein Sci 25(2):442–455
66. Chen L, Cohen J, Song X, Zhao A, Ye Z, Feulner CJ, Doonan P, Somers W, Lin L, Chen PR (2016) Improved variants of SrtA for site-specific conjugation on antibodies and proteins with high efficiency. Sci Rep 6:31899
67. Lyon RP, Bovee TD, Doronina SO, Burke PJ, Hunter JH, Neff-LaFord HD, Jonas M, Anderson ME, Setter JR, Senter PD (2015) Reducing hydrophobicity of homogeneous antibody-drug conjugates improves pharmacokinetics and therapeutic index. Nat Biotech 33(7):733–735
68. Kalia J, Raines RT (2007) Catalysis of imido group hydrolysis in a maleimide conjugate. Bioorg Med Chem Lett 17(22):6286–6289
69. Tumey LN, Charati M, He T, Sousa E, Ma D, Han X, Clark T, Casavant J, Loganzo F, Barletta F, Lucas J, Graziani EI (2014) Mild method for succinimide hydrolysis on ADCs: impact on ADC potency, stability, exposure, and efficacy. Bioconjug Chem 25:1871
70. Fontaine SD, Reid R, Robinson L, Ashley GW, Santi DV (2015) Long-term stabilization of maleimide-thiol conjugates. Bioconjug Chem 26:145
71. Lyon RP, Setter JR, Bovee TD, Doronina SO, Hunter JH, Anderson ME, Balasubramanian CL, Duniho SM, Leiske CI, Li F, Senter PD (2014) Self-hydrolyzing maleimides improve the stability and pharmacological properties of antibody-drug conjugates. Nat Biotechnol 32:1059
72. Shen BQ, Xu K, Liu L, Raab H, Bhakta S, Kenrick M, Parsons-Reponte KL, Tien J, Yu SF, Mai E, Li D, Tibbitts J, Baudys J, Saad OM, Scales SJ, McDonald PJ, Hass PE, Eigenbrot C, Nguyen T, Solis WA, Fuji RN, Flagella KM, Patel D, Spencer SD, Khawli LA, Ebens A, Wong WL, Vandlen R, Kaur S, Sliwkowski MX, Scheller RH, Polakis P, Junutula JR (2012) Conjugation site modulates the in vivo stability and therapeutic activity of antibody-drug conjugates. Nat Biotechnol 30:184
73. Alley SC, Benjamin DR, Jeffrey SC, Okeley NM, Meyer DL, Sanderson RJ, Senter PD (2008) Contribution of linker stability to the activities of anticancer immunoconjugates. Bioconjug Chem 19(3):759–765
74. Badescu G, Bryant P, Swierkosz J, Khayrzad F, Pawlisz E, Farys M, Cong Y, Muroni M, Rumpf N, Brocchini S, Godwin A (2014) A new reagent for stable thiol-specific conjugation. Bioconjug Chem 25(3):460–469
75. Toda N, Asano S, Barbas CF (2013) Rapid, stable, chemoselective labeling of thiols with Julia–Kocieński-like reagents: a serum-stable alternative to maleimide-based protein conjugation. Angew Chem Int Ed 52(48):12592–12596
76. Bernardim B, Cal PMSD, Matos MJ, Oliveira BL, Martínez-Sáez N, Albuquerque IS, Perkins E, Corzana F, Burtoloso ACB, Jiménez-Osés G, Bernardes GJL (2016) Stoichiometric and irreversible cysteine-selective protein modification using carbonylacrylic reagents. Nat Commun 7:13128
77. Chari RVJ, Martell BA, Gross JL, Cook SB, Shah SA, Blättler WA, McKenzie SJ, Goldmacher VS (1992) Immunoconjugates containing novel maytansinoids: promising anticancer drugs. Cancer Res 52(1):127–131
78. Hamblett KJ, Senter PD, Chace DF, Sun MMC, Lenox J, Cerveny CG, Kissler KM, Bernhardt SX, Kopcha AK, Zabinski RF, Meyer DL, Francisco JA (2004) Effects of drug

loading on the antitumor activity of a monoclonal antibody drug conjugate. Clin Cancer Res 10(20):7063–7070

79. Maruani A, Richards DA, Chudasama V (2016) Dual modification of biomolecules. Org Biomol Chem 14(26):6165–6178
80. Levengood MR, Zhang X, Hunter JH, Emmerton KK, Miyamoto JB, Lewis TS, Senter PD (2017) Orthogonal cysteine protection enables homogeneous multi-drug antibody–drug conjugates. Angew Chem Int Ed 56(3):733–737
81. Ariyasu S, Hayashi H, Xing B, Chiba S (2017) Site-specific dual functionalization of cysteine residue in peptides and proteins with 2-azidoacrylates. Bioconjug Chem 28(4):897–902
82. Maruani A, Smith MEB, Miranda E, Chester KA, Chudasama V, Caddick S (2015) A plug-and-play approach to antibody-based therapeutics via a chemoselective dual click strategy. Nat Commun 6:6645
83. Li X, Patterson JT, Sarkar M, Pedzisa L, Kodadek T, Roush WR, Rader C (2015) Site-specific dual antibody conjugation via engineered cysteine and selenocysteine residues. Bioconjug Chem 26(11):2243–2248
84. Tang F, Yang Y, Tang Y, Tang S, Yang L, Sun B, Jiang B, Dong J, Liu H, Huang M, Geng M-Y, Huang W (2016) One-pot N-glycosylation remodeling of IgG with non-natural sialylglycopeptides enables glycosite-specific and dual-payload antibody-drug conjugates. Org Biomol Chem 14(40):9501–9518
85. Yurkovetskiy AV, Yin M, Bodyak N, Stevenson CA, Thomas JD, Hammond CE, Qin L, Zhu B, Gumerov DR, Ter-Ovanesyan E, Uttard A, Lowinger TB (2015) A polymer-based antibody–vinca drug conjugate platform: characterization and preclinical efficacy. Cancer Res 75(16):3365–3372
86. Burke PJ, Hamilton JZ, Pires TA, Setter JR, Hunter JH, Cochran JH, Waight AB, Gordon KA, Toki BE, Emmerton KK, Zeng W, Stone IJ, Senter PD, Lyon RP, Jeffrey SC (2016) Development of novel quaternary ammonium linkers for antibody–drug conjugates. Mol Cancer Ther 15:938
87. Pillow TH (2017) Novel linkers and connections for antibody–drug conjugates to treat cancer and infectious disease. Pharm Patent Anal 6(1):25–33
88. Jeffrey SC, Andreyka JB, Bernhardt SX, Kissler KM, Kline T, Lenox JS, Moser RF, Nguyen MT, Okeley NM, Stone IJ, Zhang X, Senter PD (2006) Development and properties of β-glucuronide linkers for monoclonal antibody−drug conjugates. Bioconjug Chem 17(3):831–840
89. Zhao RY, Wilhelm SD, Audette C, Jones G, Leece BA, Lazar AC, Goldmacher VS, Singh R, Kovtun Y, Widdison WC, Lambert JM, Chari RVJ (2011) Synthesis and evaluation of hydrophilic linkers for antibody–maytansinoid conjugates. J Med Chem 54(10):3606–3623
90. Kern JC, Cancilla M, Dooney D, Kwasnjuk K, Zhang R, Beaumont M, Figueroa I, Hsieh S, Liang L, Tomazela D, Zhang J, Brandish PE, Palmieri A, Stivers P, Cheng M, Feng G, Geda P, Shah S, Beck A, Bresson D, Firdos J, Gately D, Knudsen N, Manibusan A, Schultz PG, Sun Y, Garbaccio RM (2016) Discovery of pyrophosphate diesters as tunable, soluble, and bioorthogonal linkers for site-specific antibody–drug conjugates. J Am Chem Soc 138(4):1430–1445
91. Mendelsohn BA, Barnscher SD, Snyder JT, An Z, Dodd JM, Dugal-Tessier J (2017) Investigation of hydrophilic auristatin derivatives for use in antibody drug conjugates. Bioconjug Chem 28(2):371–381
92. Buck PM, Kumar S, Wang X, Agrawal NJ, Trout BL, Singh SK (2012) Computational methods to predict therapeutic protein aggregation. Methods Mol Biol 899:425
93. Jain T, Sun T, Durand S, Hall A, Houston NR, Nett JH, Sharkey B, Bobrowicz B, Caffry I, Yu Y, Cao Y, Lynaugh H, Brown M, Baruah H, Gray LT, Krauland EM, Xu Y, Vásquez M, Wittrup KD (2017) Biophysical properties of the clinical-stage antibody landscape. Proc Natl Acad Sci 114(5):944–949
94. Lee CC, Perchiacca JM, Tessier PM (2013) Toward aggregation-resistant antibodies by design. Trends Biotechnol 31(11):612–620

95. Sharma VK, Patapoff TW, Kabakoff B, Pai S, Hilario E, Zhang B, Li C, Borisov O, Kelley RF, Chorny I, Zhou JZ, Dill KA, Swartz TE (2014) In silico selection of therapeutic antibodies for development: viscosity, clearance, and chemical stability. Proc Natl Acad Sci 111(52):18601–18606
96. Tomar DS, Kumar S, Singh SK, Goswami S, Li L (2016) Molecular basis of high viscosity in concentrated antibody solutions: strategies for high concentration drug product development. MAbs 8(2):216–228
97. Beckley NS, Lazzareschi KP, Chih H-W, Sharma VK, Flores HL (2013) Investigation into temperature-induced aggregation of an antibody drug conjugate. Bioconjug Chem 24(10):1674–1683
98. Guo J, Kumar S, Prashad A, Starkey J, Singh SK (2014) Assessment of physical stability of an antibody drug conjugate by higher order structure analysis: impact of thiol- maleimide chemistry. Pharm Res 31(7):1710–1723
99. Li W, Prabakaran P, Chen W, Zhu Z, Feng Y, Dimitrov D (2016) Antibody aggregation: insights from sequence and structure. Antibodies 5(3):19
100. Voynov V, Chennamsetty N, Kayser V, Wallny HJ, Helk B, Trout BL (2010) Design and application of antibody cysteine variants. Bioconjug Chem 21:385
101. Tumey LN, Li F, Rago B, Han X, Loganzo F, Musto S, Graziani EI, Puthenveetil S, Casavant J, Marquette K, Clark T, Bikker J, Bennett EM, Barletta F, Piche-Nicholas N, Tam A, O'Donnell CJ, Gerber HP, Tchistiakova L (2017) Site selection: a case study in the identification of optimal cysteine engineered antibody drug conjugates. AAPS J 19(4):1123–1135
102. Tiller KE, Tessier PM (2015) Advances in antibody design. Annu Rev Biomed Eng 17(1):191–216
103. Polu KR, Lowman HB (2014) Probody therapeutics for targeting antibodies to diseased tissue. Expert Opin Biol Ther 14(8):1049–1053
104. Marshall DJ, Harried SS, Murphy JL, Hall CA, Shekhani MS, Pain C, Lyons CA, Chillemi A, Malavasi F, Pearce HL, Thorson JS, Prudent JR (2016) Extracellular antibody drug conjugates exploiting the proximity of two proteins. Mol Ther 24(10):1760–1770
105. Brinkmann U, Kontermann RE (2017) The making of bispecific antibodies. MAbs 9(2):182–212
106. Sheridan C (2016) Despite slow progress, bispecifics generate buzz. Nat Biotechnol 34:1215
107. Metz S, Haas AK, Daub K, Croasdale R, Stracke J, Lau W, Georges G, Josel H-P, Dziadek S, Hopfner K-P, Lammens A, Scheuer W, Hoffmann E, Mundigl O, Brinkmann U (2011) Bispecific digoxigenin-binding antibodies for targeted payload delivery. Proc Natl Acad Sci 108(20):8194–8199
108. Rossi EA, Goldenberg DM, Chang C-H (2012) The dock-and-lock method combines recombinant engineering with site-specific covalent conjugation to generate multifunctional structures. Bioconjug Chem 23(3):309–323
109. Li JY, Perry SR, Muniz-Medina V, Wang X, Wetzel LK, Rebelatto MC, Hinrichs MJ, Bezabeh BZ, Fleming RL, Dimasi N, Feng H, Toader D, Yuan AQ, Xu L, Lin J, Gao C, Wu H, Dixit R, Osbourn JK, Coats SR (2016) A biparatopic HER2-targeting antibody-drug conjugate induces tumor regression in primary models refractory to or ineligible for HER2-targeted therapy. Cancer Cell 29:117
110. Trail PA, Dubowchik GM, Lowinger TB (2018) Antibody drug conjugates for treatment of breast cancer: novel targets and diverse approaches in ADC design. Pharmacol Therap 181:126–142
111. de Goeij BECG, Vink T, ten Napel H, Breij ECW, Satijn D, Wubbolts R, Miao D, Parren PWHI (2016) Efficient payload delivery by a bispecific antibody–drug conjugate targeting HER2 and CD63. Mol Cancer Ther 15(11):2688–2697
112. de Goeij BECG, Satijn D, Freitag CM, Wubbolts R, Bleeker WK, Khasanov A, Zhu T, Chen G, Miao D, van Berkel PHC, Parren PWHI (2015) High turnover of tissue factor enables efficient intracellular delivery of antibody–drug conjugates. Mol Cancer Ther 14(5):1130–1140

113. Andreev J, Thambi N, Perez Bay AE, Delfino F, Martin J, Kelly MP, Kirshner JR, Rafique A, Kunz A, Nittoli T, MacDonald D, Daly C, Olson W, Thurston G (2017) Bispecific antibodies and antibody–drug conjugates (ADCs) bridging HER2 and prolactin receptor improve efficacy of HER2 ADCs. Mol Cancer Ther 16(4):681–693
114. DeVay RM, Delaria K, Zhu G, Holz C, Foletti D, Sutton J, Bolton G, Dushin R, Bee C, Pons J, Rajpal A, Liang H, Shelton D, Liu S-H, Strop P (2017) Improved lysosomal trafficking can modulate the potency of antibody drug conjugates. Bioconjug Chem 28(4):1102–1114
115. Ducry L (2012) Challenges in the development and manufacturing of antibody–drug conjugates. In: Voynov V, Caravella JA (eds) Therapeutic proteins: methods and protocols. Humana Press, Totowa, pp 489–497
116. Rohrer T (2012) Consideration for the safe and effective manufacturing of antibody drug conjugates. Chim Oggi 30(5):76
117. Denk R, Flückiger A (2017) ADCs: Anforderungen an GMP und Arbeitsschutz. TechnoPharm 7(1):32–37
118. Ducry L, Suhartono M, Rohrer T (2016) Manufacturing ADCs utilizing full-disposable system. World ADC Summit, Berlin, Hanson Wade
119. Stanton D (2014) ADC pipelines drive single-use expansion at Lonza's clinical facility. 2017
120. Han T (2017) Utilize disposable technologies for ADC manufacture. World ADC Summit, Berlin, Hanson Wade
121. Boedeker B, Jones Seymor K (2015) A single-use ADC process: from development to clinical. World ADC Summit, San Diego, Hanson Wade
122. Czapkowski B, Steen J, Bortell E, Patel V, Seo YS, Jiang J, Lagliva J, Di Grandi D, Kozlov M (2017) Trial of high efficiency TFF capsule prototype for ADC purification. ADC Rev J Antibody-Drug Conjug. https://doi.org/10.14229/jadc.2017.11.04.001
123. Dunny E, O'Connor I, Bones J (2017) Containment challenges in HPAPI manufacture for ADC generation. Drug Discov Today 22(6):947–951
124. ISPE Baseline Guide: Volume 7 – Risk-based manufacture of pharmaceutical products (Risk-MaPP). International Society for Pharmaceutical Engineering (2017)
125. Hensgen MI, Stump B (2013) Safe handling of cytotoxic compounds in a biopharmaceutical environment. In: Ducry L (ed) Antibody-drug conjugates. Humana Press, Totowa, pp 133–143
126. Marcq O (2017) Robustly outsource and transfer ADC technology. World ADC Summit, Berlin, Hanson Wade
127. Marcq O (2017) ADC safety and toxicity: technology choices and importance of process development to control safety related CQAs. In: 5th antibody industrial symposium, Tours
128. Turula V (2016) Manufacturing support for antibody drug conjugates: clinical and commercial scenarios. World ADC Summit, Berlin, Hanson Wade
129. Krummen L (2013) Lessons learned from two case studies in the FDA QbD biotech pilot. CMC Forum Europe, Prague
130. Galush WJ, Wakankar AA (2013) Formulation development of antibody–drug conjugates. In: Ducry L (ed) Antibody-drug conjugates. Humana Press, Totowa, pp 217–233
131. Roberts SA, Andrews PA, Blanset D, Flagella KM, Gorovits B, Lynch CM, Martin PL, Kramer-Stickland K, Thibault S, Warner G (2013) Considerations for the nonclinical safety evaluation of antibody drug conjugates for oncology. Regul Toxicol Pharmacol 67(3):382–391
132. Hinrichs MJM, Dixit R (2015) Antibody drug conjugates: nonclinical safety considerations. AAPS J 17(5):1055–1064
133. Kumar S, King LE, Clark TH, Gorovits B (2015) Antibody–drug conjugates nonclinical support: from early to late nonclinical bioanalysis using ligand-binding assays. Bioanalysis 7(13):1605–1617
134. Brachet G, Respaud R, Arnoult C, Henriquet C, Dhommee C, Viaud-Massuard MC, Heuze-Vourc'h N, Joubert N, Pugniere M, Gouilleux-Gruart V (2016) Increment in drug loading on an antibody-drug conjugate increases its binding to the human neonatal Fc receptor in vitro. Mol Pharm 13:1405

135. ICH (2009) S9 Nonclinical evaluation for anticancer pharmaceuticals. http://www.ich.org/products/guidelines/safety/safety-single/article/nonclinical-evaluation-for-anticancer-pharmaceuticals.html
136. Kelley B, Cromwell M, Jerkins J (2016) Integration of QbD risk assessment tools and overall risk management. Biologicals 44(5):341–351
137. Lacoste E (2016) Optimization of ADC process development. World ADC Summit, Berlin, Hanson Wade
138. Nilapwar S (2016) Development of robust, scalable site-specific conjugation for monoclonal and bispecific mAbs: a DOE approach. World ADC Summit, San Diego, Hanson Wade
139. Agten SM, Dawson PE, Hackeng TM (2016) Oxime conjugation in protein chemistry: from carbonyl incorporation to nucleophilic catalysis. J Pept Sci 22(5):271–279
140. Rashidian M, Mahmoodi MM, Shah R, Dozier JK, Wagner CR, Distefano MD (2013) A highly efficient catalyst for oxime ligation and hydrazone–oxime exchange suitable for bioconjugation. Bioconjug Chem 24(3):333–342
141. Botzanowski T, Erb S, Hernandez-Alba O, Ehkirch A, Colas O, Wagner-Rousset E, Rabuka D, Beck A, Drake PM, Cianférani S (2017) Insights from native mass spectrometry approaches for top- and middle- level characterization of site-specific antibody-drug conjugates. MAbs 9(5):801–811
142. Pan LY, Salas-Solano O, Valliere-Douglass JF (2014) Conformation and dynamics of interchain cysteine-linked antibody-drug conjugates as revealed by hydrogen/deuterium exchange mass spectrometry. Anal Chem 86(5):2657–2664
143. Chizkov RR, Million RP (2015) Trends in breakthrough therapy designation. Nat Rev Drug Discov 14(9):597
144. Shea M, Ostermann L, Hohman R, Roberts S, Kozak M, Dull R, Allen J, Sigal E (2016) Impact of breakthrough therapy designation on cancer drug development. Nat Rev Drug Discov 15:152
145. Dye E, Sturgess A, Maheshwari G, May K, Ruegger C, Ramesh U, Tan H, Cockerill K, Groskoph J, Lacana E, Lee S, Miksinski SP (2016) Examining manufacturing readiness for breakthrough drug development. AAPS PharmSciTech 17(3):529–538
146. Dye ES, Groskoph J, Kelley B, Millili G, Nasr M, Potter CJ, Thostesen E, Vermeersch H (2015) CMC considerations when a drug development project is assigned breakthrough therapy status. Pharm Eng 35(1):1–11
147. Jacobson F (2016) Antibody drug conjugates – introduction to a new EBE initiative. CMC Strategy Forum – EBE Satellite Session. Paris

HER2-Targeted ADCs: At the Forefront of ADC Technology Development

Kevin J. Hamblett

Abstract Ado-trastuzumab emtansine, referred to as trastuzumab-MCC-DM1 or T-DM1, was the first antibody drug conjugate (ADC) approved for HER2 positive metastatic breast cancer. This chapter reviews the development of trastuzumab-MCC-DM1, summarizes novel anti-HER2 antibody drug conjugate technologies in clinical trials, and discusses future directions of these technologies beyond targeting HER2. In an effort to improve the efficacy of trastuzumab a panel of drug linkers were conjugated to the anti-HER2 antibody and compared in preclinical experiments. In the hallmark phase III EMILIA trial treatment with trastuzumab-MCC-DM1 led to significantly longer median survival compared to the standard of care lapatinib and capecitabine in patients with 2nd line HER2 positive metastatic breast cancer. Subsequently, multiple anti-HER2 ADCs were generated with different ADC platforms allowing a comparison of different drug linkers, drug to antibody ratios, site-specific antibody drug conjugates, and biparatopic antibody drug conjugates. Anti-HER2 antibody drug conjugates currently in clinical testing are described. Promising early clinical data are emerging from some of the ADCs employing novel technologies. Future directions including bispecific antibody drug conjugates directed against HER2 and another target are discussed. Ultimately the goal is to generate clinical candidate ADCs that can improve patient outcomes. Comparison of anti-HER2 ADCs will inform how novel ADC technologies can be applied beyond HER2 to other cancer associated antigens.

Keywords Antibody drug conjugate · HER2 · ERBB2 · Kadcyla · trastuzumab emtansine · T-DM1, DM1

K. J. Hamblett (✉)
Zymeworks Biopharmaceuticals Inc., Seattle, WA, USA
e-mail: kevin.hamblett@zymeworks.com

M. Damelin (ed.), *Innovations for Next-Generation Antibody-Drug Conjugates*, Cancer Drug Discovery and Development,
https://doi.org/10.1007/978-3-319-78154-9_7

Introduction

Receptor tyrosine kinases are transmembrane proteins that regulate cell growth, metabolism, survival, and differentiation. The human epidermal growth factor receptor (HER) family contains four receptor tyrosine kinase members: HER1 (Erb-B1, also known as epidermal growth factor receptor [EGFR]), HER2 (Erb-B2), HER3 (Erb-B3), and HER4 (Erb-B4). Each HER family protein consists of four extracellular domains (ECD) numbered 1–4, for example HER2, as shown in Fig. 1. A specific conformation of HER family receptor ECDs is required for receptor dimerization. Upon HER family receptor dimerization the cytoplasmic kinase domain auto-phosphorylates which subsequently signals downstream proteins. Overexpression or amplification of receptor tyrosine kinases can lead to cancer [1]. HER2 is overexpressed and amplified in a subset of patients with breast, gastric, ovarian, and other cancers [2].

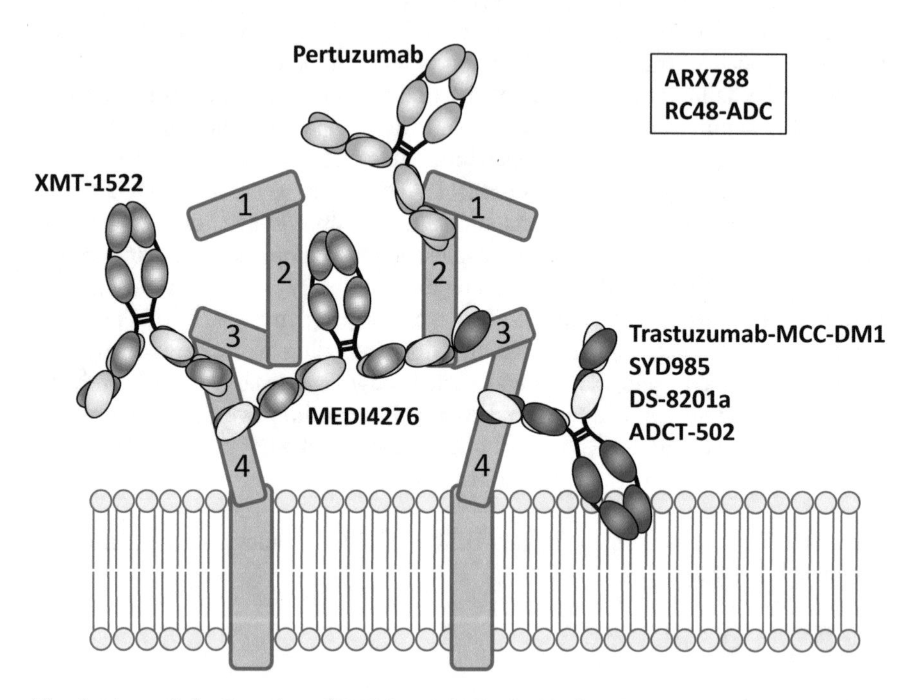

Fig. 1 Extracellular Domains of HER2 and Antibody Binding. Each extracellular domain of HER2 is labelled 1–4. Trastuzumab-based ADCs, trastuzumab-MCC-DM1, SYD985, DS-8201a, and ADCT-502 bind to ECD4 of HER2. Pertuzumab binds to ECD2 of HER2. XMT-1522 binds to an ECD4 epitope different than trastuzumab. MEDI4276 is a bispecific antibody, scFv arm binds to ECD4 (same as trastzumab) and Fab arm binds to ECD2 (distinct from pertuzumab). ARX788 and RC48-ADC binding location is unknown

Approved Anti-HER2 Antibodies

Two anti-HER2 antibodies are approved for cancer treatment: pertuzumab and trastuzumab. Pertuzumab is an anti-HER2 antibody that binds to the second extracellular domain (ECD2) of HER2 and is approved for the treatment of HER2 positive breast cancer [3]. Pertuzumab's primary mechanism of action is antagonism of HER2 homo- and hetero-dimerization and blockade of downstream signaling [3]. Trastuzumab, binds to the fourth extracellular domain (ECD4) of HER2 and is approved for the treatment of HER2 positive breast and gastric cancer [4]. Trastuzumab's mechanisms of action include antibody dependent cellular cytotoxicity and ligand independent blockade of HER2 dimerization, leading to reduced downstream signaling [5, 6]. HER2 is internalized in the presence or absence of trastuzumab [7, 8]. HER2 internalization provides a route to deliver drug into HER2 expressing cancer cells with an antibody drug conjugate (ADC). HER2 is a cell surface candidate for an ADC because the gene is overexpressed in breast and gastric cancers compared to normal tissues and HER2 internalizes.

ADC Components

ADCs contain three components (1) antibody, (2) linker, and (3) drug. The antibody recognizes a cell surface antigen on specific cancer cells. The linker connects the drug to the antibody. Common drugs used in ADCs are often too toxic for use as chemotherapy including agents targeting tubulin or DNA. Drugs are typically conjugated to native antibody amino acids lysines or cysteines to generate an ADC. Conjugation of drugs to native antibody lysines or cysteines generates a distribution of species with different numbers of drug per antibody. Lysine linked conjugates can contain species with 0, 1, 2, 3, 4, 5, 6, 7, or more drugs per antibody. Maytansine based drugs including DM1 and DM4 are commonly conjugated to lysines. Conjugation to the inter-chain disulfide cysteines can yield antibody with 0, 2, 4, 6, and 8 drugs per antibody depending on the level of reducing agent for an IgG1 antibody. Auristatin based drugs including monomethyl auristatin E (MMAE) and monomethyl auristatin F (MMAF) are commonly conjugated to cysteines. The average drug antibody ratio (DAR) is commonly 3–4 for both maytansine and auristatin based ADCs. DAR 4 was selected for MMAE based ADCs due to the larger therapeutic index of DAR 4 compared to DAR 8 [9]. Maytansine based ADCs with DARs above 9 distribute to the liver reducing the efficacy compared to DAR 2–6 [10].

Linkers are classified into either cleavable (i.e. valine-citrulline) or non-cleavable (i.e. maleimide-caproyl). Cleavable linkers activate following a pH change, enzyme recognition, or disulfide reduction to liberate a specific drug [11–13]. S-methyl-DM4, MMAE, pyrrolobenzodiazepines, and other drugs that employ cleavable linkers are typically membrane permeable and can enter adjacent cells and mediate cell death, a process referred to as bystander killing [13–15]. Non-cleavable linkers are not broken following ADC internalization and catabolism, the drug remains attached to the amino acid it was conjugated to, generating the catabolite amino acid-linker-drug. To be an effective ADC, the non-cleavable linker catabolite must be capable of arriving at and binding to the drug's intracellular target [16, 17]. Non-cleavable linker catabolites such as cysteine-mcMMAF and lysine-MCC-DM1 do not exhibit bystander activity as they are more polar and significantly less potent than free drugs liberated with cleavable linkers such as MMAE and DM1 [13, 18].

ADC Mechanism of Action

The mechanism of action of an antibody drug conjugate is a multi-step process and dependent on the specific linkers and drugs. First, the antibody part of the ADC binds to a cell surface antigen and the antigen-ADC complex is internalized into endosomes. Endosome acidification decreases the pH from 7.4 to approximately pH 5.5–6.0 [19]. Late endosomes and their contents ultimately fuse with lysosomes wherein the pH drops to 5.0–5.5 activating lysosomal proteases. Along the endolysosomal pathway pH-sensitive linkers are cleaved to release drug. For example, the pH-sensitive benzyl carbonate linker in the anti-TROP2-CL2A-SN38 conjugate IMMU-132 is hydrolyzed with a half-life of 10.2 h at pH 5.0 to yield SN-38, and thus presumably some SN-38 release occurs in the late endosome and lysosome [20, 21]. Lysosomal function is required for activity of ADCs containing disulfide and protease-sensitive linkers as lysosomal inhibitors, including bafilomycin, and gene knock-down of lysosomal ATPase subunits abolish ADC potency [17, 22–24]. Within the lysosome the antibody component of the ADC is catabolized into amino acids to generate amino acid-linker-drug [17, 22]. The only catabolites identified with the non-cleavable linker ADCs Ab-MCC-DM1 and Ab-mcMMAF were amino acid-linker-drug lysine-MCC-DM1 and cysteine-mcMMAF, respectively [16, 17]. Maytansine-based non-cleavable linker catabolites including lysine-MCC-DM1 exit the lysosome via the lysosomal transporter SLC46A3 [24]. For ADCs with cleavable disulfide linkers such as the SPDB, lysine-SPDB-DM4 is formed. Next, the disulfide linker is cleaved by reduction to form DM4 with a free sulfhydryl, which is methylated to form S-methyl-DM4 [17]. Cleavable MMAE auristatin ADCs use dipeptide linkers such as valine-citrulline (vc) recognized by lysosomal proteases [11, 25]. After valine-citrulline peptide bond cleavage the adjacent para-amino benzyloxycarbonyl (PABC) spacer self-immolates to generate MMAE.

Selection of a cleavable or non-cleavable linker can depend on many factors including antigen expression homo- or heterogeneity, internalization of the ADC into the cell, and tolerability. Some antigens are expressed in a heterogeneous fashion within a tumor, Kovtun et al. modeled this with a mixture of antigen positive and negative cells [13]. Cleavable DM1 ADC was efficacious in the mixed cell tumors with heterogeneous antigen expression, whereas the non-cleavable DM1 ADC was not efficacious. The catabolites of non-cleavable linker ADCs, e.g. lysine-MCC-DM1 liberated from Ab-MCC-DM1, typically have poor cell potency due to restricted cell membrane permeability, in the hundred nM range or higher, three to four orders of magnitude less potent than drugs liberated from cleavable linkers [18]. Polson et al. observed that robust antigen internalization is necessary for the function of non-cleavable linker ADCs, but not cleavable linker ADCs [26].

Trastuzumab-MCC-DM1 Preclinical Development

Trastuzumab based ADCs were explored to determine if an anti-HER2 ADC could improve the efficacy of trastuzumab. Lewis Philips et al. conjugated maytansinoids to the lysines of trastuzumab with hetero-bifunctional linkers with an approximate drug to antibody ratio of 3.5. The cleavable linkers SPDP and SPP were used to couple DM1, cleavable SSNPP to couple either DM3 or DM4, and the non-cleavable SMCC linker to couple DM1 [27]. The four cleavable linker conjugates contain disulfide bonds with adjacent methyl substitutions that provide steric hindrance to protect or expose the disulfide bond. The location and orientation of the methyl substitutions impact the rate of disulfide reduction and correlates with linker stability [28]. SSNPP is chemically similar to the SPDB linker, with SSNPP containing a methyl substituent adjacent to the disulfide on the antibody side. Conjugation of DM1 to trastuzumab via the non-cleavable linker SMCC generated trastuzumab-MCC-DM1, also referred to as T-DM1, ado-trastuzumab emtansine, or Kadcyla. Comparison of the four cleavable linker and one non-cleavable linker trastuzumab conjugates in BT-474 and SK-BR-3, two HER2 3+ cell lines, yielded similar potency. The serum concentration profiles of trastuzumab conjugated to SMCC-DM1 and SSNPP-DM4 were similar and significantly longer than SSNPP-DM3, SPP-DM1 and SPDP-DM1 conjugates. In contrast to the conjugate serum concentration profiles, the total antibody serum concentrations of trastuzumab-MCC-DM1 and trastuzumab-SPP-DM1 were similar indicating that DM1 was released from trastuzumab-SPP-DM1 faster than trastuzumab-MCC-DM1, which was subsequently confirmed by Erickson et al. [29]. Trastuzumab-MCC-DM1 treatment of animals bearing MMTV-HER2 Fo5 tumor transplant model was more efficacious than either trastuzmab-SPP-DM1 or trastuzumab-SSNPP-DM4. Interestingly, in the BT-474EEI, model the efficacy of trastuzumab-MCC-DM1 and trastzumab-SPP-DM1 were similar despite an approximate twofold difference in conjugate serum concentration exposure [29]. Despite the serum concentration differences, similar concentrations of radiolabeled DM1 catabolites were observed in the BT-474EEI tumors for trastuzumab-MCC-DM1 and trastuzumab-SPP-DM1 which likely contributed to the similar efficacy in this model. Trastuzumab-MCC-DM1 was tolerated in rats at 25 mg/kg (1632 μg/m^2 DM1) with no difference in percent weight change from the day of dosing compared to vehicle (15.9% vs. 16.3%, respectively) and a 6.7% increase in weight when administered with 50 mg/kg

(3264 μg/m^2 DM1). In contrast, 22 mg/kg (1632 μg /m^2 DM1) trastuzumab-SPP-DM1 led to a 10% decrease in weight over the course of the study. Trastuzumab-MCC-DM1 was selected for additional investigation based on the improved efficacy and tolerability, and thus therapeutic index, as compared to trastuzumab-SPP-DM1, similar to the findings with CD22 antibody drug conjugates with non-cleavable and cleavable linkers [26].

Trastuzumab-MCC-DM1 was evaluated in preclinical efficacy and toxicity studies prior to filing an investigational new drug application. Conjugation of DM1 did not attenuate the innate mechanisms of trastuzumab: antibody dependent cellular cytotoxicity, and inhibition of downstream signaling [18]. Trastuzumab-MCC-DM1 treatment of multiple HER2 positive (IHC 3+) breast cancer and gastric cancer xenografts was more efficacious than the unconjugated antibody trastuzumab [27, 30]. Trastuzumab does not cross-react with rat HER2, nevertheless the toxicology assessment of trastuzumab-MCC-DM1 included studies in both rats and non-human primates [31]. Trastuzumab-MCC-DM1 was tolerated at 40 mg/kg (~4400 μg/m^2 DM1) in rats when administered as a single intravenous (IV) dose, whereas 60 mg/kg (~6800–7800 μg/m^2 DM1) was not tolerated. Rats tolerated 11 mg/kg of trastuzumab-MCC-DM1 once weekly for three total doses, however, 22 mg/kg was not tolerated. Histopathology revealed dose-dependent effects on the liver, bone marrow, and lymphoid organs after trastuzumab-MCC-DM1 administration in rats.

Four doses of trastuzumab-MCC-DM1 administered IV once every 3 weeks to cynomolgus monkeys was tolerated at 30 mg/kg (6000 μg/m^2 DM1). Treatment related findings in cynomolgus monkeys were similar to the rat with hepatic, bone marrow, and lymphoid organ findings. Trastuzumab-MCC-DM1 related findings were also observed in epithelial and phagocytic cells in cynomolgus monkeys. Decreased platelets and red cell parameters correlated with the histopathology findings in the bone marrow. Increased transaminase elevations (AST and ALT) correlated with histopathology findings in the liver. Conjugated trastuzumab-MCC-DM1 clearance was more rapid than total antibody clearance in cynomolgus monkeys, similar to observations in mice [29]. Trastuzumab-MCC-DM1 was advanced to clinical testing based on the preclinical evidence including efficacy in multiple xenograft models and the tolerability profile in cynomolgus monkeys.

Trastuzumab-MCC-DM1 Clinical Development: Second Line Metastatic HER2 Positive Breast Cancer

A phase I clinical trial (NCT00932373/TMD3569g) evaluated trastuzumab-MCC-DM1 in HER2 positive metastatic breast cancer patients that relapsed following a trastuzumab regimen. Two dosing strategies were evaluated, once every 3 weeks

[32] and once weekly [33]. Doses ranged from 0.3 to 4.8 mg/kg in the once three weekly dosing regimen. Dose limiting transient grade 4 thrombocytopenia was observed in two of three patients dosed at 4.8 mg/kg every 3 weeks leading to dose de-escalation. Fifteen patients were administered 3.6 mg/kg, the maximum tolerated dose (MTD), and clinical responses were observed in five of the fifteen patients based on RECIST criteria. In humans, the pharmacokinetic profiles of total trastuzumab and trastuzumab-MCC-DM1 diverged indicating loss of DM1 following administration, similar to the pre-clinical data [29]. Trastuzumab-MCC-DM1 half-life in humans at 3.6 mg/kg, the MTD, was approximately 4 days across multiple studies, similar to the half-life observed in cynomolgus monkeys at the highest non-severely toxic dose [31, 34]. Weekly dosing had a lower MTD of 2.4 mg/kg compared to the once every 3 week regimen. The weekly dosing schedule had a twofold higher exposure than the once every 3 week dosing schedule. Nevertheless, no difference between the two dosing schedules was observed in the clinical benefit rate, which is the combination of complete responses, partial responses and stable disease >6 months. Next, a single arm phase II study evaluating trastuszumab-MCC-DM1 once every 3 weeks at 3.6 mg/kg was initiated (NCT00509769/TDM4258g) [35]. Trastuzumab-MCC-DM1 generated a response rate of 25.9% in HER2 positive metastatic breast cancer patients that had relapsed on HER2 therapy.

Trastuzumab-MCC-DM1 was directly compared to standard of care in a randomized phase III registration study, referred to as EMILIA [36]. In total 991 patients previously treated with trastuzumab and a taxane were administered either trastuzumab-MCC-DM1 or the combination of lapatinib and capecitabine. Trastuzumab-MCC-DM1 at 3.6 mg/kg, once every 3 weeks increased progression free survival (9.6 vs. 6.4 months) and overall survival (30.9 months vs. 25.1 months) compared to lapatinib and capecitabine. Forty-three percent of patients treated with trastuzumab-MCC-DM1 achieved a complete or partial response in contrast to 30.8% of patients treated with lapatinib and capecitabine. Fewer grade 3 or 4 adverse events were observed with trastuzumab-MCC-DM1 (40.8%) as compared to lapatinib and capecitabine (57.0%). The types of grade 3 and 4 adverse events were different amongst the treatment arms. Thrombocytopenia and increased liver transaminases were the most frequently observed adverse events in trastuzumab-MCC-DM1 treated patients. Diarrhea, hand-foot syndrome, and vomiting were the most frequently observed adverse events in lapatinib and capecitabine treated patients. The EMILIA trial demonstrated that trastuzumab-MCC-DM1 is more efficacious and safer than the combination of lapatinib and capecitabine. Trastuzumab-MCC-DM1 was approved by the FDA in February 2013 for the treatment of HER2 positive metastatic breast cancer in patients that have relapsed following trastuzumab and taxane. To reduce confusion with trastuzumab prescriptions the conjugated form trastuzumab-MCC-DM1 was given the USAN name ado-trastuzumab emtansine and trade name Kadcyla.

Trastuzumab-MCC-DM1 Clinical Development: First Line Metastatic HER2 Positive Breast Cancer

Clinical trials with trastuzumab-MCC-DM1 as a single agent and in combination were initiated to explore its utility in earlier treatment. Trastuzumab, pertuzumab, and taxanes are the first line drugs approved for HER2 positive breast cancer. Taxanes stabilize microtubules, in contrast maytansine based molecules, including lysine-MCC-DM1, inhibit microtubule polymerization. The mechanisms of trastuzumab-MCC-DM1 and taxanes are in opposition and thus not suitable for combination. Trastuzumab would likely compete for HER2 positive cells and could reduce the efficacy of trastuzumab-MCC-DM1 if combined. Pertuzumab binds to ECD2 of HER2, a distinct epitope different from trastuzumab's epitope, ECD4, Fig. 1, and thus pertuzumab can be combined with a trastuzumab containing molecule. Thus, the combination of pertuzumab and trastuzumab-MCC-DM1 was explored in preclinical models. Combination of trastuzumab-MCC-DM1 and pertuzumab improved the potency and efficacy as compared to either agent alone in MDA-175 (HER2 1+) *in vitro* and *in vivo* [37]. The effect of combining trastuzumab-MCC-DM1 and pertuzumab in HER2 expressing (3+) cell lines was variable with some lines demonstrating additivity or synergy in the presence of heregulin, a ligand for HER3 and HER4. Yet, in the absence of heregulin the addition of pertuzumab did not increase the *in vitro* potency of trastuzumab-MCC-DM1 in multiple HER2 3+ cell lines, including KPL-4. Efficacy of the trastuzumab-MCC-DM1 and pertuzumab combination modestly improved the time to tumor volume doubling compared to the single agents in the KPL-4 xenograft model. The MARIANNE trial evaluated the utility of trastuzumab-MCC-DM1 in previously untreated metastatic breast cancer patients as both a single agent and in combination with pertuzumab compared to the standard of care trastuzumab plus a taxane [38]. Progression free survival and response rates of trastuzumab-MCC-DM1 alone or in combination with pertuzumab were non-inferior as compared to trastuzumab plus taxane. Patients treated with trastuzumab-MCC-DM1 alone (45.4%) and in combination with pertuzumab (46.2%) had fewer grade 3 and higher adverse events than trastuzumab plus taxane (54.1%). Amongst patients that responded to treatment the duration of response was longer in patients administered trastuzumab-MCC-DM1 as compared to trastuzumab plus taxane. The disconnect between the preclinical data and clinical findings could be due to the patient population tested as the greatest combination benefit was observed in the HER2 1+ MDA-MB-175 model.

Trastuzumab-MCC-DM1 Clinical Development: Non-Breast HER2 Positive Malignancies

Approximately 20% of gastric cancer patients overexpress HER2 and are eligible for trastuzumab combination therapy [39]. Trastuzumab-MCC-DM1 preclinical efficacy correlates with HER2 expression in gastric cancer cell lines [30]. The GATSBY trial (NCT01641939/BO27952) was performed to assess the efficacy of trastuzumab-MCC-DM1 in metastatic gastric cancer patients compared to a taxane [40]. Two dosing regimens of trastuzumab-MCC-DM1 were evaluated in separate study arms, 3.6 mg/kg once every 3 weeks and 2.4 mg/kg once weekly. Overall survival of both trastuzumab-MCC-DM1 regimens (7.9 months) was similar to taxane (8.6 months). HER2 expression in gastric cancer is heterogeneous more frequently than breast cancer which leads to different scoring systems in the two indications and could have contributed to the lack of preclinical to clinic translation in gastric cancer [41]. Trastuzumab-MCC-DM1 lacks bystander activity which could limit efficacy in malignancies with heterogeneous expression of HER2, such as gastric cancer.

HER2 ADCs Following Trastuzumab-MCC-DM1

The treatment paradigm for second line HER2 positive metastatic breast cancer now includes trastuzumab-MCC-DM1 establishing HER2 as a clinically validated targeted for ADCs. Building on trastuzumab-MCC-DM1 several anti-HER2 ADCs are at the preclinical stage, some of which may enter the clinic in the future [42–45]. Seven anti-HER2 ADCs are currently in clinical trials, each molecule has modified one or more components of trastzumab-MCC-DM1: the antibody, linker, drug, or method of conjugation (Table 1).

ADC Technology: Cleavable Linker

Remegen developed an anti-HER2 ADC with a cleavable linker to explore how an ADC with bystander activity compared to trastuzumab-MCC-DM1. Remegen immunized mice with the HER2 ECD and generated the antibody hertuzumab, also referred to as RC48 [46, 47]. Hertuzumab does not compete with trastuzumab and binds with higher affinity to HER2 [47]. Hertuzumab was conjugated to the cleavable mc-vc-PABC-MMAE with an average DAR of 4 to generate hertuzumab-vc-MMAE. Hertuzumab-vc-MMAE efficacy was similar to trastuzumab-MCC-DM1 in BT474 xenografts. Hertuzumab-vc-MMAE was more efficacious than

Table 1 Anti-HER2 ADCs in clinical development

Clinical candidate	Epitope ECD (if known) [antibody]	Linker class	Drug/Class	Notes
Trastuzumab-MCC-DM1	Anti-ECD4 [trastuzumab]	Non-cleavable	DM1/Maytansine	Approved
RC48-ADC	Anti-HER2 Hertuzumab	Cleavable	MMAE/Auristatin	
ARX788	Anti-HER2 Unknown	Non-cleavable	AS269/Auristatin	Site-specific, DAR = 2
SYD985	Anti-ECD4 [trastuzumab]	Cleavable	DUBA/Duocarmycin	Fractionated, DAR2 and DAR4
DS-8201a	Anti-ECD4 [trastuzumab]	Cleavable	DXd/Topoisomerase I Inhibitor	Complete cysteine loading, DAR = 8
ADCT-502	Anti-ECD4 [trastuzumab]	Cleavable	Tesirine/ Pyrrolobenzodiazepine dimer (PBD)	Site-specific, DAR = 2
XMT-1522	Anti-ECD4 [HT19]	Cleavable	Auristatin F-HPA/ Auristatin	Polymer-linker-drug, DAR~15
MEDI4276	Anti-ECD2 [39S] x anti-ECD4 [trastuzumab scFv]	Cleavable	AZ13599185/Tubulysin	Site-Specific, DAR = 4

trastuzumab-MCC-DM1 in BT474/T721 cell line xenografts, which were developed to be lapatinib and trastuzumab resistant. Hertuzumab-vc-MMAE was more efficacious than trastuzumab-MCC-DM1 in SK-OV-3 ovarian cancer xenografts [46]. RC48-ADC is currently in multiple phase I clinical trials for HER2 expressing malignancies (NCT02881138/NCT02881190). RC-48 contains a different antibody than trastuzumab-MCC-DM1 and uses a cleavable linker with the auristatin MMAE.

ADC Technology Improvements: Site-Specific Antibody Drug Conjugates

Junutula et al. introduced cysteine mutations into an antibody sequence at different amino acid locations, referred to as Thiomabs, to site-specifically conjugate with two drugs per antibody [48]. A site-specific anti-MUC16 thiomab drug conjugate (TDC) maintained efficacy and improved the tolerability, and thus the therapeutic index, as compared to a heterogeneous ADC. Location of the site-specific cysteine influences the stability of the ADC which can impact the efficacy and tolerability

[49, 50]. Recently, an anti-MUC16 TDC escalated to a dose of 5.6 mg/kg in patients, approximately twofold higher than the ADC version [51]. Thiomab versions of trastuzumab with either a non-cleavable DM1 or cleavable MMAE recapitulated that a site-specific conjugate can increase the therapeutic index compared to a heterogeneous ADC in preclinical models [48, 50]. Cysteine mutation represents one way to generate a homogeneous site-specific antibody conjugate. Alternative methods to generate homogeneous site-specific antibody drug conjugates include introduction of non-natural amino acids or selenocysteine, chemical bridging of the four inter-chain native disulfide cysteines, enzyme modification of amino acid side chains contained within a specific recognized protein sequence, and glycan modification [42, 52–54]. Introduction of non-natural amino acids, such as a para-azidomethyl-L-phenylalanine or para-acetylphenylalanine, into a protein sequence permits bio-orthogonal chemistry to be performed [53, 54]. Bio-orthogonal chemistry approaches to generate site-specific ADCs do not modify the native amino acid side chains, in contrast to the standard methods of cysteine and lysine conjugation.

Ambrx generated an anti-HER2 antibody that contains the non-natural amino acid para acetyl phenylalanine (pAcF) [55]. Early preclinical work utilized trastuzumab with pAcF, however, it is not clear if trastuzumab is the anti-HER2 antibody employed in the final clinical candidate ARX788 [56]. ARX788 is an anti-HER2 antibody with two pAcF amino acids conjugated to AS269 with a DAR of 1.9. AS269 is the auristatin MMAF with a non-cleavable hydroxyl amino PEG linker. ARX788 was more potent than trastuzumab-MCC-DM1 in three cell lines with moderate HER2 expression (153-fold in JIMT-1, 30-fold in MDA-MB-453, and 8.7-fold in MDA-MB-175). ARX788 potency was similar to trastuzumab-MCC-DM1 in four cell lines with high HER2 expression (SKBR3, HCC1954, NCI-N87 and SKOV-3) and 4–8-fold more potent in two cell lines with high HER2 expression (Calu-3 and BT474). Non-cleavable conjugates containing either the auristatin MMAF or maytansine DM1 targeting CD79b had similar efficacy suggesting that use of the non-cleavable MMAF would have similar potency and efficacy compared to non-cleavable DM1 conjugates [57]. The potency differences observed could be due to binding a different epitope than trastuzumab if a different antibody was used, or differences in the trafficking, potency, or cellular retention of pAcF-AS269 compared to lysine-MCC-DM1. ARX788 was efficacious in mice bearing HER2 expressing NCI-N87, SKOV-3, HCC-1954, and JIMT-1 xenografts. ARX788 was more efficacious than trastuzumab-MCC-DM1 in JIMT-1 and NCI-N87 at both dose levels. However, in SKOV-3 ARX788 was more efficacious than trastuzuzmab-MCC-DM1 only at the low dose. In HCC-1954 the efficacy of ARX788 and trastuzumab-MCC-DM1 was similar at both dose levels. ARX788 conjugate serum concentration was similar to total antibody in non-human primates indicating that the drug linker was stable through 20 days. Thus part of the efficacy improvement of ARX788 over trastuzumab-MCC-DM1 could be because of higher conjugate serum concentration exposure. A Phase I study investigating ARX788 in advanced cancers expressing HER2 is underway (NCT02512237).

ADC Technology Improvements: Novel Drug-Linkers

A DNA alkylating agent, duocarmycin, was conjugated to trastuzumab to evaluate the effect of a different mechanism of action on ADC properties. Duocarmycins are DNA alkylating agents that exhibit potent activity and toxicity [58]. However, the potency of duocarmycins led to toxicity in humans prior to reaching efficacious doses. ADC technology using duocarmycins was explored to augment the therapeutic index of duocarmycin [59]. Seco-duocarmycin-hydroxybenzamide-azaindole (DUBA) was conjugated to trastuzumab cysteines using the cleavable valine-citrulline linker and a self-immolative spacer to generate SYD983. As a cysteine conjugate SYD983 contains DAR 0, 2, 4, 6, and 8. Hydrophobic interaction chromatography fractionated SYD983 to primarily contain DAR 2 and DAR 4 species for the clinical candidate molecule SYD985, which has an average DAR of 2.7 [60]. SYD985 had similar binding and internalization compared to unconjugated trastuzumab. SYD985 in vitro potency was similar to trastuzumab-MCC-DM1 in the HER2 3+ cell lines SK-BR-3, UACC-93 and NCI-N87 [61]. SYD985 was approximately 10–100 fold more potent than trastuzumab-MCC-DM1 in cell lines with lower HER2 expression SK-OV-3 (2+), MDA-MB-175-VII (1+), and ZR-75-1 (1+). After dipeptide linker cleavage and spacer self-immolation SYD985 releases seco-DUBA, a cell membrane permeable compound. In contrast to trastuzumab-MCC-DM1, SYD985 is capable of bystander activity after exposure to HER2 expressing cells. SYD985 was more efficacious than trastuzumab-MCC-DM1 in the BT-474 xenograft model and several patient derived xenograft models with HER2 expression ranging from 3+ down to 1+. An isotype control antibody-vc-seco-DUBA conjugate demonstrated efficacy in some patient derived xenograft models, typically similar efficacy to approximately 1/3 the dose of SYD985. Part of the efficacy of the isotype control conjugate in mouse xenograft models may be due to the poor conjugate stability of antibody-vc-seco-DUBA conjugates in mouse plasma [60]. A mouse-specific carboxylestease, cCES1c was identified as a contributor to the poor mouse plasma stability. The poor plasma stability may account for some of the efficacy observed with SYD985 and the isotype control conjugate. Alternatively it is possible that in species lacking cCES1c SYD985 may be more efficacious due to greater exposure of intact ADC as compared to mice where ADC exposure is attenuated because of poor conjugate stability. A component of SYD985 efficacy was demonstrated to be antibody targeted by pre-treating xenograft models with tenfold excess trastuzumab which attenuated SYD985 efficacy. The highest non-severely toxic dose of SYD983, the SYD985 parent, was 30 mg/kg administered every 3.5 weeks for two doses in non-human primates. SYD985 is currently in a phase I clinical trial for HER2 expressing malignancies (NCT02277717).

SYD985 was administered once every 3 weeks to all solid tumor patients in the phase I dose escalation and patients with either breast, gastric, urothelial or endometrial cancers with at least HER2 1+ in the dose expansion phase. Dose limiting toxicity was observed at the 2.4 mg/kg dose [62]. Eye disorders were observed in 3 out of the 39 patients and appeared to be dose dependent. Out of 34 patients nine responses were observed (26.5%). Twenty-two patients treated with SYD985 had breast cancer, eight of which had a response (36.4%). Fourteen breast cancer patients were HER2 positive (IHC 3+), responses were observed in five of these patients (35.7%). The remaining eight breast cancer patients were HER2 negative (IHC 2+ or lower), three of which had a response (37.5%). SYD985 generated responses at tolerated doses and advanced to the second part of its phase I trial.

Topoisomerase I inhibitors are another class of DNA agents explored in clinical trials [63]. Exatecan mesylate, a potent inhibitor was explored in clinical trials as a free compound (DX-8951) and in a pro-drug form (DE-310) [64, 65]. DE-310 consists of DX-8951 conjugated to a tetrapeptide glycine-glycine-phenylalanine-glycine (GGFG) peptidyl moiety attached to a carboxymethyldextran polyalcohol polymer. The peptide spacer of DE-310 is catabolized in lysosomes to yield DX-8951 [66, 67]. To generate the ADC DS-8201a, trastuzumab was conjugated to the cleavable GGFG peptide linker attached to a derivative of DX-8951, referred to as DXd or MAAA-1181 [68]. In contrast to other drug linker technologies DS-8201a is conjugated to DXd at all eight native cysteines of trastuzumab's four inter-chain disulfide bonds to yield a DAR of 8. DXd maintained the DNA topoisomerase activity of DX-8951 with an IC_{50} of 0.31 μM, about an order of magnitude more potent than SN-38. Cell growth inhibition ranged from 6.7–26.8 ng/mL, approximately 0.04–0.18 nM of ADC in three HER2 positive cell lines. Conjugation of DXd did not change trastuzumab's innate mechanisms of action, antibody dependent cellular cytotoxicity or downstream signaling blockade. DS-8201a demonstrated DNA damage effects similar to DXd as assessed by phosphorylation of Chk1 and H2A.X. Minimal separation of DS-8201a total antibody and conjugate serum concentrations were observed through 28 days in mice, suggesting that the drug linker is stable. However, additional assays are needed to confirm the in vivo drug-linker stability of DS-8201a. Regressions were observed after a single dose of DS-8201a at 4 mg/kg in the HER2 3+ NCI-N87 xenograft model. DS-8201a delayed tumor growth after two 10 mg/kg doses 1 week apart in the HER2 moderate, trastuzumab-MCC-DM1 resistant, JIMT-1 xenograft model. DS-8201a with DAR 8 was more efficacious compared to the same ADC with a DAR of 3.4 when dosed at the same protein dose (10 mg/kg) in the HER2 low model Capan-1. DS-8201a was more efficacious than trastuzumab-MCC-DM1 in the JIMT-1, Capan-1, and CFPAC-1 xenograft models. A tenfold excess of trastuzumab abolished the efficacy of DS-8201a in the HER2 low CFPAC-1 model. DS-8201a generated regressions in four patient derived xenograft (PDX) models ranging from HER2 1+ to 3+ after a single dose of 10 mg/kg. In contrast, trastuzumab-MCC-DM1 was efficacious in only one PDX model, ST225. To determine the role of bystander activity on the efficacy of DS-8201a a modified form of the DXd drug with less cell membrane permeability was generated, referred to as DXd(2). DS-8201a was capable of killing antigen positive and negative co-cultured cells in vitro and in vivo, whereas the anti-HER2 antibody conjugate with the non-cell membrane permeable DXd(2) did not affect the HER2 negative cells [69]. The highest non-severely toxic dose of DS-8201a administered once every 3 weeks to cynomolgus monkeys was 30 mg/kg. At 78.8 mg/kg bone marrow, intestinal, and pulmonary toxicity was observed with

DS-8201a. DS-8201a is being explored in a phase I treatment for the treatment of breast and gastric cancer patients in the dose escalation (NCT02564900).

DS-8201a was administered once every 3 weeks between 0.8 and 8 mg/kg. The highest dose administered was 8 mg/kg, yet the maximum tolerated dose was not reached [70]. Seven of twenty patients achieved a response (35%) in the dose escalation phase, two patients with gastric cancer and five with breast cancer. Patients in the dose expansion were administered either 5.4 or 6.4 mg/kg DS-8201a every 3 weeks [71]. Nineteen of fifty (38%) evaluable patients achieved a complete or partial response in the dose expansion. Four of fourteen patients (29%) with low HER2 achieved a response. Nausea (62%), anorexia (56%), and platelet decreases (28%) were the most common adverse events. A phase II study is planned to further evaluate DS-8201a.

Pyrrolobenzodiazepine dimers (PBD) bind to DNA and lead to DNA breaks and inhibition of DNA-protein interactions. Trastuzumab was site-specifically conjugated to the PBD tesirine to generate ADCT-502 [72, 73]. ADCT-502 generated complete regressions in the HER2 1+ HBCx-10 breast cancer PDX model after a single dose of 0.2 mg/kg. No efficacy was observed in the HBCx-10 model following a single dose of trastuzumab-MCC-DM1 at 30 mg/kg. ADCT-502 is being explored in a phase I trial for the patients with HER2 expressing breast, gastric, non-small cell lung and bladder cancer (NCT03125200).

ADC Technology Improvements: Increased Drug Loading

To increase the number of drugs conjugated to an antibody more than lysine or cysteine conjugation, Mersana developed a polymer, referred to as a Fleximer, each of which contains four to five drugs. Three to five Fleximers are attached to antibody cysteines with maleimide chemistry [74]. The anti-HER2 antibody HT19, which binds to ECD4 of HER2, was conjugated to approximately fifteen auristatin F hydroxypropylamide (AF-HPA) drugs per antibody with Fleximer technology, to generate XMT-1522 [75]. HT19 and trastuzumab both bind to ECD4 of HER2, however, they do not block each other indicating that they bind distinct epitopes. Within lysosomes the Fleximer polymer is hypothesized to be degraded into glycerol and glycolate and AF-HPA is released from the Fleximer by carboxylesterases [76, 77]. AF-HPA is capable of bystander activity, presumably because its ability to cross cell membranes. However, AF-HPA is subsequently metabolized into auristatin F (AF) in vivo which is less cell permeable than AF-HPA [78]. Free AF-HPA concentration peaks in NCI-N87 xenograft bearing animals approximately 2 days after ADC administration and declines thereafter. Free AF continues to increase in concentration peaking between 7 and 14 days. XMT-1522 was between 3 and 2500-fold more potent than trastuzumab-MCC-DM1 in vitro in HER2 expressing cell lines. XMT-1522 achieved complete regressions at a dose of 1 mg/kg in the NCI-N87 xenograft model. In contrast, trastuzumab-MCC-DM1 generated complete regressions at a dose of 10 mg/kg in the NCI-N87 xenograft model. XMT-1522 demonstrated superior efficacy to trastuzumab-MCC-DM1 in cell line xenograft models JIMT-1 (HER2 2+) and SNU5 (HER2 1+). Efficacy of XMT-1522 was observed in multiple PDX models with a range of HER2 expression [79]. Trastuzumab conjugated to the Fleximer-AF-HPA was administered at 0.67, 1.34, and 2.68 mg/kg to non-human primates which led to a decrease in platelet levels and increases in AST and ALT levels [80]. XMT1522 likely has a similar toxicology profile to trastuzumab-Fleximer-AF-HPA as the antibodies bind to ECD2 of HER2. XMT-1522 is currently in a phase I clinical trial in advanced breast cancer patients with HER2 of 1+ or higher (NCT02952729).

ADC Technology Improvements: Enhanced Internalization

Bispecific antibody technology is being explored to treat cancer by redirecting and activating T-cells, blocking two ligands, blocking two receptors, or increased receptor crosslinking [81]. Bispecific antibodies designed to improve internalization and lysosomal routing could enhance the potency of ADCs. The anti-HER2 antibody 39S binds to a distinct epitope of HER2 that does not block trastuzumab or pertuzumab. MEDI4276 consists of the single-chain variable fragment of trastuzumab fused to the fully human anti-HER2 antibody 39S, to generate a biparatopic anti-HER2 antibody [82]. The biparatopic anti-HER2 antibody internalized into BT-474 cells more rapidly than trastuzumab, pertuzumab or the combination. Cysteine mutations were introduced into the anti-HER2 biparatopic antibody at serines 239 and 442 for site specific conjugation. A leucine to phenylalanine mutation at position 234 was also introduced into the bispecific anti-HER2 antibody. Mutation of serine 239 and leucine 234 reduced binding to Fcγ receptors. Fcγ receptor binding led to uptake of trastuzumab-MCC-DM1 in megakaryocytes and their subsequent destruction was hypothesized to be the cause of thrombocytopenia [83]. Reduced binding of MEDI4276 to Fcγ receptors was intended to prevent thrombocytopenia caused by ADC depletion of megakaryocytes. The drug linker AZ13601508 is comprised of the tubulysin AZ13599185 linked to a maleimidocaproyl by a lysine protease cleavable linker [84]. To generate MEDI4276, AZ13601508 was conjugated to the site-specific cysteines of the anti-HER2 biparatopic antibody. MEDI4276 was significantly more potent than trastuzumab-MCC-DM1 in all HER2 expressing cell lines tested. Weekly dosing of 3 mg/kg of MEDI4276 for four doses led to complete regressions in JIMT-1 and a trastuzumab-MCC-DM1 resistant NCI-N87 xenograft model, whereas no response was observed after trastuzumab-MCC-DM1 treatment. MEDI4276 generated regressions in twelve of seventeen (70%) PDX models with HER2 0, 1+, or 2+ expression. Cynomolgus monkeys treated with MEDI4276 experienced impacts to tissues similar to the tubulin inhibitor mechanism of action, presumably myelosuppression, as well as gastrointestinal toxicity. MEDI4276 is in a phase I clinical trial for patients with advanced HER2 expressing breast or gastric cancer (NCT02576548).

Trastuzumab-MCC-DM1 Resistance and Potential Impact

There are at least seven anti-HER2 antibody drug conjugates currently in clinical trials (Table 1). All of the ADCs described herein were observed to be more efficacious than trastuzumab-MCC-DM1 in specific settings. Mechanisms of acquired trastuzumab-MCC-DM1 resistance include reduction of HER2 levels on the cell surface, increased levels of multi-drug resistance transporters, modified ADC intracellular trafficking, and modulation of signaling pathways [85–87]. Each technology and new clinical candidate may be able to address distinct components of trastuzumab-MCC-DM1 resistance. MMAE used in RC48 could be less susceptible than lysine-MCC-DM1 to specific multi-drug resistant transporters. RC48 demonstrated superior efficacy against a lapatinib and trastuzumab resistant BT-474 cell line compared to trastuzumab-MCC-DM1, suggesting that MMAE could be less susceptible to downstream signaling mutation resistance [47]. ARX788 and trastuzumab-MCC-DM1 both employ non-cleavable linkers and generate the amino acid-linker-drug catabolites pAF-AS269 and lysine-MCC-DM1, respectively. After antibody catabolism in the lysosome lysine-MCC-DM1 is transported into the cytoplasm by SLC46A3, however, auristatin non-cleavable catabolites do not require SLC46A3 [24]. Thus, ARX788 with the auristatin based catabolite pAF-AS269 could overcome trastuzumab-MCC-DM1 resistant cells due to aberrant SLC46A3 function or expression. Presumably some multi-drug-resistant transporters that could mediate trastuzumab-MCC-DM1 resistance might not recognize pAF-AS269 as a substrate, however, there is evidence that ABCC1 recognized both maytansine and auristatin based non-cleavable linker catabolites [87]. RC48-ADC, SYD985, DS-8201a, XMT-1522, and MEDI4276 all report some bystander activity which could overcome innate trastuzumab-MCC-DM1 resistance, HER2 expression heterogeneity, and trastuzmab-MCC-DM1 induction of decreased HER2 expression. The drugs MMAE, AS269, DUBA, DXd, AF-HPA, and tubulysin are structurally distinct from the maytansine lysine-MCC-DM1 which could allow the respective ADCs to overcome trastuzumab-MCC-DM1 induction of multi-drug resistant transporter expression. The improved drug-linker stability of ARX788 and DS-8201a thus higher serum conjugate concentration compared to trastuzumab-MCC-DM1 could overcome reduced HER2 expression. Each of the anti-HER2 ADCs in the clinic could overcome some of the reported trastuzumab-MCC-DM1 resistance mechanisms.

Future of HER2 Therapy and ADCs

Preliminary clinical data from the anti-HER2 ADCs currently in clinical trials is on the horizon. Responses were observed with SYD985 and DS-8201a in phase I trials. Advanced clinical trials will reveal if the ADC modifications will improve clinical treatment of cancer patients expressing HER2. SYD985, DS-8201a, and ADCT-502 represent changes in the linker-drug, but use the same antibody as trastuzumab-MCC-DM1, which will allow direct comparison of the ADC technologies. ARX788, ADCT-502, and MEDI4276 are site-specific conjugates, which in preclinical experiments were shown to improve the therapeutic index compared to heterogeneous ADCs, such as trastuzumab-MCC-DM1. Each of these ADCs has multiple differences from trastuzumab-MCC-DM1 complicating the interpretation of site-specific technology impact. RC48-ADC, XMT-1522, and MEDI4276 evaluate a different antibody and linker-drug system, which introduce additional variables which will complicate the interpretation of which factors are critical for ADCs.

MEDI4276's biparatopic antibody with significantly improved internalization compared to trastuzumab is a unique antibody approach distinct from the other candidates. A different way to employ a bispecific antibody conjugate is to pair an anti-HER2 antibody with an antibody targeting another receptor. Prolactin receptor (PRLR) is efficiently trafficked to lysosomes, in contrast to HER2. To exploit PRLR's lysosomal trafficking property a bispecific anti-HER2 x anti-PRLR antibody was generated [88]. A bispecific antibody targeting HER2 and CD63, also referred to as LAMP3, a receptor that traffics to endosomes and lysosomes employs a similar strategy [89]. Both strategies demonstrated improved potency compared to the mono-specific ADCs, however, additional studies are necessary to learn the pharmacological impact. CD63 is expressed at much higher levels and across multiple tissues than PRLR, albeit the majority of the expression is anticipated to be within endosomes and lysosomes and not at the cell surface. A low affinity anti-CD63 antibody was generated to ensure that HER2 binding was required to facilitate CD63 binding. However, as antibodies are circulated throughout the body they are pinocytosed into cells lining the vascular endothelium and trafficked to endosomes where IgG antibodies bind to FcRn. Binding of IgG to FcRn is pH specific and FcRn recycles IgG back into circulation rescuing antibodies from catabolism in lysosomes [90]. It is unclear how a bispecific antibody targeting CD63 or another broadly expressed protein that traffics to lysosomes will behave in the context of FcRn within normal vascular endothelial cells. In normal cells bispecific binding to FcRn and CD63 could lead to enhanced trafficking to lysosomes, if so this can lead to faster antibody clearance and greater toxicity of a bispecific ADC [91].

While these and other advances in the future will benefit patients with HER2 expression, the question remains: is HER2 a unique target for ADC technology in solid tumors? Currently there are over 60 ADCs in clinical trials for the treatment of hematological and solid cancers [92]. In the past 20 years dozens of solid tumor targeted ADCs have failed in clinical trials, fueling the debate as to the uniqueness of HER2. Recently, encouraging data with the solid tumor anti-DLL3 ADC rovalpituzumab tesirine suggests that HER2 is not unique as an ADC target for solid tumors [93]. HER2 is a validated ADC target and will likely continue for some time as a preferred cell surface target to evaluate new antibody and ADC technologies. Emerging data with DS-8201a indicate that the HER2 patient population may expand and include treatment of patients with lower HER2 levels. The impact of current and future HER2 ADCs will inform the ADC field of new directions to explore for targets beyond HER2. Continued ADC technology advances will generate optimized ADCs for the treatment of HER2 expressing cancers to expand the patient population, improve patient survival, and reduce adverse events.

References

1. Yarden Y, Pines G (2012) The ERBB network: at last, cancer therapy meets systems biology. Nat Rev Cancer 12:553–563
2. Martin V, Cappuzzo F, Mazzucchelli L, Frattini M (2014) HER2 in solid tumors: more than 10 years under the microscope; where are we now? Future Oncol 10:1469–1486
3. Franklin MC, Carey KD, Vajdos FF, Leahy DJ, de Vos AM, Sliwkowski MX (2004) Insights into ErbB signaling from the structure of the ErbB2-pertuzumab complex. Cancer Cell 5:317–328
4. Cho HS, Mason K, Ramyar KX, Stanley AM, Gabelli SB, Denney DW Jr et al (2003) Structure of the extracellular region of HER2 alone and in complex with the Herceptin fab. Nature 421:756–760
5. Hudis CA (2007) Trastuzumab — mechanism of action and use in clinical practice. N Engl J Med 357:39–51
6. Junttila TT, Akita RW, Parsons K, Fields C, Lewis Phillips GD, Friedman LS et al (2009) Ligand-independent HER2/HER3/PI3K complex is disrupted by trastuzumab and is effectively inhibited by the PI3K inhibitor GDC-0941. Cancer Cell 15:429–440
7. De Santes K, Slamon D, Anderson SK, Shepard M, Fendly B, Maneval D et al (1992) Radiolabeled antibody targeting of the HER-2/neu oncoprotein. Cancer Res 52:1916–1923
8. Austin CD, De Maziere AM, Pisacane PI, van Dijk SM, Eigenbrot C, Sliwkowski MX et al (2004) Endocytosis and sorting of ErbB2 and the site of action of cancer therapeutics trastuzumab and geldanamycin. Mol Biol Cell 15:5268–5282
9. Hamblett KJ, Senter PD, Chace DF, Sun MM, Lenox J, Cerveny CG et al (2004) Effects of drug loading on the antitumor activity of a monoclonal antibody drug conjugate. Clin Cancer Res 10:7063–7070
10. Sun X, Ponte JF, Yoder NC, Laleau R, Coccia J, Lanieri L et al (2017) Effects of drug-antibody ratio on pharmacokinetics, biodistribution, efficacy, and tolerability of antibody-Maytansinoid conjugates. Bioconjug Chem 28:1371–1381
11. Doronina SO, Toki BE, Torgov MY, Mendelsohn BA, Cerveny CG, Chace DF et al (2003) Development of potent monoclonal antibody auristatin conjugates for cancer therapy. Nat Biotechnol 21:778–784
12. Hamann PR, Hinman LM, Hollander I, Beyer CF, Lindh D, Holcomb R et al (2002) Gemtuzumab ozogamicin, a potent and selective anti-CD33 antibody-calicheamicin conjugate for treatment of acute myeloid leukemia. Bioconjug Chem 13:47–58
13. Kovtun YV, Audette CA, Ye Y, Xie H, Ruberti MF, Phinney SJ et al (2006) Antibody-drug conjugates designed to eradicate tumors with homogeneous and heterogeneous expression of the target antigen. Cancer Res 66:3214–3221
14. Flynn M, Zammarchi F, Tyrer PC, Akarca AU, Janghra N, Britten CE et al (2016) ADCT-301, a Pyrrolobenzodiazepine (PBD) dimer-containing antibody drug conjugate (ADC) targeting CD25-expressing hematological malignancies. Mol Cancer Ther 15:2709
15. Okeley NM, Miyamoto JB, Zhang X, Sanderson RJ, Benjamin DR, Sievers EL et al (2010) Intracellular activation of SGN-35, a potent anti-CD30 antibody-drug conjugate. Clin Cancer Res 16:888–897
16. Doronina SO, Mendelsohn BA, Bovee TD, Cerveny CG, Alley SC, Meyer DL et al (2006) Enhanced activity of monomethylauristatin F through monoclonal antibody delivery: effects of linker technology on efficacy and toxicity. Bioconjug Chem 17:114–124
17. Erickson HK, Park PU, Widdison WC, Kovtun YV, Garrett LM, Hoffman K et al (2006) Antibody-maytansinoid conjugates are activated in targeted cancer cells by lysosomal degradation and linker-dependent intracellular processing. Cancer Res 66:4426–4433
18. Junttila TT, Li G, Parsons K, Phillips GL, Sliwkowski MX (2011) Trastuzumab-DM1 (T-DM1) retains all the mechanisms of action of trastuzumab and efficiently inhibits growth of lapatinib insensitive breast cancer. Breast Cancer Res Treat 128:347–356

19. Maxfield FR (2014) Role of endosomes and lysosomes in human disease. Cold Spring Harb Perspect Biol 6:a016931
20. Cardillo TM, Govindan SV, Sharkey RM, Trisal P, Goldenberg DM (2011) Humanized anti-Trop-2 IgG-SN-38 conjugate for effective treatment of diverse epithelial cancers: preclinical studies in human cancer Xenograft models and monkeys. Clin Cancer Res 17:3157–3169
21. Govindan SV, Cardillo TM, Sharkey RM, Tat F, Gold DV, Goldenberg DM (2013) Milatuzumab–SN-38 conjugates for the treatment of CD74⁺ cancers. Mol Cancer Ther 12:968–978
22. Rock BM, Tometsko ME, Patel SK, Hamblett KJ, Fanslow WC, Rock DA (2015) Intracellular catabolism of an antibody drug conjugate with a noncleavable linker. Drug Metab Dispos 43:1341–1344
23. Sutherland MS, Sanderson RJ, Gordon KA, Andreyka J, Cerveny CG, Yu C et al (2006) Lysosomal trafficking and cysteine protease metabolism confer target-specific cytotoxicity by peptide-linked anti-CD30-auristatin conjugates. J Biol Chem 281:10540–10547
24. Hamblett KJ, Jacob AP, Gurgel JL, Tometsko ME, Rock BM, Patel SK et al (2015) SLC46A3 is required to transport Catabolites of noncleavable antibody Maytansine conjugates from the lysosome to the cytoplasm. Cancer Res 75:5329–5340
25. Jeffrey SC, Andreyka JB, Bernhardt SX, Kissler KM, Kline T, Lenox JS et al (2006) Development and properties of beta-glucuronide linkers for monoclonal antibody-drug conjugates. Bioconjug Chem 17:831–840
26. Polson AG, Calemine-Fenaux J, Chan P, Chang W, Christensen E, Clark S et al (2009) Antibody-drug conjugates for the treatment of non-Hodgkin's lymphoma: target and linker-drug selection. Cancer Res 69:2358–2364
27. Lewis Phillips GD, Li G, Dugger DL, Crocker LM, Parsons KL, Mai E et al (2008) Targeting HER2-positive breast cancer with trastuzumab-DM1, an antibody-cytotoxic drug conjugate. Cancer Res 68:9280–9290
28. Kellogg BA, Garrett L, Kovtun Y, Lai KC, Leece B, Miller M et al (2011) Disulfide-linked antibody-maytansinoid conjugates: optimization of in vivo activity by varying the steric hindrance at carbon atoms adjacent to the disulfide linkage. Bioconjug Chem 22:717–727
29. Erickson HK, Lewis Phillips GD, Leipold DD, Provenzano CA, Mai E, Johnson HA et al (2012) The effect of different linkers on target cell catabolism and pharmacokinetics/pharmacodynamics of trastuzumab maytansinoid conjugates. Mol Cancer Ther 11:1133–1142
30. Barok M, Tanner M, Koninki K, Isola J (2011) Trastuzumab-DM1 is highly effective in preclinical models of HER2-positive gastric cancer. Cancer Lett 306:171–179
31. Poon KA, Flagella K, Beyer J, Tibbitts J, Kaur S, Saad O et al (2013) Preclinical safety profile of trastuzumab emtansine (T-DM1): mechanism of action of its cytotoxic component retained with improved tolerability. Toxicol Appl Pharmacol 273:298–313
32. Krop IE, Beeram M, Modi S, Jones SF, Holden SN, Yu W et al (2010) Phase I study of trastuzumab-DM1, an HER2 antibody-drug conjugate, given every 3 weeks to patients with HER2-positive metastatic breast cancer. J Clin Oncol 28:2698–2704
33. Beeram M, Krop IE, Burris HA, Girish SR, Yu W, Lu MW et al (2012) A phase 1 study of weekly dosing of trastuzumab emtansine (T-DM1) in patients with advanced human epidermal growth factor 2-positive breast cancer. Cancer 118:5733–5740
34. Girish S, Gupta M, Wang B, Lu D, Krop IE, Vogel CL et al (2012) Clinical pharmacology of trastuzumab emtansine (T-DM1): an antibody-drug conjugate in development for the treatment of HER2-positive cancer. Cancer Chemother Pharmacol 69:1229–1240
35. Burris HA 3rd, Rugo HS, Vukelja SJ, Vogel CL, Borson RA, Limentani S et al (2011) Phase II study of the antibody drug conjugate trastuzumab-DM1 for the treatment of human epidermal growth factor receptor 2 (HER2)-positive breast cancer after prior HER2-directed therapy. J Clin Oncol 29:398–405
36. Verma S, Miles D, Gianni L, Krop IE, Welslau M, Baselga J et al (2012) Trastuzumab emtansine for HER2-positive advanced breast cancer. N Engl J Med 367:1783–1791

37. Lewis Phillips GD, Fields CT, Li G, Dowbenko D, Schaefer G, Miller K et al (2014) Dual targeting of HER2-positive cancer with trastuzumab emtansine and pertuzumab: critical role for neuregulin blockade in antitumor response to combination therapy. Clin Cancer Res 20:456–468
38. Perez EA, Barrios C, Eiermann W, Toi M, Im YH, Conte P et al (2017) Trastuzumab Emtansine with or without Pertuzumab versus Trastuzumab plus Taxane for human epidermal growth factor receptor 2-positive, advanced breast cancer: primary results from the phase III MARIANNE study. J Clin Oncol 35:141–148
39. Van Cutsem E, Bang YJ, Feng-Yi F, Xu JM, Lee KW, Jiao SC et al (2015) HER2 screening data from ToGA: targeting HER2 in gastric and gastroesophageal junction cancer. Gastric Cancer 18:476–484
40. Thuss-Patience PC, Shah MA, Ohtsu A, Van Cutsem E, Ajani JA, Castro H et al (2017) Trastuzumab emtansine versus taxane use for previously treated HER2-positive locally advanced or metastatic gastric or gastro-oesophageal junction adenocarcinoma (GATSBY): an international randomised, open-label, adaptive, phase 2/3 study. Lancet Oncol 18:640
41. Ruschoff J, Hanna W, Bilous M, Hofmann M, Osamura RY, Penault-Llorca F et al (2012) HER2 testing in gastric cancer: a practical approach. Mod Pathol 25:637–650
42. Behrens CR, Ha EH, Chinn LL, Bowers S, Probst G, Fitch-Bruhns M et al (2015) Antibody-drug conjugates (ADCs) derived from Interchain cysteine cross-linking demonstrate improved homogeneity and other pharmacological properties over conventional heterogeneous ADCs. Mol Pharm 12:3986–3998
43. Bryant P, Pabst M, Badescu G, Bird M, McDowell W, Jamieson E et al (2015) In vitro and in vivo evaluation of cysteine Rebridged Trastuzumab-MMAE antibody drug conjugates with defined drug-to-antibody ratios. Mol Pharm 12:1872–1879
44. Kudirka RA, Barfield RM, McFarland JM, Drake PM, Carlson A, Banas S et al (2016) Site-specific tandem Knoevenagel condensation-Michael addition to generate antibody-drug conjugates. ACS Med Chem Lett 7:994–998
45. Ma D, Narayanan B, Marquette K, Graziani E, Loganzo F, Charati M, Prashad N, Tumey N, Golas J, Hosselet C, Hu G, Barletta F, Betts A, Lucas J, O'Donnell C, Tchistiakova L, Gerber H, Sapra P (2016) Creating a superior, site-specific anti-HER2 antibody-drug conjugate (NG-HER2 ADC) for treatment of solid tumors. AACR Annual Meeting, New Orleans, LA
46. Jiang J, Dong L, Wang L, Wang L, Zhang J, Chen F et al (2016) HER2-targeted antibody drug conjugates for ovarian cancer therapy. Eur J Pharm Sci 93:274–286
47. Yao X, Jiang J, Wang X, Huang C, Li D, Xie K et al (2015) A novel humanized anti-HER2 antibody conjugated with MMAE exerts potent anti-tumor activity. Breast Cancer Res Treat 153:123–133
48. Junutula JR, Flagella KM, Graham RA, Parsons KL, Ha E, Raab H et al (2010) Engineered thio-trastuzumab-DM1 conjugate with an improved therapeutic index to target human epidermal growth factor receptor 2-positive breast cancer. Clin Cancer Res 16:4769–4778
49. Strop P, Liu SH, Dorywalska M, Delaria K, Dushin RG, Tran TT et al (2013) Location matters: site of conjugation modulates stability and pharmacokinetics of antibody drug conjugates. Chem Biol 20:161–167
50. Shen BQ, Xu K, Liu L, Raab H, Bhakta S, Kenrick M et al (2012) Conjugation site modulates the in vivo stability and therapeutic activity of antibody-drug conjugates. Nat Biotechnol 30:184–189
51. Liu JFM, Moore KN, Wang JS, Patel M, Birrer MJ, Hamilton E, Barroilhet L, Flanagan WM, Wang Y, Garg A, Lu X, Vaze A, Amin D, Leipold D, Commerford SR, Humke EW, Burris HA (2017) CT009 - Targeting MUC16 with the THIOMABTM-drug conjugate DMUC4064A in patients with platinum-resistant ovarian cancer: a Phase I escalation study. AACR Annual Meeting, Washington, DC
52. Badescu G, Bryant P, Bird M, Henseleit K, Swierkosz J, Parekh V et al (2014) Bridging disulfides for stable and defined antibody drug conjugates. Bioconjug Chem 25:1124–1136

53. Tian F, Lu Y, Manibusan A, Sellers A, Tran H, Sun Y et al (2014) A general approach to site-specific antibody drug conjugates. Proc Natl Acad Sci 111:1766–1771
54. Zimmerman ES, Heibeck TH, Gill A, Li X, Murray CJ, Madlansacay MR et al (2014) Production of site-specific antibody-drug conjugates using optimized non-natural amino acids in a cell-free expression system. Bioconjug Chem 25:351–361
55. Humphreys RC, Kirtely J, Hewit A, Biroc S, Knudsen N, Skidmore L et al (2015) Abstract 639: site specific conjugation of ARX-788, an antibody drug conjugate (ADC) targeting HER2, generates a potent and stable targeted therapeutic for multiple cancers. Cancer Res 75:639
56. Jackson D, Atkinson J, Guevara CI, Zhang C, Kery V, Moon SJ et al (2014) In vitro and in vivo evaluation of cysteine and site specific conjugated herceptin antibody-drug conjugates. PLoS One 9:e83865
57. Polson AG, Yu SF, Elkins K, Zheng B, Clark S, Ingle GS et al (2007) Antibody-drug conjugates targeted to CD79 for the treatment of non-Hodgkin lymphoma. Blood 110:616–623
58. Pravin CP, Vijay S, Moses L (2015) A short review on the synthetic strategies of Duocarmycin analogs that are powerful DNA alkylating agents. Anti Cancer Agents Med Chem 15:616–630
59. Elgersma RC, Coumans RG, Huijbregts T, Menge WM, Joosten JA, Spijker HJ et al (2015) Design, synthesis, and evaluation of linker-Duocarmycin payloads: toward selection of HER2-targeting antibody-drug conjugate SYD985. Mol Pharm 12:1813–1835
60. Dokter W, Ubink R, van der Lee M, van der Vleuten M, van Achterberg T, Jacobs D et al (2014) Preclinical profile of the HER2-targeting ADC SYD983/SYD985: introduction of a new duocarmycin-based linker-drug platform. Mol Cancer Ther 13:2618–2629
61. van der Lee MM, Groothuis PG, Ubink R, van der Vleuten MA, van Achterberg TA, Loosveld EM et al (2015) The preclinical profile of the Duocarmycin-based HER2-targeting ADC SYD985 predicts for clinical benefit in low HER2-expressing breast cancers. Mol Cancer Ther 14:692–703
62. Koper N (2016) Development Update on SYD985, a Duocarmycin-based ADC. World ADC Summit; 2016 October 12, San Diego, CA
63. Cuya SM, Bjornsti M-A, van Waardenburg RCAM (2017) DNA topoisomerase-targeting chemotherapeutics: what's new? Cancer Chemother Pharmacol 80:1–14
64. Abou-Alfa GK, Letourneau R, Harker G, Modiano M, Hurwitz H, Tchekmedyian NS et al (2006) Randomized phase III study of Exatecan and gemcitabine compared with gemcitabine alone in untreated advanced pancreatic cancer. J Clin Oncol 24:4441–4447
65. Soepenberg O, de Jonge MJA, Sparreboom A, de Bruin P, Eskens FALM, de Heus G et al (2005) Phase I and pharmacokinetic study of DE-310 in patients with advanced solid tumors. Clin Cancer Res 11:703–711
66. Kumazawa E, Ochi Y (2004) DE-310, a novel macromolecular carrier system for the camptothecin analog DX-8951f: potent antitumor activities in various murine tumor models. Cancer Sci 95:168–175
67. Ochi YK, Kumazawa E, Shiose Y, Kuga H, Inoue, K (2003) DE-310, a novel macro-molecular carrier system for the camptothecin analog DX-8951f [IV]: a pos-sible drug release mechanism for antitumor activity. AACR Annual Meeting, p 395
68. Ogitani Y, Aida T, Hagihara K, Yamaguchi J, Ishii C, Harada N et al (2016) DS-8201a, a novel HER2-targeting ADC with a novel DNA topoisomerase I inhibitor, demonstrates a promising antitumor efficacy with differentiation from T-DM1. Clin Cancer Res 22:5097–5108
69. Ogitani Y, Hagihara K, Oitate M, Naito H, Agatsuma T (2016) Bystander killing effect of DS-8201a, a novel anti-human epidermal growth factor receptor 2 antibody-drug conjugate, in tumors with human epidermal growth factor receptor 2 heterogeneity. Cancer Sci 107:1039–1046
70. Honda T (2016) Preclinical profiles of topoisomerase I inhibitor Exatecan derivative-based HER2 targeting ADC. World ADC Summit, 2016 Ocober 12
71. Doi TI, Iwata H, Tsurutani J, Takahashi S, Park H, Redfern CH, Shitara K, Shimizu C, Taniguchi H, Iwasa T, Taira S, Lockhart AC, Fisher JM, Jikoh T, Fujisaki Y, Lee CC, Yver

A, Tamura K (2017) Single agent activity of DS-8201a, a HER2-targeting antibody-drug conjugate, in heavily pretreated HER2 expressing solid tumors. Abstract 108. ASCO Annual Meeting, Chicago, Illinois

72. Tiberghien AC, Levy J-N, Masterson LA, Patel NV, Adams LR, Corbett S et al (2016) Design and synthesis of Tesirine, a clinical antibody–drug conjugate Pyrrolobenzodiazepine dimer payload. ACS Med Chem Lett 7:983–987
73. van Berkel P (2016) Building a diversified product portfolio of PBD-based antibody drug conjugates. World ADC Summit. San Diego, CA
74. Bergstrom DA, Bodyak N, Yurkovetskiy A, Park PU, DeVit M, Yin M, et al (2015) A novel, highly potent HER2-targeted antibody-drug conjugate (ADC) for the treatment of low HER2-expressing tumors and combination with trastuzumab-based regimens in HER2-driven tumors. AACR Annual Meeting, 75:LB–231
75. Bodyak N, Yurkovetskiy A, Gumerov DR, Xiao D, Joshua DTDT, Poling LL, Qin LY, Yin M, DeVit MJ, et al (2016) Optimization of lead antibody selection for XMT-1522, a novel, highly potent HER2-targeted antibody-drug conjugate (ADC). AACR Annual Meeting, p 596
76. Lowinger TB (2015) Fleximer ADCs: advancing to the clinic. World ADC Summit, 21 Oct 2015, San Diego, CA
77. Yurkovetskiy AV, Yin M, Bodyak N, Stevenson CA, Thomas JD, Hammond CE et al (2015) A polymer-based antibody–Vinca drug conjugate platform: characterization and preclinical efficacy. Cancer Res 75:3365–3372
78. Bergstrom DA (2017) ADCs with diverse payloads of tumor-killing agents. 15th international congress on targeted anticancer therapies, March 7, 2017, Paris, France
79. Bergstrom D, Bodyak N, Park P, Yurkovetskiy A, DeVit M, Yin M, et al (2016) XMT-1522 induces tumor regressions in pre-clinical models representing HER2-positive and HER2 low-expressing breast cancer. San Antonio Breast Cancer Symposium, San Antonio, TX. p P4–14-28
80. Bodyak N, Yurkovetskiy A, Park PU, Gumerov DR, DeVit M, Yin M, et al (2015) Abstract 641: Trastuzumab-dolaflexin, a highly potent Fleximer-based antibody-drug conjugate, demonstrates a favorable therapeutic index in exploratory toxicology studies in multiple species. AACR Annual Meeting, p 641
81. Kontermann RE (2012) Dual targeting strategies with bispecific antibodies. MAbs 4:182–197
82. Li JY, Perry SR, Muniz-Medina V, Wang X, Wetzel LK, Rebelatto MC et al (2016) A Biparatopic HER2-targeting antibody-drug conjugate induces tumor regression in primary models refractory to or ineligible for HER2-targeted therapy. Cancer Cell 29:117–129
83. Uppal H, Doudement E, Mahapatra K, Darbonne WC, Bumbaca D, Shen B-Q et al (2015) Potential mechanisms for thrombocytopenia development with Trastuzumab Emtansine (T-DM1). Clin Cancer Res 21:123–133
84. Li J, Toader D, Perry SR, Muniz-Medina V, Wetzel L, Rebelatto MC, Masson Hinrichs MJ, Fleming R, Bezabeh B, Thompson P, Dimasi N, Lam B, Yu X, Gao C, Dixit R, Coats S, Osbourn J, Wu H (2016) MEDI4276, a HER2-targeting antibody tubulysin conjugate, displays potent in vitro and in vivo activity in preclinical studies. AACR Annual Meeting, New Orleans, LA
85. Barok M, Joensuu H, Isola J (2014) Trastuzumab emtansine: mechanisms of action and drug resistance. Breast Cancer Res 16:209
86. Lewis Phillips GD (2011) Mechanisms of acquired resistance to Trastuzumab Emtansine (T-DM1). World ADC Summit
87. Loganzo F, Tan X, Sung M, Jin G, Myers JS, Melamud E et al (2015) Tumor cells chronically treated with a trastuzumab-maytansinoid antibody-drug conjugate develop varied resistance mechanisms but respond to alternate treatments. Mol Cancer Ther 14:952–963
88. Andreev J, Thambi N, Perez Bay AE, Delfino F, Martin J, Kelly MP et al (2017) Bispecific antibodies and antibody-drug conjugates (ADCs) bridging HER2 and prolactin receptor improve efficacy of HER2 ADCs. Mol Cancer Ther 16:681–693

89. de Goeij BE, Vink T, Ten Napel H, Breij EC, Satijn D, Wubbolts R et al (2016) Efficient payload delivery by a Bispecific antibody-drug conjugate targeting HER2 and CD63. Mol Cancer Ther 15:2688–2697
90. Roopenian DC, Akilesh S (2007) FcRn: the neonatal fc receptor comes of age. Nat Rev Immunol 7:715–725
91. Hamblett KJ, Le T, Rock BM, Rock DA, Siu S, Huard JN et al (2016) Altering antibody-drug conjugate binding to the neonatal fc receptor impacts efficacy and tolerability. Mol Pharm 13:2387–2396
92. Beck A, Goetsch L, Dumontet C, Corvaia N (2017) Strategies and challenges for the next generation of antibody-drug conjugates. Nat Rev Drug Discov 16:315–337
93. Saunders LR, Bankovich AJ, Anderson WC, Aujay MA, Bheddah S, Black K et al (2015) A DLL3-targeted antibody-drug conjugate eradicates high-grade pulmonary neuroendocrine tumor-initiating cells in vivo. Sci Transl Med 7:302ra136

Next Generation Payloads for ADCs

L. Nathan Tumey

Abstract The clinical success of gemtuzumab ozogamicin, brentuximab vedotin and ado-trastuzumab emtansine has spurred significant investment into new ADC payloads that may expand the utility of ADC technology. Innovations in the past 5–10 years have resulted in the identification of new payloads that are overcoming resistance mechanisms, showing efficacy against slow growing tumors, and enabling the use of biomarkers to better understand ADC PK/PD relationships. Moreover, ADC technology is now enabling the delivery of steroids, anti-inflammatory agents, and anti-infectives to specific cell types.

Keywords Antibody drug conjugate · Targeted drug delivery · ADC payload · Oncology · Tubulin · Calicheamicin · Spliceosome · RNA-polymerase · Glucocorticoid

Introduction

As the clinical ADC pipeline continues to grow, so does the optimism that perhaps the long-sought promise of "magic bullet" therapeutics is finally coming to pass. The concept of antibody-delivered drugs goes back over five decades [1], but clinical success has only been realized through the persistent efforts of a few research groups, most notably those at Wyeth, Seattle Genetics, Genentech and ImmunoGen. Antibody drug conjugates (ADCs) typically consist of a targeting moiety (the antibody) tethered to a cytotoxic payload (the drug) via a cleavable or noncleavable linker. The ADC itself is essentially a prodrug which is catabolized at the site of action thereby resulting in the localized release of a payload of interest. The linker moiety is typically attached to the payload at some point during the synthesis (manufacture) of the "linker-payload" and then subsequently attached to

---

L. N. Tumey (✉)
Binghamton University, Binghamton, NY, USA
e-mail: ntumey@Binghamton.edu

M. Damelin (ed.), *Innovations for Next-Generation Antibody-Drug Conjugates*, Cancer Drug Discovery and Development,
https://doi.org/10.1007/978-3-319-78154-9_8

the antibody in a so-called "conjugation" reaction. The resulting ADC linker is designed to be stable in circulation but readily cleaved upon antigen-mediated uptake into the lysosome. This catabolic process typically releases the payload directly inside the target tissue, thus circumventing metabolic and permeability issues that are sometimes associated with the parent payload.

In a simplistic sense, the biochemical efficacy of the ADC is driven by the payload while the safety of the ADC is driven by the tissue selectivity imparted by the antibody. As such, a consistent theme of ADC research over the past 20 years has been the "redeployment" of efficacious but poorly tolerated drugs as ADC payloads. While there is certainly merit in this idea, researchers quickly observed that many chemotherapeutic drugs (such as methotrexate and doxorubicin) were not sufficiently potent to serve as effective ADC payloads. Clinical success was finally realized through the incorporation of ultra-potent payloads such as calicheamicin, maytansinoids, and auristatins. (Fig. 1) The regulatory approval of gemtuzumab ozogamicin (Mylotarg, **1**) in 2000 [2], brentuximab vedotin (Adcetris, **2**) in 2011 [3], and ado-trastuzumab emtansine (Kadcyla, **3**) in 2013 [4] has spurred on significant investment that has fueled an increasingly diverse clinical and preclinical ADC pipeline. While DNA damaging agents and inhibitors of tubulin polymerization continue to be significant areas of exploration, a steady outpouring of research has resulted in the introduction of a variety of ADC payloads that target other essential cellular processes, such as RNA polymerization and splicing, kinesin mediated protein transport, and regulation of apoptosis. Unlike currently approved ADCs, these emerging payload classes are beginning to overcome PGP-efflux and other

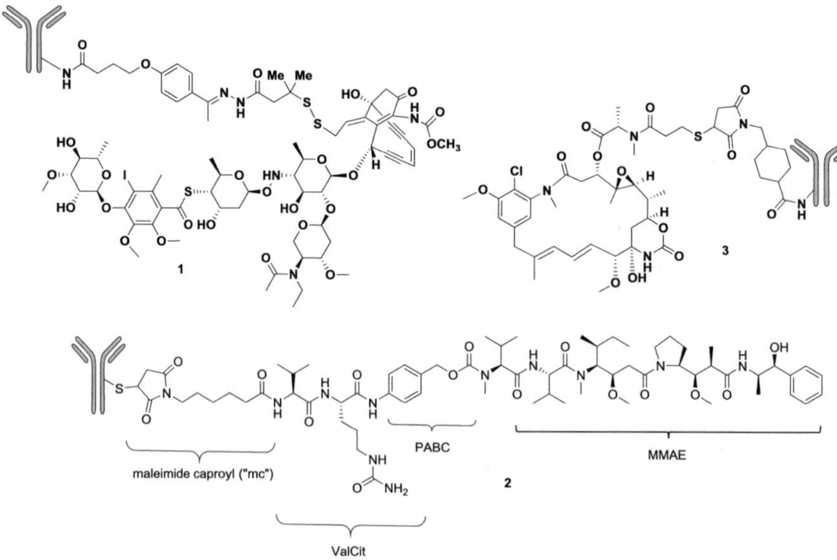

Fig. 1 The structure of gemtuzumab ozogamicin (Mylotarg, **1**), brentuximab vedotin (Adcetris, **2**), and ado-trastuzumab emtansine (Kadcyla, **3**). The linker-payload name of compound **2** is shown in detail for reference purposes

mechanisms of ADC resistance, exhibit efficacy against slow growing and quiescent tumors, and enable the use of mechanistic biomarkers. Moreover, the recent success of ADCs in oncology is paving the way for the antibody-mediated delivery of other therapeutic agents such as anti-inflammatory agents and anti-infectives. In this chapter, we will review recent progress made in the identification of these new payloads for use in up-and-coming ADC programs.

Tubulin Binding Payloads

Tubulin polymerization is essential for many cellular processes such as mitosis, intracellular transport, and maintaining structural integrity. Blockage of tubulin polymerization by agents such as auristatins and maytansines have formed the basis for the recent renaissance of ADCs entering clinical development. Clinical-stage conjugates that employ such agents include polatuzumab vedotin, indatuximab ravtansine, mirvetuximab soravtansine, and glembatumumab vedotin. Both maytansines and auristatins bind to the vinca binding site on tubulin and typically have sub-nM potency in a variety of tumor cell proliferation assays. Due to the success of this payload class in the clinic, a variety of new tubulin binders have been explored in recent years. Goals of these efforts often include increased safety, efficacy, and structural novelty.

Auristatins

The structure of Dolastatin 10 has served as the basis for numerous auristatin ADC payloads. (Fig. 2) In particular, variations of the C-terminal amine have resulted in multiple well-known ADC payloads such as MMAE (**4**), MMAD (**5**), and MMAF

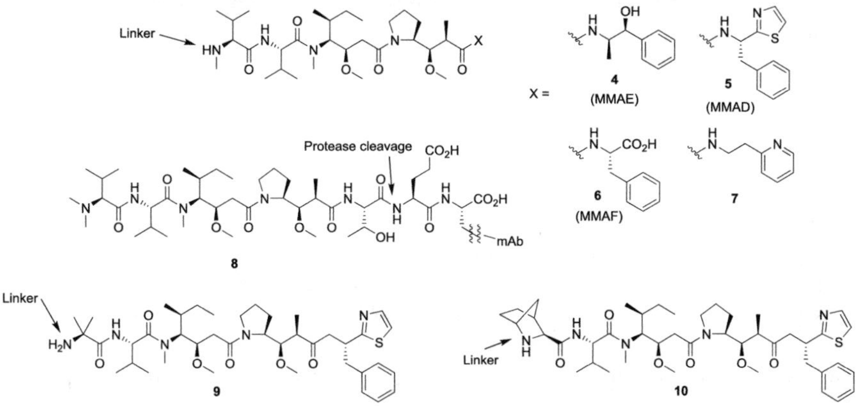

Fig. 2 Structures of auristatin payloads

(**6**). It has been widely recognized that changes to the C-terminal residue can be used to modulate the ADC hydrophobicity. For example, Mendelsohn recently reported a set of new C-terminal modifications specifically designed result in payloads with decreased LogD as compared to MMAE. Unfortunately, the most polar analogs were only weakly active in cytotoxicity assays. It was unclear whether this was due to decreased permeability or decreased affinity for tubulin. However, incorporation of an amino pyridine (**7**) resulted in a slightly more polar payload (logD = 2.54 vs. 2.99) which retained activity in tumor cell proliferation assays [5]. Unfortunately, no data was provided to show that the increased polarity of this payload provided any distinct advantage over MMAE. A similar strategy was employed by Lyon in 2015 [6]. In this case, the authors moved the site of linker attachment to C-terminal end of the molecule (**8**) thus allowing the entire elimination of the phenyl moiety from the payload. Moreover, the linker attachment could now be performed directly through a cathepsin cleavable amide linkage thereby eliminating the need for the hydrophobic PABC immolation element. This allowed the loading to be increased to a drug antibody ratio (DAR) of 8, rather than the typical loading of 4. The resulting ADC (**8**) was significantly more polar than corresponding mcValCitPABC-MMAF and mcMMAF ADCs and exhibited improved PK exposure and efficacy.

Efforts have also been made to introduce changes to the N-terminal end of auristatins. For example, Maderna reported the introduction of α,α disubstituted amino acids resulting in structures such as **9** (PF-06380101) [7]. These auristatins were shown to have increased intrinsic clearance in human liver hepatocytes as compared to monosubstituted analogs such as MMAD (**5**). The authors speculate that increased rates of clearance may result in improved safety, as any prematurely released payload would be cleared from the bloodstream more quickly. While no head-to-head comparison of either safety or PK was reported, this payload (with a ValCitPABC linker) has been used in multiple clinical programs [8–10] and has shown acceptable efficacy and safety. In a similar approach, a patent from Novartis describes the preparation of auristatins that incorporate a bicyclic amino acid at the N-terminus (i.e. **10**) [11]. Potential advantages imparted by this moiety have not been reported.

Tubulysin Analogs

Tubulysins belong to a class of structurally related tetrapeptides that are produced by myxobacteria [12]. Like auristatins, they bind to the vinca binding site of tubulin and potently inhibit tumor cell proliferation. However, unlike auristatins, most tubulysins are not PGP substrates and therefore may offer an advantage in overcoming resistance to auristatin-based payloads. This has attracted significant interest in targeted delivery approaches. Indeed, small-molecule drug conjugates

(SMDCs) targeting the folate receptor and prostate-specific membrane antigen (PSMA) have employed tubulysin as a payload [13, 14]. However, only recently have antibody-directed approaches been reported.

Traditionally, most cleavable ADC linker strategies require a primary or secondary amine for payload attachment, a feature which is not available in naturally occurring tubulysins. In order to obtain tubulysin analogs with a suitable conjugation handles, a team from Pfizer undertook a significant SAR study of both the N-terminal and C-terminal variants [15]. Payload **11** was found to retain potency against a variety of cancer cell lines, including a line with high expression of PGP (KB 8.5). An anti-Her2 ADC using this payload (**12**) was found to have excellent *in vitro* potency, but unexpected plasma metabolism of the C-11 position (giving **13**) rendered the ADC inactive. The team found that the metabolism could be blocked by use of an ester isostere (**14**) or by site-specific attachment of the payload to "hidden" sites on the antibody [16]. A patent from Novartis has also reported similar strategies for addressing metabolism of the C-11 acetate in tubulysin ADCs [17].

A team from MedImmune has reported the use of a tubulysin warhead (AZ13599185) in a biparatopic Her2 ADC (**15**) that recently entered clinical trials. The payload was attached via a proteolytically cleavable linker to two engineered cysteine residues in the Fc domain (239C and 442C). Interestingly, the ADC was shown to cause regression in T-DM1 resistant tumor models. However, it is unclear whether this activity is due to the ability of tubulysin to evade PGP or to some other mechanism. ADC **15** was also shown to have activity in low Her2 expressing lines, including so called "triple negative" tumor xenografts which are negative in diagnostic tests for Her2 expression. It remains to be seen whether this activity against low expressing cell lines is due to properties of the payload or due to properties of the biparatopic antibody. ADC **15** was evaluated for safety in cynomolgus monkeys and the DLT was found to be epithelial degeneration in the gastrointestinal (GI) tract [18] (Fig. 3).

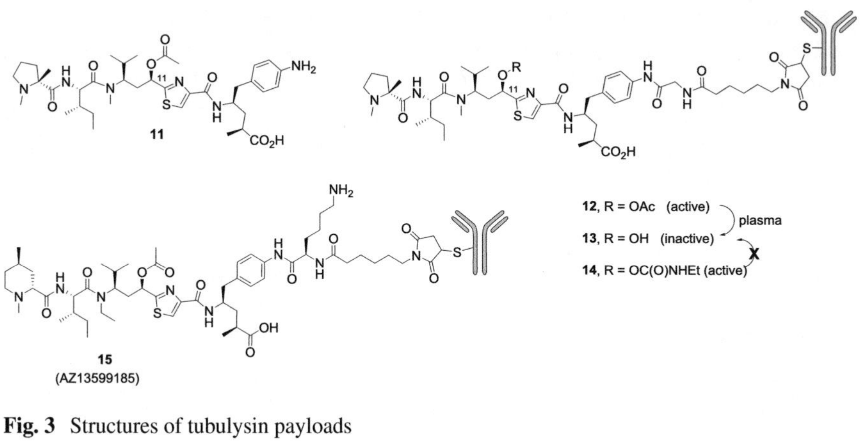

11

15
(AZ13599185)

12, R = OAc (active)
13, R = OH (inactive)
14, R = OC(O)NHEt (active)
plasma

Fig. 3 Structures of tubulysin payloads

Other Tubulin Binding Agents

We would be remiss at this point not to mention recent innovations around maytansine ADCs. While the payload structure has been largely unchanged over the past 10 years, a number of important innovations with respect to conjugation and linker technologies have been reported. For example, Kovtun has shown that the incorporation of polar functionalities such as sulfate and PEG in the linkers can enable maytansinoid ADCs to evade PGP pumps [19] and Pillow has demonstrated that site-specific linkage of maytansinoid payloads can improve the efficacy of the resulting ADCs [20]. A report by Widdison has described an anilino-linked maytansinoid that was shown to have improved bystander activity as compared to traditional disulfide-linked maytansinoids [21].

Finally, two other tubulin binding agents (cryptophycin [22] and cemadotin [23]) have been reported as ADC payloads. However, little supporting data has been published to-date and the advantages that may be offered by these payloads are unclear at this time.

DNA-Damaging Payloads

The widespread use of tubulin binding agents is due, in part, to the fact that they are modestly selective for rapidly dividing cells. This provides an added measure of safety and is no-doubt a reflection of the importance of tubulin in the process of mitosis. However, this feature can also be a drawback as some tumor types and some cell types (such as tumor initiating cells) are inherently slow growing. Moreover, most mouse xenograft models consist of tumors which grow much faster than typical human tumors, thereby perhaps giving a false indication of efficacy for an agent that is highly specific for rapidly dividing cells. For these reasons, there has been a tremendous growth in interest in DNA damaging ADC payloads over the past 5–10 years. These agents have the benefit of being exquisitely potent against both dividing and non-dividing cells. DNA damaging agents fall into roughly three mechanistic categories: DNA double strand breakers, DNA alkylators, and DNA intercalators. The prototypical example of the first class, DNA double strand breakers, are enediyne antibiotics such as calicheamicin and uncialamycin. DNA alkylators include benzodiazepine dimers and duocarmycin-like payloads, each of which may be designed as a bis-alkylator (DNA-cross linker) or a mono-alkylator. Finally, DNA-intercalators include the therapeutically important camptothecin and anthracycline agents. Examples of new developments in each of these structural classes will be given below.

Calicheamicin and Uncialamycin

Calicheamicin is an enediyne antibiotic that was originally isolated from the soil microorganism *M. echinospora*. The natural product is a trisulfide that binds to the minor groove of DNA and is activated by reductive cleavage followed by a so-called "Bergman cyclization" resulting in a diradical that abstracts protons from the DNA backbone [24]. Calicheamicin-based ADCs are typically linked through a hindered disulfide and undergo an analogous activation process, as shown in Fig. 4. The hydrazide-linked calicheamicin known as AcButDMH-calich (**1**, Fig. 4) has been extensively used as a warhead on a variety of ADCs including an anti-EFNA4 ADC (PF-06647263) [25] and an anti-CD22 ADC (Inotuzumab ozogamicin) [26]. Mylotarg, an anti-CD33 conjugate of this linker-payload, was approved for the treatment of acute myeloid leukemia (AML) but was voluntarily withdrawn from the market due to safety and efficacy concerns. However, recent studies have shown that a fractionated dosing regimen may improve the therapeutic window [27]. Many of the safety concerns with this payload are thought to result from premature

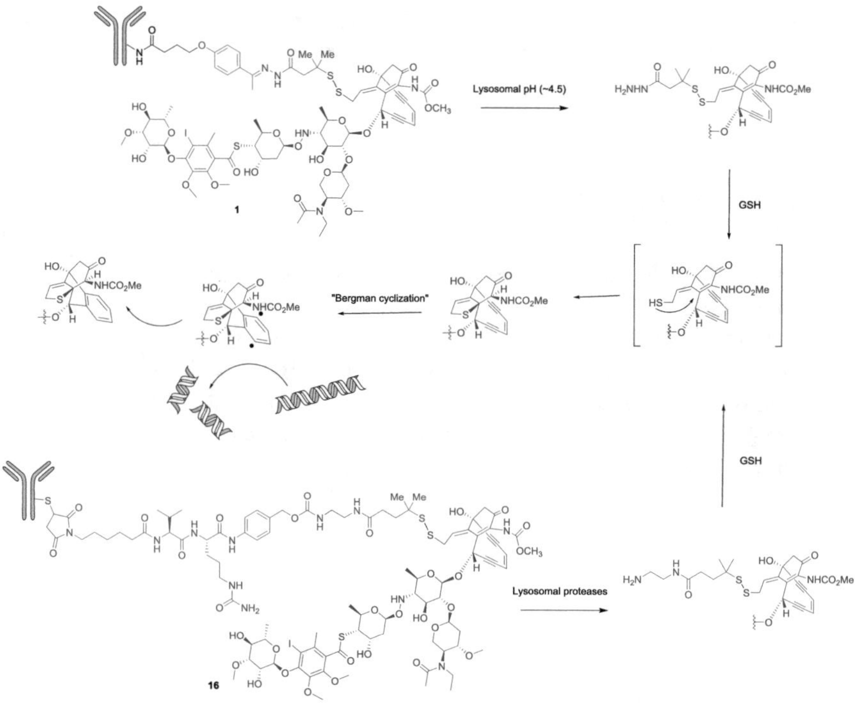

Fig. 4 Activation of calicheamicin ADCs typically begins with a lysosomal activation followed by a reductive step that results in the formation of a diradical that abstracts hydrogen atoms from DNA, thereby causing strand scission. For clarity, the linker is shown in red and the payload is shown in blue. The activation mechanism of both AcButDMH-calicheamicin (top, **1**) and mcValCitPABC-DMAE-calicheamicin (bottom, **16**) is shown

hydrolytic cleavage of the hydrazide, thereby slowly releasing a non-targeted calicheamicin payload.

In order to alleviate this premature cleavage, a team from StemCentrx devised an alternate activation process involving a proteolytically cleavable linker [28] (**16**). The linker-payloads of interest were conjugated to an engineered cysteine on an anti-CD46 antibody. While the specific structure of interest was not revealed, an exemplar ADC was shown to be active in several xenograft models at 0.6–1 mg/kg (qdx4) and was tolerated in mice at up to 8 mg/kg (single dose) and in cynomolgus monkeys at up to 2.5 mg/kg. While no head-to-head comparisons were reported, AcButDMH-calicheamicin (**1**) ADCs have been reported to exhibit human MTDs of 1.8–9 mg/m^2 in humans [29], which corresponds roughly to ~0.05–0.25 mg/kg. This suggests a possible safety advantage to the use of proteolytically cleavable calicheamicin payloads. In addition to the revived interest in calicheamicin, this work potentially provides an impetus for the evaluation of a myriad of other enediyne natural products as possible ADC payloads. For example, Bristol Myers Squibb reported a limited set of data on an uncialamycin linker-payload (**17**) [30]. Naturally occurring uncialamycin does not have an appropriate handle for linker attachment so the team introduced an amino group on the anthraquinone core from which they were able to attach a ValCitPABC linker. An anti-CD70 conjugate of this molecule exhibited low pM activity against numerous cancer cell lines. However, no *in vivo* data was reported (Fig. 5).

Benzodiazepine Dimers

Pyrrolo[2,1-c][1,4]benzodiazepines (PBDs) are a class of antitumor agents that function by binding into the minor groove of DNA and subsequently alkylating the amino group on bases, typically guanines. This, of course, leads to problems in both DNA replication and transcription. Historically, most PBDs have been homodimeric, thus forming inter-strand or intra-strand cross-links in the DNA, often at sequences containing GXXC. (Fig. 6) However, recent innovations reported by ImmunoGen have moved away from bis-alkylators and towards mono-alkylating PBDs (*vide*

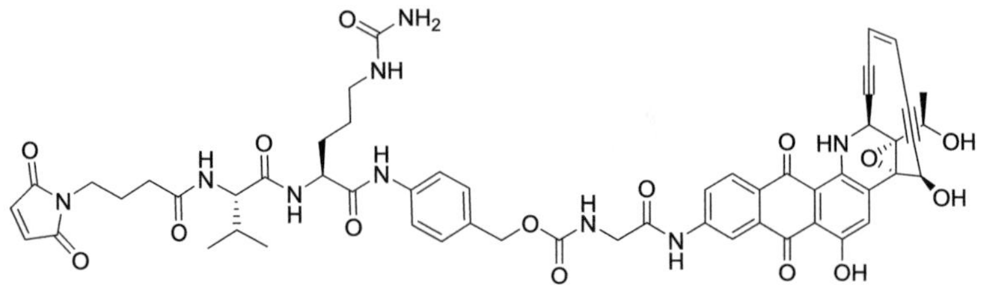

17

Fig. 5 An uncialamycin linker-payload recently reported by Bristol Myers Squib

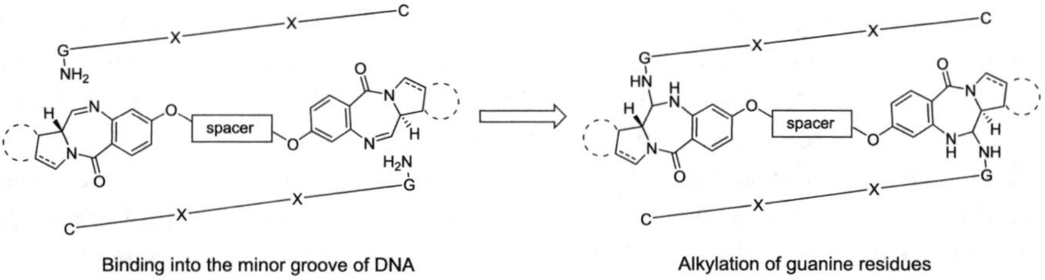

Fig. 6 Typical mode of action of PBD dimers

infra). For a detailed discussion of this payload class, the reader is directed to an excellent review was recently published describing both the SAR of the core payload and its use as an ADC payload [31].

Seattle Genetics and Spirogen (now AstraZeneca) developed an innovative approach for the attachment of a PBD dimer to an antibody via the introduction of an anilino handle on one of the C-2 aryl moieties. (**18**) A protease cleavable mcVa-lAla linker was used to link the payload to an engineered cysteine residue, S239C. While a systematic study of the conjugation site has not been reported, the authors note that stochastic hinge-cysteine ADCs with this payload were prone to rapid aggregation and contamination with significant amounts of unconjugated antibody. Limiting the DAR to 2 was necessary in order to control the aggregation thus mitigating these manufacturing liabilities [32]. Preparation of the S239C site-specific conjugate proved challenging as the linker-payload was quite insoluble and required the conjugation to be performed in 50% propylene glycol. In spite of these difficulties, this PBD linker-payload (known as Talirine) was quickly advanced onto multiple clinical programs. An anti-CD33 conjugate (SGN33A, vadastuximab talirine) was recently in phase III clinical trials for AML, but trials were halted due to safety concerns. Early studies of this ADC demonstrated that it is effective in AML tumor models at doses as low as 30 μg/kg, thus showing activity at doses 3–10 fold below that of gemtuzumab ozogamicin (Mylotarg). Moreover, unlike Mylotarg, SGN33A exhibited activity in drug resistant and low antigen-expressing cell lines such as TF1-α and HEL 92.1.7 [33]. In human trials, this ADC was found to have an MTD of 40 μg/kg. Dose limiting toxicities (DLTs) included pulmonary embolism and hypocellular marrow [31]. The early success of this ADC has led to the advancement of corresponding anti-CD70 [32], anti-CD123 [34], and anti-CD352A [35] conjugates into the clinic. Importantly, these talirine ADCs have shown activity in a wide variety of models that overexpress PGP-1. In contrast, calicheamicin-based ADCs (such as gemtuzumab ozogamicin) have been shown to be susceptible to PGP-mediated resistance mechanisms in both *in vitro* models and in clinical studies [36, 37].

The success of talirine-based conjugates (**18**) has prompted considerable interest in next-generation PBD payloads. The team from Spirogen/AstraZeneca, therefore, undertook an effort specifically aimed at addressing the hydrophobicity of the first-generation bis-aryl PBD dimer. The C2-anisole and C2'-anilino groups were eliminated resulting in loss of potency. The potency loss was offset by extension of the 3-carbon spacer, a feature that the authors speculate allows for greater flexibility thus allowing greater opportunity for contact with the minor groove. Given the removal of the anilino attachment site, the team creatively trapped the reactive imine in its carbinolamine form using a ValAlaPABC linker. Finally, an 8-unit PEG chain was introduced between the maleimide and the dipeptide linker. Combined, these features resulted in a reduction in the clogD from 4.71 (talirine, **18**) to 2.11 (tesirine, **19**) [38]. The increased polarity translated to improvements in solubility and conjugation efficiency. The conjugation, previously performed in 50% propylene glycol, could now be accomplished in 10% DMSO. Moreover, stochastic hinge conjugates could now be prepared using TCEP reduction of the native antibody. A Her2 conjugate of tesirine exhibited activity against SKBR3 cells at ~5 ng/mL while a non-targeted control ADC was 100–1000 fold less active. An anti-DLL3 conjugate of this payload (Rovalpituzumab tesirine, or "Rova-T") is currently in a pivotal clinical trial for small cell lung carcinoma (SCLC). This agent specifically targets tumor initiating cells (TICs) and was shown to exhibit excellent activity against a panel of SCLC and large cell neuroendocrine carcinoma (LCNEC) patient derived xenograft (PDX) models [39]. A CD25 conjugate of the same linker-payload (ADCT-301) was recently advanced into the clinic by ADC Therapeutics and is being evaluated for activity in various types of lymphoma and leukemia [40]. Interestingly, in spite of the increased polarity of the payload, ADCT-301 was shown to exhibit significant so-called "bystander" activity, in that the payload released from CD25 expressing cells is able to diffuse into and kill nearby cells that do not express CD25. This is thought to be an important feature for many ADCs because antigen expression in tumors is notoriously heterogeneous.

Further evolution of the PBD-dimer structure is illustrated in recent work from ImmunoGen. Rather than attaching a linker to the PBD core itself, a 1,3-substituted aryl group was introduced within the spacer element. (**20**) This allowed for direct attachment of the payload to lysine residues via a noncleavable linker [41]. Treatment with 2.5 mg/kg of an anti-folate receptor α (FRα) conjugate of this linker-payload (**20**) resulted in nearly complete tumor regression in a epidermoid carcinoma cell line (KB). However, when the conjugate was dosed at 3.75 mg/kg, prolonged body weight loss and delayed lethality was observed. Fascinatingly and unexpectedly, the authors found that one of the two imine reactive groups could be reduced with only a marginal loss in potency. The resulting ADC was shown to be efficacious at doses as low as 1 mg/kg (tumor regression observed at 5 mg/kg) and was tolerated in mice at doses of up to 10 mg/kg without any loss of body weight. Not surprisingly, no bystander activity was observed for the noncleavable ADC (**20**). However, the introduction of a hindered disulfide linkage resulted in robust activity against co-cultured antigen negative cells [41]. Finally, a sulfate group was incorporated into the linker in order to minimize PGP-mediated efflux of the initially released lysosomal catabolite [42]. An anti-CD33 conjugate of the resulting linker payload (IMGN779, **21**) is currently undergoing clinical evaluation (Fig. 7).

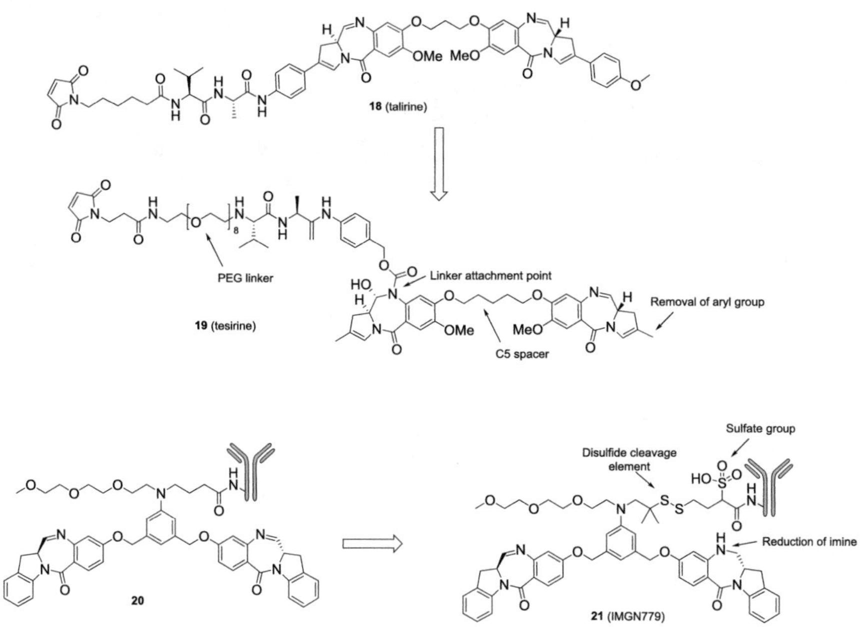

Fig. 7 Structures of PBD linker payloads

One unique feature of PBD dimer payloads is the fact that the DNA alkylation is technically reversible, albeit not under physiological conditions. A group from Genentech takes advantage of this feature in order to quantitate the amount of a PBD payload that had become bound to DNA. Upon antigen-mediated internalization, the PBD ADC (**22**) is catabolized and reduced resulting in the release of the free PBD (**23**) which subsequently alkylates (cross links) DNA as shown. The tumor samples are homogenized and the DNA is isolated, treated with nuclease, and then heated to 90 °C in order to release the PBD (**23**), which, in turn, is quantitated by LC-MS/MS. This serves as an effective biomarker, allowing the team to correlate plasma exposure of the ADC with on-target and off-target tissue exposure [43]. For example, 96 h after dosing (5 mg/kg, i.v.), the concentration of PBD in tumor was found to be ~200 pmol per gram of tissue while the concentration in liver, kidney, and lung was found to be <3 pmol per gram of tissue. This type of analysis opens the door for studying the mechanism of both efficacy and toxicity of ADCs in a way that has not been possible for most other payload classes. The use of DNA-alkylation as a biomarker has been reported previously [44], and it is likely that examples of this type of approach will continue to be reported as DNA-damaging payloads are advancing through clinical evaluation (Fig. 8).

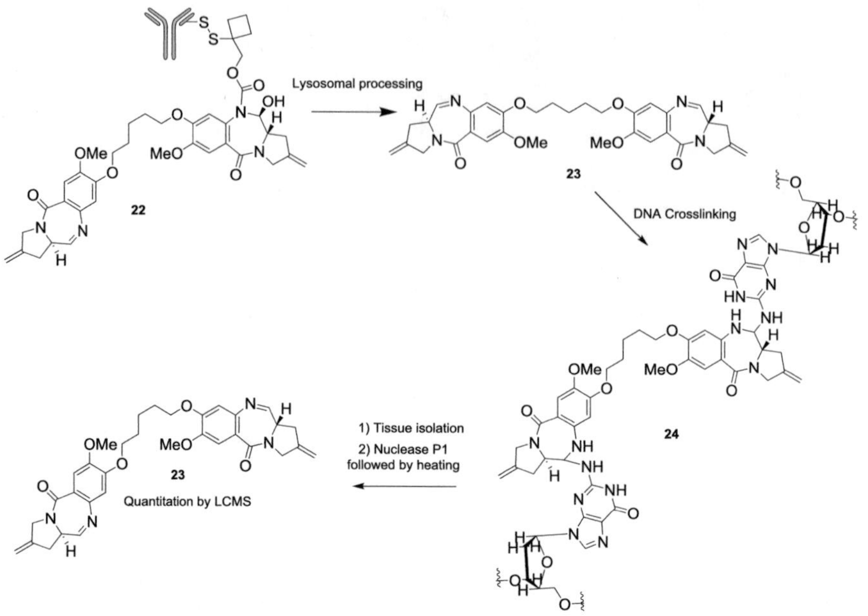

Fig. 8 Quantitation of DNA-bound PBD by LCMS

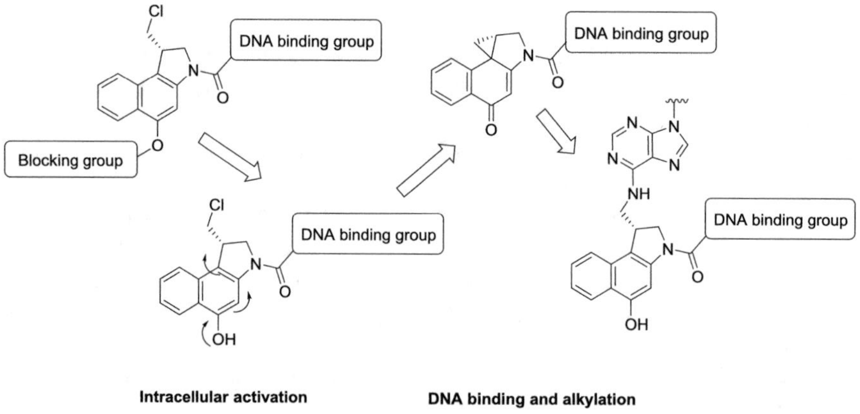

Fig. 9 Typical mechanism of duocarmycin DNA alkylation

Duocarmycin Based Payloads

Duocarmycins are a class of DNA-damaging natural products isolated from Streptomyces. Most duocarmycins contain a cyclopropabenzindole (CBI) or related pharmacophore that binds to the minor groove of DNA and alkylates adenine residues, as shown in Fig. 9. Typically, this process involves a 2-step process: Removal

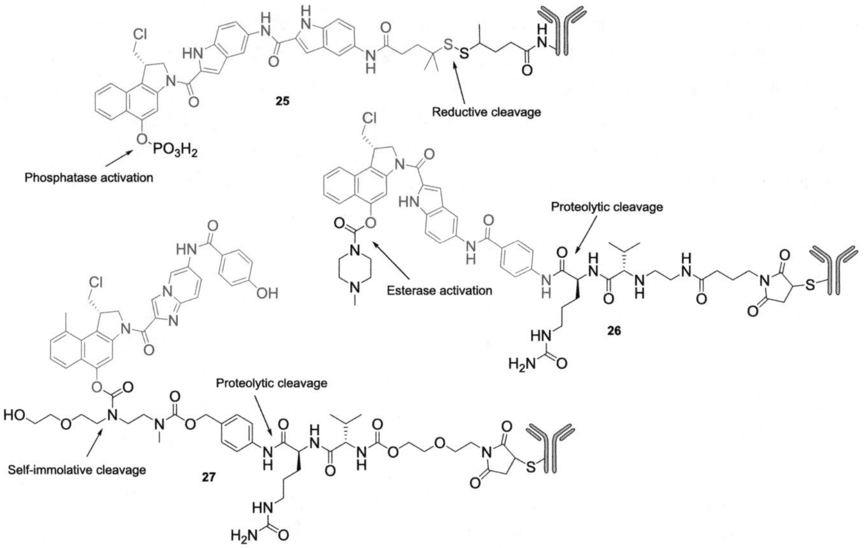

Fig. 10 Structures of duocarmycin linker-payloads

of a phenolic blocking group followed by an elimination of HCl resulting in the formation of an electrophilic cyclopropyl moiety. Some duocarmycins have been reported to exhibit delayed toxicity in animal models, perhaps related to their mechanistic similarity to PBDs. However, several compounds of this class have overcome this liability and have been advanced into clinical and late-stage preclinical studies [45, 46].

A variety of attachment strategies have been used to link duocarmycin payloads to ADCs. Building on their seminal work in this field [46], Zhao and team from ImmunoGen blocked the phenolic activation group with a phosphate moiety and linked the DNA-binding group to an antibody via a hindered disulfide linker, as shown in Fig. 10 [47] (**25**). Both anti-CanAg and anti-CD19 ADCs of this molecule exhibited single-digit pM activity against antigen expressing cells and over 3–4 orders of magnitude lower activity against a non-antigen expressing cell line. Cellular activity of the corresponding S-methyl capped linker-payload (as a small molecule) was dependent upon pre-treatment with phosphatase. However, the ADC did not require phosphatase pre-treatment for activity, thereby showing that the phenolic phosphate is cleaved from the ADC during the internalization process, likely in the lysosome or late endosome. The anti-CD19 ADC of **25** was found to be highly active in a mouse xenograft model of Burkitt's lymphoma while the linker-payload alone was found to be inactive at the same dose (payload dose = 75 μg/kg, qdx5).

A closely related anti-CD70 duocarmycin ADC (**26**, MDX-1203) has been evaluated preclinically and clinically by Medarex (now Bristol-Myers Squibb). In this case, a carbamoyl prodrug guards against premature activation of the CBI warhead while the DNA binding motif is attached to the antibody via a proteolytically cleavable linker [44]. The phenolic carbamate is susceptible to premature cleavage in plasma, perhaps via esterases, thereby rendering the payload susceptible to enzymatic inactivation via serum proteases [48]. In spite of the stability challenges, MDX-1203 (**26**) was highly active at doses as low as 4 mg/kg in a variety of renal cell carcinoma (RCC) and B cell lymphoma (BCL) xenograft models and was tolerated in cynomolgus monkeys at doses as high as 100 mg/kg. Based on these findings, MDX-1203 was advanced into human clinical trials in patients with advanced RCC or BCL. At the highest dose (15 mg/kg), 11 of 16 patients were found to achieve stable disease. Unexpectedly, however, this dose also elicited delayed toxicities (facial edema, pleural effusion and pericardial effusion) in 50% of the patients beginning approximately 14–56 days after the final dose [49]. Delayed toxicity was not noted at lower doses and the MTD was thus determined to be 8 mg/kg. It is unclear whether the delayed toxicity observed in the clinic is mechanistically related to the delayed toxicity that had been observed for other DNA-damaging ADCs in murine preclinical safety models. In spite of the challenges associated with this molecule, an interesting report in 2013 describes a bioanalytical method for the quantitation of alkylated adenine residues in tissues that have been exposed to MDX-1203 [44]. This opens the door for a possible mechanistic understanding of the efficacy and toxicity associated with this molecule.

Rather than linking the duocarmycin through the DNA binding group, Dokter and colleagues from Synthon developed an innovative approach for linking to the antibody through a self-immolative carbamoyl phenolic blocking group. (**27**) The self-immolation is triggered by the proteolytic cleavage of a ValCitPABC moiety, as shown in Fig. 10 [50]. A Her2 ADC using this payload (**27**, known as SYD985) was shown to be far more effective than T-DM1 in the killing of low Her2 expressing cells lines both *in vitro* and *in vivo*. At doses of 1–3 mg/kg, SYD985 elicited tumor stasis and regression in multiple low Her2 expressing (1+ and 2+) models, while T-DM1 was found to be generally ineffective even at doses as high as 30 mg/kg. Moreover, co-culture experiments demonstrated that SYD985 was able to kill non-Her2 expressing cells (0+) in the presence of SK-BR-3 (Her2 3+) and SK-OV-3 (Her2 2+) cells. This suggests that the released payload is sufficiently permeable that it can elicit cytotoxicity in tumors with heterogeneous antigen expression [51]. Unexpectedly, the phenolic carbamate was found to be cleaved in mouse plasma resulting in unexpectedly low plasma ADC exposure and the premature release of payload. Premature cleavage was not observed in other species (including cynomolgus monkey) and the source of instability was eventually traced to a mouse-specific esterase (Ces1C). SYD985 was well tolerated in cynomolgus monkeys at doses of 30 mg/kg (2 doses, 3.5 weeks apart). In contrast to many auristatin-based ADCs, no hepatotoxicity, thrombocytopenia, or peripheral sensory neuropathy were observed at this dose [50]. Based on these results, SYD985 is currently undergoing clinical evaluation in Her2 positive metastatic breast cancer.

Finally, Pfizer has reported a series of CBI dimer linker-payloads that are conceptually related to duocarmycin. Attached to an anti-CD33 antibody, these ADCs were shown to be effective against CD33 expressing xenograft models at doses as low as 0.3 mg/kg. Importantly, the compounds were shown to retain activity against PGP expressing TF-1 cells both *in vitro* and *in vivo* [52, 53]. No safety data has been reported to-date.

Anthracycline and Camptothecin

Unlike most other ADC payloads, anthracyclines and camptothecin (and related analogs) are widely used small-molecule chemotherapeutic agents. They act both as topoisomerase inhibitors and DNA intercalators, thereby interfering with DNA transcription and replication. The wealth of clinical data associated with these compounds combined with the success of multiple DNA-damaging ADCs makes them attractive for use as ADC payloads. However, the *in vitro* cytotoxicity of most anthracyclines and camptothecins is in a range believed to be insufficient for optimal ADC efficacy. In fact, early doxorubicin conjugates exhibited efficacy only when dosed at ~700 mg/kg [54]. Thus, most recent efforts for the advancement of these payloads have focused on ultra-potent agents that have not been evaluated clinically. For instance, Burke showed that an anti-CD70 ADC employing an ultrapotent camptothecin analog (**28**) was active in an RCC xenograft model (Caki-1) when dosed at levels as low as 3 mg/kg [55]. Camptothecin analogs have notoriously poor solubility, and thus it is interesting to note that conjugation of this payload was facilitated by the use of a highly polar glucuronide linker. Using this linker, little or no ADC aggregation was observed even at loadings of up to 8 drugs per antibody.

A water soluble camptothecin derivative known as exatecan has also been reported to result in highly active ADCs. Conjugates of this payload utilizing a GlyGlyPheGly linker that incorporate a short ether linkage between the payload and the cleavage element (**29**) have been shown to result in low aggregation and excellent cellular cytotoxicity even with a DAR of 8 [56]. In particular, anti-Her2 ADCs (such as DS-8201a) of this payload have been show exhibit excellent bystander activity and to overcome resistance that is imparted by PGP expression [57, 58]. This compound is currently undergoing clinical evaluation by Daiichi Sankyo.

An active metabolite of irinotecan (known as SN-38) has also been evaluated as an ADC payload and has shown promise in the context of anti-Trop2 [59], anti-CD74 [60] and anti-CD22 [61] conjugates. The payload is attached via a hydrolytically cleavage carbonate linkage to the sterically hindered C-20 alcohol of SN-38. (**30**) While the carbonate linker was designed to be cleaved at low pH, it is also susceptible to premature cleavage in plasma. This results in a relatively short half-life ($T_{1/2}$ of the ADC ~11 h) in PK studies and thus requires more frequent dosing in order to maintain plasma levels of the ADC [59].

In spite of these stability challenges, the anti-Trop2 conjugate of SN-38 (known as IMMU-132) has shown promise in a variety of epithelial cancer models, including Calu-3 (lung), COLO-205 (colorectal), and BxPC-3 (pancreatic) at doses as low as 0.4 mg SN-38/kg (~10 mg/kg ADC) [62]. Interestingly, and perhaps not surprisingly given the stability issue mentioned above, non-targeted SN-38 conjugates have also shown modest anti-tumor activity in some of the above models. Two doses of IMMU-132 (3 days apart) were tolerated in mice at up to 12 mg SN-38/kg (~300 mg/kg ADC) and in cynomolgus monkeys at up to 0.96 mg SN-38/kg (~23 mg/kg ADC). At higher doses (1.92 mg SN-38/kg or ~48 mg/kg ADC), significant gastrointestinal and hematological toxicity was observed. The authors believe that the dose-limiting toxicities (DLTs) observed for IMMU-132 are directly related to the free payload, which exhibits similar DLTs as a single agent [62]. IMMU-132 (Sacituzumab Govitecan) is currently being evaluated in Phase II clinical trials. Initial reports show that the conjugate is tolerated at doses up to ~10 mg/kg in humans (dosing on days 1 and 8 of a 21 day cycle) and the primary DLT is neutropenia [63].

Finally, Genentech has reported an anti-CD22 anthracycline-based ADC that is active against tumor models that have become resistant to vcMMAE conjugates [64]. The ADC, **31**, consists of a proteolytic linker attached to a doxorubicin analog (known as PNU-159682) that has a pM activity against a variety of cell lines. This conjugate was found to have *in vivo* activity against a variety of CD22 expressing cell lines at doses of 1–2 mg/kg (single dose), comparable to the activity of an anti-CD22 vcMMAE conjugate. Importantly, the doxorubicin conjugate showed activity in xenograft models that had acquired resistance to auristatin conjugates. The resistant lines were shown to have increased PGP expression, thus indicating that the doxorubicin conjugate may be useful in PGP expressing tumors. While the exact released species was not identified, the payload itself was shown not to be a substrate for PGP mediated efflux. More recently, the same payload has been reported on an anti-CD30 conjugate linked via a sortase-mediated conjugation strategy [65] (Fig. 11).

Bcl-x_L Inhibitors

Most chemotherapy agents have historically acted via direct disruption of critical cellular machinery, such as DNA replication, DNA transcription, or tubulin polymerization. However, numerous recent studies have teased out various apoptotic signaling pathways and have opened up a new mechanism for cytotoxicity: Direct induction of apoptosis. This is particularly attractive because one of the hallmarks of cancer is, in fact, insensitivity to apoptotic signaling. One mechanism by which cells become resistant towards apoptosis is through overexpression of certain anti-apoptotic Bcl-2 family members, such as Bcl-x_L. These anti-apoptotic proteins bind and block the activity of pro-apoptotic BH3-domain proteins such as Bid and Bim. Agents that block the BH3-binding domain on Bcl-x_L have been shown to restore proper apoptotic function and perhaps even induce apoptosis in malignant cells. Bcl-x_L inhibitors have been evaluated in the clinic, however significant thrombocytopenia has been a dose-limiting side effect, likely because circulating platelets are dependent upon Bcl-x_L for survival [66]. Thus, teams have begun to explore the possibility of ADC-mediated delivery of Bcl-x_L inhibitors in order to avoid these off-target activities.

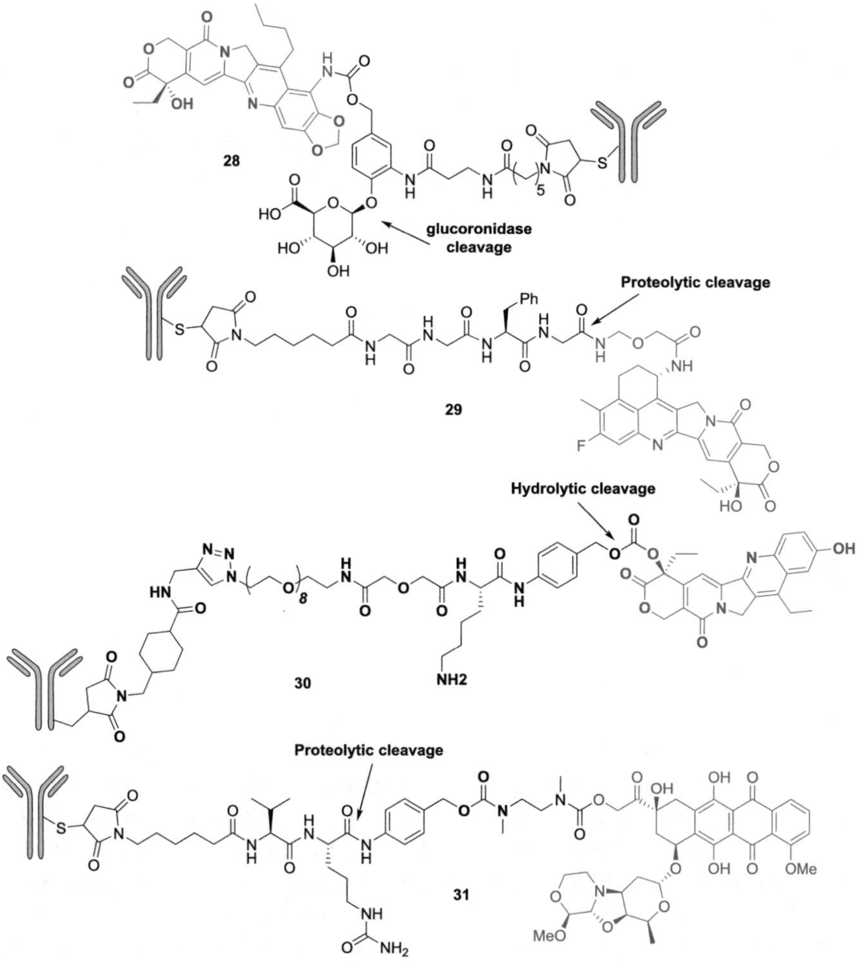

Fig. 11 Structure of anthracycline and camptothecin based ADCs

Given their clinical experience with Bcl2 and Bcl-x_L inhibitors, it is not surprising that AbbVie is leading the way in the development of this new class of ADC payload [67, 68]. While the specific details have not been reported, two examples of anti-EGFR Bcl-x_L ADCs (**32** and **33**) are shown in Fig. 12. Both compounds were shown to be active in xenograft models at doses of 3–10 mg/kg and were demonstrated to be synergistic with docetaxel. Given the previous clinical DLTs with Bcl-x_L inhibitors, it is important to note that these ADCs were tolerated in mice at doses of up to 30 mg/kg with no signs of thrombocytopenia. Many permutations of these ADCs incorporated charged moieties into the payload (i.e. **33**). While the specific role of this functionality was not disclosed, it is conceivable that it either helps the payload to evade PGP pumps or perhaps limits the permeability of the payload thereby allowing the intracellular concentration of the inhibitor to build up over the course of treatment.

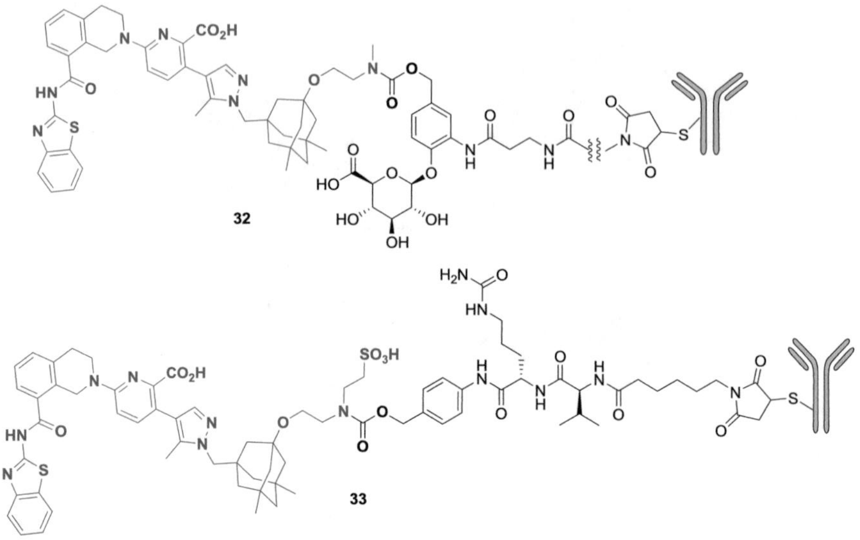

Fig. 12 Structures of Bcl-x_L inhibitor linker-payloads

Spliceosome Inhibitors

RNA splicing is a critical step in the process of DNA translation. Newly synthesized pre-mRNA is edited and processed in a large protein complex known as the spliceosome. A number of natural products are known to inhibit RNA splicing by binding to various subunits of the spliceosome. Thailanstatin A binds noncovalently to the SF3b subunit of the sliceosome with low-nM to sub-nM affinity, thereby inhibiting proper RNA splicing [69]. A team at Pfizer developed an anti-Her2 noncleavable thailanstatin ADC (**34**) that shows low nM activity in a variety of Her2 expressing cell lines, including a PGP-overexpressing line. In vivo activity was demonstrated in an N87 gastric cancer xenograft model at doses as low as 1.5 mg/kg (qdx4) and the compound was well tolerated in rats at doses of 10 mg/kg.

RNA Polymerase Inhibitors

RNA polymerase inhibitors are potent cytotoxins that directly block the transcription of DNA into mRNA. No doubt, the most well-known class of RNA polymerase inhibitors are the amatoxins, a series of macrocyclic peptides produced by a variety of mushrooms, particularly the *Amanita* genus. One natural product of this class (α-amanitin) was coupled to an anti-EpCAM antibody via lysine chemistry thereby generating a non-cleavable ADC (DAR~6) that showed pM activity against a variety of solid tumor lines. The ADC was shown to have antitumor activity in a PxPc-3

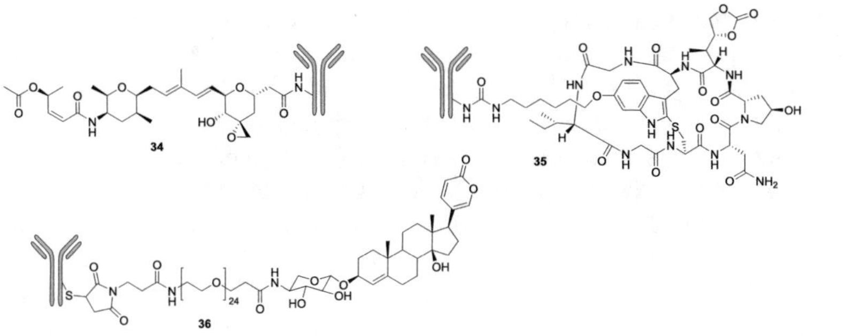

Fig. 13 Spliceosome inhibitor (34), RNA polymerase inhibitor (35), and NKA inhibitor (36) ADCs

pancreatic cancer model at doses as low as 2 mg/kg (single dose, IP) and 0.8 mg/kg (2 doses, 7 days apart, IP). Consistent with the toxicity profile of α-amanitin, severe body weight loss and pronounced liver toxicity was observed at 6 mg/kg and 12 mg/kg (single dose, IP) [70].

Building on this work, several teams have now filed patent applications on amatoxin ADCs [71–73]. For example, Heidelberg Pharma describes a method for incorporating a noncleavable lysine-reactive linker off the central 6-hydroxyindole (**35**). For reasons that are unclear, the 1,2 diol of the natural product was tied up in a cyclic carbonate as illustrated in Fig. 13. An anti-Her2 conjugate of this linker-payload was shown to have ~40 pM activity against Her2 expressing SKOV-3 and SKBR-3 cell lines and ~2 nM activity against trastuzumab-resistant JIMT-1 cells. This ADC induced complete tumor regression in a JIMT-1 xenograft model at 30 μg amatoxin/kg (~1 mg/kg ADC, single dose IV) and was tolerated in mice at up to 300 μg amatoxin/kg (~10 mg/kg ADC, single dose IV). Interestingly, a closely related conjugate lacking the cyclic carbonate was not tolerated at this dose [73].

Emerging Cytotoxic Payloads

Innovative approaches to induce antiproliferative activity continue to be reported. For example, Bayer recently filed a patent application for the use of kinesin spindle protein (KSP) inhibitors as ADC payloads [74]. KSP is an enzyme responsible for the ATP-dependent transport of cellular vesicles along cytosolic microtubules. The success of tubulin polymerization inhibitors as ADC payloads is perhaps a driver behind current interest in KSP inhibitors. While no *in vivo* activity was reported, anti-TWEAKR conjugates of KSP inhibitors exhibited low nM to sub-nM activity against a panel of cancer cell lines. Given the similarity of cellular processes dependent upon tubulin and KSP, it might be anticipated that efficacy and tolerability trends may overlap between these two classes of inhibitors.

Finally, Marshall has reported a fascinating new approach for the induction of cytotoxicity by blocking a surface membrane ion pump, Na^+/K^+-ATPase (NKA) [75]. Cardiac glycoside (CG) is a potent NKA inhibitor that that induces increased intracellular sodium concentration and can trigger apoptosis. Unlike other cytotoxic agents mentioned above, CG binds to a cell surface protein and thus does not require internalization. A CG conjugate (**36**) with antibodies that target cell various surface proteins resulted in potent cytotoxicity. In contrast, control CG conjugates that target a non-expressed antigen are >100 fold less toxic. Moreover, conjugated CG is ~350 fold more potent (mol/mol) than unconjugated CG. Two particular features may render these so-called "extracellular drug conjugates" (EDCs) advantageous as compared to many of the aforementioned mechanisms: (1) Lysosomal processing is not required and thus complications associated with lysosomal release and catabolism are avoided and (2) PGP efflux pumps and related resistance mechanisms are not likely to influence the activity of EDCs. While *in vivo* efficacy was demonstrated with an anti-CD20 EDC, it remains to be seen whether sufficient safety and efficacy can be achieved in order to warrant clinical development.

Non-oncology Payloads

The vast majority of ADC technology developed to-date has been aimed at oncology applications. However, the increasing success of clinical ADCs in oncology have prompted a flurry of interest in the targeted delivery of non-oncology payloads.

Anti-Inflammatory ADC Payloads

Anti-inflammatory ADCs are of particular interest due both to the unmet medical need for many diseases (in particular autoimmune disorders) and to the large portfolio of antibodies that have been designed to target specific lymphocytes. For example, pioneering work by Soren Moestrup showed that dexamethasone could be specifically targeted to macrophages by an anti-CD163 conjugate (**37**) [76]. This ADC was shown to block LPS-induced TNF-α in *ex-vivo* rat spleen at concentrations of ~10 ng/mL while a cognate non-targeted ADC was approximately 500-fold less active. It was also able to block the release of LPS induced TNF-α and IL-1 in Lewis rats at doses as low as 0.02 mg/kg [76] and has exhibited efficacy in a variety of autoimmune disease models [77–79].

More recently, Kern and colleagues at Merck have developed an innovative strategy for linking dexamethasone and other glucocorticoid receptor (GR) modulators to antibodies through a phosphatase-cleavable linkage. (**38–39**) Anti-CD70 conjugates were generated in order to specifically target the dexamethasone to T-cells. However, the resulting conjugate (**38**) did not activate 786-O cells (CD70+) as well as might be expected based on the activity of dexamethasone alone. Conjugation of a more potent glucocorticoid modulator (fluticasone, **39**) resulted in an ADC that was active at ~15-fold lower concentration and exhibited a 2–3 fold higher E_{max} [80]. A related series of protease-cleavable GR modulator ADCs has also been described [81].

Numerous selective kinase inhibitors have been developed in the past two decades as immunomodulators. While tremendous strides have been made at designing highly selective inhibitors, the sheer number of homologous kinases makes the identification of an exquisitely selective kinase inhibitor a daunting prospect. For this reason, there is increasing interest in having "dual selectivity" imparted by delivering the small molecule (a selective kinase inhibitor) via a tissue-specific delivery vehicle (selective tissue targeting). For example, Peter Schultz describes the delivery of dasatinib directly to T-cells via conjugation with an antibody against CXCR4, a protein expressed selectively on the surface of human T-cells . The efficacy of dasatinib is believed to be driven by inhibition of Bcr-Abl and Src family kinases in T-cells, but exposure in other tissues likely leads to the well-studied cardiovascular and dermatological side effects. Thus, selective delivery of dasatinib to T-cells may impart an improved therapeutic window for this agent. The resulting anti-CXCR4-dasatinib conjugate (**40**) was shown to block cytokine release from human T-cells with an IC_{50} of ~12 nM. In contrast, a control ADC (anti-Her2) with the same linker payload did not block cytokine release at concentrations of up to 200 nM [82].

Lymphocyte function-associated antigen-1 (LFA-1) is an integrin that is ubiquitously expressed on leukocytes including monocytes, macrophages, and granulocytes. Antibodies targeting the alpha chain of LFA-1 (CD11a) have been used to direct both phosphodiesterase 4 (PDE4) inhibitors and liver X receptor (LXR) agonists to cells of the immune system. PDE4 inhibitors are known for their GI toxicity and thus methods of selectively targeting these agents in ways that avoid GI exposure may prove therapeutically valuable. An anti-CD11a PDE4 conjugate (**41**) was shown to block TNFα release from mouse peritoneal cells with an IC_{50} of ~60 nM. Dosed at 5 mg/kg in mice, this ADC was shown to block recruitment of T-cells to the site of inflammation in a carrageenan-induced air pouch inflammation model [82]. A similar strategy was employed for the delivery of a LXR agonist to T-cells in hopes of avoiding hepatocyte-mediated side effects. While no in vivo data was reported, the conjugate (a protease cleavable ADC) was shown to be internalized into THP-1 cells but not into heptatocytes [83]. Combined, these studies provide a potential path forward for anti-inflammatory compounds that have been underutilized or deprioritized due to off-target side effects (Fig. 14).

Anti-Infective ADC Payloads

Bacteria and viruses do not possess mechanisms to directly internalize an ADC and therefore the development of an anti-infective ADC may seem rather counter-intuitive. However, a team from Genentech made the insightful observation that

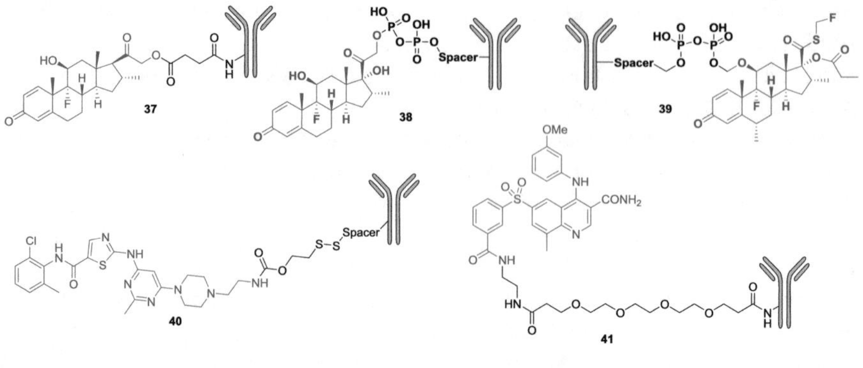

Fig. 14 Structures of recently reported anti-inflammatory ADCs

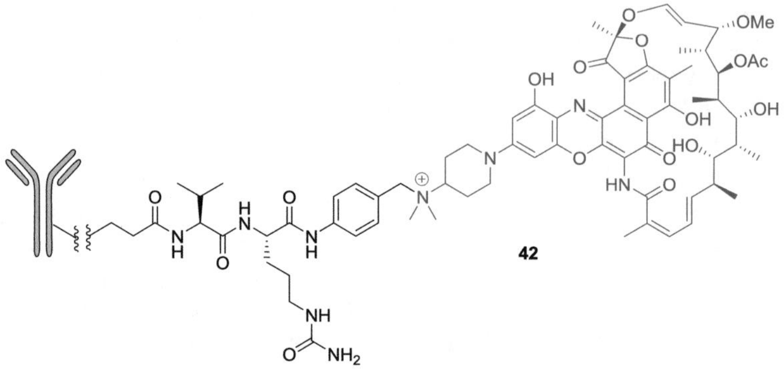

Fig. 15 An antibody-antibiotic drug conjugate

Staphylococcus aureus are known to evade the host immune system by residing in various intracellular compartments of the host macrophages. With this in mind, the team generated a proteolytically released rifampicin analog conjugated to an anti-S. *aureus* antibody (**42**). Conceptually, the ADC would coat (opsonize) the bacteria before being internalized into a host cell macrophage. Once inside the macrophage lysosome, the ADC would undergo lysosomal processing thereby releasing the antibiotic which, in turn, would kill the bacteria that are hiding out in the host cell. The ADC (**42**) was shown to opsonize and kill methicillin resistant *Staph aureus* (MRSA) inside macrophages while a control ADC with a non-cleavable linker did not. At 50 mg/kg, the conjugate was shown to be more effective at eradicating a murine MRSA infection than vancomycin [84]. While this may be a niche application, it is a timely reminder that many creative uses of ADCs remain to be explored (Fig. 15).

siRNA Delivery

Lastly, an interesting and perhaps groundbreaking study by Sugo describes the use of an anti-CD71 (transferrin) Fab for the delivery of short-interfering RNA (siRNA) into muscles. siRNA technology holds tremendous therapeutic promise, but has generally been limited by the inability to selectively deliver siRNA to tissues of interest. However, liver targeting using GalNAc as a targeting ligand has enjoyed some success. As an alternative approach, the team from Takeda designed an anti-CD71 maleimide conjugate with a ~12-mer siRNA. When dosed at 10 mg/kg, an anti-CD71 siApoB conjugate was found to reduce the amount of ApoB mRNA by 44% 24 h post-dose. A related conjugate (anti-CD71 siHPRT) was shown to reduce the amount of HPRT mRNA by 65% even 7 days after dosing [85]. While these results are certainly preliminary, they demonstrate that ADC delivery of siRNA is a feasible goal. Importantly, this study demonstrates that delivery of siRNA may require subtle changes to the targeting moiety, as antibody-mediated delivery of siRNA has proven challenging [86]. The authors suggest that the monovalent Fab used in this study may provide either more efficient lysosomal trafficking or more efficient endosomal release as compared to the previously reported antibody-directed approach.

Conclusions

While the ADC pipeline has grown considerably over the past 5 years, few have reached late stage trials. Since the inception of ADC technology, approximate 80 conjugates have entered clinical development. Approximately 30% of these have been discontinued and only four agents are actively being pursued in phase III clinical trials. While the high rate of clinical failure cannot be attributed to any single factor, it is interesting to note the lack of diversity of payload technology in the current clinical pipeline [87]. Developments described in this chapter are hopefully paving the way for an increasingly diverse clinical pipeline with greater chances of clinical success. Of particular interest are emerging payloads that address liabilities in current ADC technology, such as overcoming PGP-efflux and other mechanisms of ADC resistance, the ability to kill slow growing or quiescent tumors, and the ability to use biomarkers to develop a mechanistic understanding of ADC toxicity. In parallel with these advances, we have now seen a steady flow of new reports describing linker-payloads for use in non-oncology ADC applications. In fact, corporate presentations suggest that both antibacterial and anti-inflammatory ADCs will be entering the clinic in 2018–2019. In summary, the ADC research community has made tremendous strides over the past 10 years and the field is now in a position of anxiously awaiting clinical results that will, hopefully, validate many of the emerging technologies described in this chapter.

References

1. Perez HL, Cardarelli PM, Deshpande S et al (2014) Antibody-drug conjugates: current status and future directions. Drug Discov Today 19:869–881. https://doi.org/10.1016/j.drudis.2013.11.004
2. Ricart AD (2011) Antibody-drug conjugates of calicheamicin derivative: Gemtuzumab ozogamicin and inotuzumab ozogamicin. Clin Cancer Res 17:6417–6427. https://doi.org/10.1158/1078-0432.CCR-11-0486
3. Terriou L, Bonnet S, Debarri H et al (2013) Brentuximab vedotin: new treatment for CD30+ lymphomas. Bull Cancer 100:775–779. https://doi.org/10.1684/bdc.2013.1778
4. Corrigan PA, Cicci TA, Auten JJ, Lowe DK (2014) Ado-trastuzumab emtansine: a HER2-positive targeted antibody-drug conjugate. Ann Pharmacother 48:1484–1493
5. Mendelsohn BA, Barnscher SD, Snyder JT et al (2017) Investigation of hydrophilic Auristatin derivatives for use in antibody drug conjugates. Bioconjug Chem 28:371–381. https://doi.org/10.1021/acs.bioconjchem.6b00530
6. Lyon RP, Bovee TD, Doronina SO et al (2015) Reducing hydrophobicity of homogeneous antibody-drug conjugates improves pharmacokinetics and therapeutic index. Nat Biotechnol 33:733–736. https://doi.org/10.1038/nbt.3212
7. Maderna A, Doroski M, Subramanyam C et al (2014) Discovery of cytotoxic Dolastatin 10 analogues with N-terminal modifications. J Med Chem 57:10527–10543. https://doi.org/10.1021/jm501649k
8. Damelin M, Bankovich A, Bernstein J et al (2017) A PTK7-targeted antibody-drug conjugate reduces tumor-initiating cells and induces sustained tumor regressions. Sci Transl Med 9:1–12. https://doi.org/10.1126/scitranslmed.aag2611
9. Tumey LN, Li F, Rago B et al (2017) Site selection: a case study in the identification of optimal cysteine engineered antibody drug conjugates. AAPS J 19:1123–1135. https://doi.org/10.1208/s12248-017-0083-7
10. Strop P, Tran T-T, Dorywalska M et al (2016) RN927C, a site-specific Trop-2 antibody-drug conjugate (ADC) with enhanced stability, is highly efficacious in preclinical solid tumor models. Mol Cancer Ther 15:2698–2708. https://doi.org/10.1158/1535-7163.MCT-16-0431
11. Geierstanger J, Grunewald B, Yunho OW, et al (2015) Cytotoxic Peptides and Conjugates Thereof. WO2015/95301
12. Murray BC, Peterson MT, R a F (2015) Chemistry and biology of tubulysins: antimitotic tetrapeptides with activity against drug resistant cancers. Nat Prod Rep 32:654. https://doi.org/10.1039/C4NP00036F
13. Reddy JA, Dorton R, Dawson A et al (2009) In vivo structural activity and optimization studies of folate-tubulysin conjugates. Mol Pharm 6:1518–1525. https://doi.org/10.1021/mp900086w
14. Kularatne SA, Venkatesh C, Santhapuram HK et al (2010) Synthesis and biological analysis of prostate-specific membrane antigen-targeted anticancer prodrugs. J Med Chem 53:7767–7777. https://doi.org/10.1021/jm100729b
15. Leverett CA, Sukuru SCK, Vetelino BC et al (2016) Design, synthesis, and cytotoxic evaluation of novel Tubulysin analogs as ADC payloads. ACS Med Chem Lett. acsmedchemlett.6b00274. https://doi.org/10.1021/acsmedchemlett.6b00274
16. Nathan Tumey L, Leverett CA, Vetelino B et al (2016) Optimization of Tubulysin antibody-drug conjugates: a case study in addressing ADC metabolism. ACS Med Chem Lett 7:977–982. https://doi.org/10.1021/acsmedchemlett.6b00195
17. Cong Q, Cheng H, Gangwar S (2014) Preparation of antimitotic compounds structurally related to tubulysins and their conjugates for targeted delivery and their use for treating cancers. US2014/0227295
18. Li JY, Perry SR, Muniz-Medina V et al (2016) A Biparatopic HER2-targeting antibody-drug conjugate induces tumor regression in primary models refractory to or ineligible for HER2-targeted therapy. Cancer Cell 29:117–129. https://doi.org/10.1016/j.ccell.2015.12.008

19. Kovtun YV, Audette CA, Mayo MF et al (2010) Antibody-maytansinoid conjugates designed to bypass multidrug resistance. Cancer Res 70:2528–2537. https://doi.org/10.1158/0008-5472.CAN-09-3546
20. Pillow TH, Tien J, Parsons-Reponte KL et al (2014) Site-specific trastuzumab maytansinoid antibody-drug conjugates with improved therapeutic activity through linker and antibody engineering. J Med Chem 57:7890–7899. https://doi.org/10.1021/jm500552c
21. Widdison WC, Ponte JF, Coccia JA et al (2015) Development of Anilino-Maytansinoid ADCs that efficiently release cytotoxic metabolites in cancer cells and induce high levels of bystander killing. Bioconjug Chem 26:2261–2278. https://doi.org/10.1021/acs.bioconjchem.5b00430
22. Steinkuhler MC, Gallinari MP, Osswald B et al (2016) Cryptophycin-based antibody-drug conjugates with novel self-immolative linkers. WO2016146638A1
23. Bernardes Goncalo JL, Casi G, Trussel S et al (2012) A traceless vascular-targeting antibody-drug conjugate for cancer therapy. Angew Chem Int Ed Engl 51:941–944
24. Liang ZX (2010) Complexity and simplicity in the biosynthesis of enediyne natural products. Nat Prod Rep 27:499–528. https://doi.org/10.1039/b908165h
25. Damelin M, Bankovich A, Park A et al (2015) Anti-EFNA4 calicheamicin conjugates effectively target triple-negative breast and ovarian tumor-initiating cells to result in sustained tumor regressions. Clin Cancer Res 21:4165–4173. https://doi.org/10.1158/1078-0432.CCR-15-0695
26. Jain N, O'Brien S, Thomas D, Kantarjian H (2014) Inotuzumab ozogamicin in the treatment of acute lymphoblastic leukemia. Front Biosci (Elite Ed) 6:40–45
27. Pilorge S, Rigaudeau S, Rabian F et al (2014) Fractionated gemtuzumab ozogamicin and standard dose cytarabine produced prolonged second remissions in patients over the age of 55 years with acute myeloid leukemia in late first relapse. Am J Hematol 89:399–403. https://doi.org/10.1002/ajh.23653
28. Gavrilyuk J, Sisodiya, Vikram N (2016) Calicheamicin Constructs and Methods of Use. WO/2016/172273
29. Donaghy H (2016) Effects of antibody, drug and linker on the preclinical and clinical toxicities of antibody-drug conjugates. MAbs 8:659–671. https://doi.org/10.1080/19420862.2016.1156829
30. Chowdari NS, Gangwar S, Sufi B (2013) Enediyne compounds, conjugates thereof, and uses and methods thereof. WO/2013/122823
31. Mantaj J, Jackson PJM, Rahman KM, Thurston DE (2017) From Anthramycin to Pyrrolobenzodiazepine (PBD)-containing antibody–drug conjugates (ADCs). Angew Chem Int Ed 56:462–488. https://doi.org/10.1002/anie.201510610
32. Jeffrey SC, Burke PJ, Lyon RP et al (2013) A potent anti-CD70 antibody-drug conjugate combining a Dimeric Pyrrolobenzodiazepine drug with site-specific conjugation technology. Bioconjug Chem 24:1256–1263. https://doi.org/10.1021/bc400217g
33. Sutherland MSK, Walter RB, Jeffrey SC et al (2013) SGN-CD33A: a novel CD33-targeting antibody-drug conjugate using a pyrrolobenzodiazepine dimer is active in models of drug-resistant AML. Blood 122:1455–1463. https://doi.org/10.1182/blood-2013-03-491506
34. Sutherland MSK, Yu C, Walter RB et al (2015) SGN-CD123A, a Pyrrolobenzodiazepine dimer linked anti-CD123 antibody drug conjugate, demonstrates effective anti-leukemic activity in multiple preclinical models of AML. Blood 126:330
35. Lewis T, Olson DJ, Gordon KA et al (2016) Abstract 1195: SGN-CD352A: a novel humanized anti-CD352 antibody-drug conjugate for the treatment of multiple myeloma. Cancer Res 76:1195–1195. https://doi.org/10.1158/1538-7445.AM2016-1195
36. Takeshita A (2013) Efficacy and resistance of gemtuzumab ozogamicin for acute myeloid leukemia. Int J Hematol 97:703–716. https://doi.org/10.1007/s12185-013-1365-1
37. Cianfriglia M (2013) The biology of MDR1-P-glycoprotein (MDR1-Pgp) in designing functional antibody drug conjugates (ADCs): the experience of gemtuzumab ozogamicin. Ann Ist Super Sanita 49:150–168. https://doi.org/10.4415/ann_13_02_07

38. Tiberghien AC, Levy JN, Masterson LA et al (2016) Design and synthesis of Tesirine, a clinical antibody-drug conjugate Pyrrolobenzodiazepine dimer payload. ACS Med Chem Lett 7:983–987. https://doi.org/10.1021/acsmedchemlett.6b00062
39. Saunders LR, Bankovich AJ, Anderson WC et al (2015) A DLL3-targeted antibody-drug conjugate eradicates high-grade pulmonary neuroendocrine tumor-initiating cells in vivo HHS public access. Sci Transl Med 7:302–136. https://doi.org/10.1126/scitranslmed.aac9459
40. Flynn MJ, Zammarchi F, Tyrer PC et al (2016) ADCT-301, a Pyrrolobenzodiazepine (PBD) dimer-containing antibody-drug conjugate (ADC) targeting CD25-expressing hematological malignancies. Mol Cancer Ther 15:2709–2721. https://doi.org/10.1158/1535-7163.MCT-16-0233
41. Miller ML, Fishkin NE, Li W et al (2016) A new class of antibody-drug conjugates with potent DNA alkylating activity. Mol Cancer Ther 15:1870–1878. https://doi.org/10.1158/1535-7163.MCT-16-0184
42. Zhao RY, Wilhelm SD, Audette C et al (2011) Synthesis and evaluation of hydrophilic linkers for antibody-Maytansinoid conjugates. J Med Chem 54:3606–3623. https://doi.org/10.1021/jm2002958
43. Ma Y, Khojasteh SC, Hop CECA et al (2016) Antibody drug conjugates differentiate uptake and DNA alkylation of pyrrolobenzodiazepines in tumors from organs of xenograft mice. Drug Metab Dispos 44:1958–1962. https://doi.org/10.1124/dmd.116.073031
44. Thevanayagam L, Bell A, Chakraborty I et al (2013) Novel detection of DNA-alkylated adducts of antibody-drug conjugates with potentially unique preclinical and biomarker applications. Bioanalysis 5:1073–1081. https://doi.org/10.4155/bio.13.57
45. Carter CA, Waud WR, Li LH et al (1996) Preclinical antitumor activity of bizelesin in mice. Clin Cancer Res 2:1143–1149
46. Chari RVJ, Jackel KA, Bourret LA et al (1995) Enhancement of the selectivity and antitumor efficacy of a CC-1065 analog through immunoconjugate formation. Cancer Res 55:4079–4084
47. Zhao RY, Erickson HK, Leece BA et al (2012) Synthesis and biological evaluation of antibody conjugates of phosphate prodrugs of cytotoxic DNA alkylators for the targeted treatment of cancer. J Med Chem 55:766–782. https://doi.org/10.1021/jm201284m
48. Tumey LN, Rago B, Han X (2015) In vivo biotransformations of antibody-drug conjugates. Bioanalysis 7:1649–1664. https://doi.org/10.4155/bio.15.84
49. Owonikoko TK, Hussain A, Stadler WM et al (2016) First-in-human multicenter phase i study of BMS-936561 (MDX-1203), an antibody-drug conjugate targeting CD70. Cancer Chemother Pharmacol 77:155–162. https://doi.org/10.1007/s00280-015-2909-2
50. Dokter W, Ubink R, van der Lee M et al (2014) Preclinical profile of the HER2-targeting ADC SYD983/SYD985: introduction of a new duocarmycin-based linker-drug platform. Mol Cancer Ther 13:2618–2629. https://doi.org/10.1158/1535-7163.MCT-14-0040-T
51. van der Lee MMC, Groothuis PG, Ubink R et al (2015) The preclinical profile of the Duocarmycin-based HER2-targeting ADC SYD985 predicts for clinical benefit in low HER2-expressing breast cancers. Mol Cancer Ther 14:692–703. https://doi.org/10.1158/1535-7163.MCT-14-0881-T
52. O'Donnell CJ Discovery of Novel Linker payloads and antibody drug conjugates for the treatment of cancer. http://worldadc-usa.com/wp-content/uploads/sites/99/2016/10/Chris-ODonnell-1.pdf. Accessed 28 Mar 2017
53. Maderna A, Subramanyam C, Tumey LN, et al (2016) Preparation of bifunctional cytotoxic agents containing the CTI pharmacophore including dimers and antibody conjugates for treating cancer. WO/2016/151432
54. Trail PA, Willner D, Lasch SJ et al (1993) Cure of xenografted human carcinomas by BR96-doxorubicin immunoconjugates. Science 261:212–215. https://doi.org/10.1126/science.8327892
55. Burke PJ, Senter PD, Meyer DW et al (2009) Design, synthesis , and biological evaluation of antibody - drug conjugates comprised of potent Camptothecin analogues. Bioconjug Chem 20:1242–1250

56. Nakada T, Masuda T, Naito H et al (2016) Novel antibody drug conjugates containing exatecan derivative-based cytotoxic payloads. Bioorg Med Chem Lett 26:1542–1545. https://doi.org/10.1016/j.bmcl.2016.02.020
57. Ogitani Y, Hagihara K, Oitate M et al (2016) Bystander killing effect of DS-8201a, a novel anti-human epidermal growth factor receptor 2 antibody???Drug conjugate, in tumors with human epidermal growth factor receptor 2 heterogeneity. Cancer Sci 107:1039–1046. https://doi.org/10.1111/cas.12966
58. Tamura K, Shitara K, Naito Y et al (2016) Single agent activity of DS-8201a, a HER2-targeting antibody-drug conjugate, in breast cancer patients previously treated with T-DM1: phase 1 dose escalation. Ann Oncol 27:552–587. https://doi.org/10.1093/annonc/mdw435.7
59. Cardillo TM, Govindan SV, Sharkey RM et al (2015) Sacituzumab govitecan (IMMU-132), an anti-Trop-2/SN-38 antibody-drug conjugate: characterization and efficacy in pancreatic, gastric, and other cancers. Bioconjug Chem 26:919–931. https://doi.org/10.1021/acs.bioconjchem.5b00223
60. Govindan SV, Cardillo TM, Sharkey RM et al (2013) Milatuzumab-SN-38 conjugates for the treatment of CD74+ cancers. Mol Cancer Ther 12:968–978. https://doi.org/10.1158/1535-7163.mct-12-1170
61. Sharkey RM, Govindan SV, Cardillo TM, Goldenberg DM (2012) Epratuzumab-SN-38: a new antibody-drug conjugate for the therapy of hematologic malignancies. Mol Cancer Ther 11:224–234. https://doi.org/10.1158/1535-7163.mct-11-0632
62. Cardillo TM, Govindan SV, Sharkey RM et al (2011) Humanized anti-Trop-2 IgG-SN-38 conjugate for effective treatment of diverse epithelial cancers: preclinical studies in human cancer Xenograft models and monkeys. Clin Cancer Res 17:3157–3169. https://doi.org/10.1158/1078-0432.ccr-10-2939
63. Starodub AN, Ocean AJ, Shah MA et al (2015) First-in-human trial of a novel anti-trop-2 antibody-SN-38 conjugate, sacituzumab govitecan, for the treatment of diverse metastatic solid tumors. Clin Cancer Res 21:3870–3878. https://doi.org/10.1158/1078-0432.CCR-14-3321
64. Yu SF, Zheng B, Go M et al (2015) A novel anti-CD22 anthracycline-based antibody-drug conjugate (ADC) that overcomes resistance to auristatin-based ADCs. Clin Cancer Res 21:3298–3306. https://doi.org/10.1158/1078-0432.CCR-14-2035
65. Stefan N, Gébleux R, Waldmeier L et al (2017) Highly potent, Anthracycline-based antibody-drug conjugates generated by enzymatic, site-specific conjugation. Mol Cancer Ther 16:879–892. https://doi.org/10.1158/1535-7163.MCT-16-0688
66. Hennessy EJ (2016) Selective inhibitors of Bcl-2 and Bcl-xL: balancing antitumor activity with on-target toxicity. Bioorg Med Chem Lett 26:2105–2114. https://doi.org/10.1016/j.bmcl.2016.03.032
67. Tao Z-F, Doherty G, Wang X, et al (2016) Preparation of Bcl-xL inhibitory compounds having low cell permeability and antibody drug conjugates containing them. WO2016094509 A1
68. Ackler SL, Bennett NB, Boghaert ER, et al (2016) Bcl-xl inhibitory compounds and antibody drug conjugates including the same. US20160158377A1
69. He H, Ratnayake AS, Janso JE et al (2014) Cytotoxic spliceostatins from Burkholderia sp. and their semisynthetic analogs. J Nat Prod 77:1864–1870. https://doi.org/10.1021/np500342m
70. Moldenhauer G, Salnikov AV, Lüttgau S et al (2012) Therapeutic potential of amanitin-conjugated anti-epithelial cell adhesion molecule monoclonal antibody against pancreatic carcinoma. J Natl Cancer Inst 104:622–634. https://doi.org/10.1093/jnci/djs140
71. Grunewald J, Jin Y, Ou W, Uno T (2016) Preparation of amatoxin derivatives and their immunoconjugates as inhibitors of RNA polymerase for treating cell proliferative disorders. WO2016071856 A1
72. Mendelsohn BA, Moon SJ (2013) Amatoxin derivatives and cell-permeable conjugates thereof as inhibitors of rna polymerase. WO2014043403 A1
73. Muller C, Anderl J, Simon W, et al (2014) Amatoxin derivatives. WO/2014/135282
74. Lerchen H-G, Wittrock S, Cancho Grande Y, et al (2016) Preparation of antibody-drug conjugates (ADCS) of KSP inhibitors with aglycosylated anti-TWEAKR antibodies. WO2016096610 A1

75. Marshall DJ, Harried SS, Murphy JL et al (2016) Extracellular antibody drug conjugates exploiting the proximity of two proteins. Mol Ther 24:1760–1770. https://doi.org/10.1038/mt.2016.119
76. Graversen JH, Svendsen P, Dagnæs-Hansen F et al (2012) Targeting the hemoglobin scavenger receptor CD163 in macrophages highly increases the anti-inflammatory potency of dexamethasone. Mol Ther 20:1550–1558. https://doi.org/10.1038/mt.2012.103
77. Granfeldt A, Hvas CL, Graversen JH et al (2013) Targeting dexamethasone to macrophages in a porcine endotoxemic model. Crit Care Med 41:e309–e318. https://doi.org/10.1097/CCM.0b013e31828a45ef
78. Thomsen KL, Møller HJ, Graversen JH et al (2016) Anti-CD163-dexamethasone conjugate inhibits the acute phase response to lipopolysaccharide in rats. World J Hepatol 8:726–730. https://doi.org/10.4254/wjh.v8.i17.726
79. Moller LN, Knudsen AR, Andersen KJ et al (2015) Anti-CD163-dexamethasone protects against apoptosis after ischemia/reperfusion injuries in the rat liver. Ann Med Surg 4:331–337. https://doi.org/10.1016/j.amsu.2015.09.001
80. Kern JC, Cancilla M, Dooney D et al (2016) Discovery of pyrophosphate Diesters as tunable, soluble, and bioorthogonal linkers for site-specific antibody-drug conjugates. J Am Chem Soc 138:1430–1445. https://doi.org/10.1021/jacs.5b12547
81. Kern JC, Dooney D, Zhang R et al (2016) Novel phosphate modified Cathepsin B linkers: improving aqueous solubility and enhancing payload scope of ADCs. Bioconjug Chem 27:2081–2088. https://doi.org/10.1021/acs.bioconjchem.6b00337
82. Wang RE, Liu T, Wang Y et al (2015) An immunosuppressive antibody-drug conjugate. J Am Chem Soc 137:3229–3232. https://doi.org/10.1021/jacs.5b00620
83. Lim RKV, Yu S, Cheng B et al (2015) Targeted delivery of LXR agonist using a site-specific antibody-drug conjugate. Bioconjug Chem 26:2216–2222. https://doi.org/10.1021/acs.bioconjchem.5b00203
84. Lehar SM, Pillow T, Xu M et al (2015) Novel antibody–antibiotic conjugate eliminates intracellular S. aureus. Nature 527:323–328. https://doi.org/10.1038/nature16057
85. Sugo T, Terada M, Oikawa T et al (2016) Development of antibody-siRNA conjugate targeted to cardiac and skeletal muscles. J Control Release 237:1–13. https://doi.org/10.1016/j.jconrel.2016.06.036
86. Cuellar TL, Barnes D, Nelson C et al (2015) Systematic evaluation of antibody-mediated siRNA delivery using an industrial platform of THIOMAB-siRNA conjugates. Nucleic Acids Res 43:1189–1203. https://doi.org/10.1093/nar/gku1362
87. Chari RVJ (2016) Expanding the reach of antibody-drug conjugates. ACS Med Chem Lett 7:974–976. https://doi.org/10.1021/acsmedchemlett.6b00312

Delivering More Payload (High DAR ADCs)

Natalya Bodyak and Alexander V. Yurkovetskiy

Abstract Antibody drug conjugates (ADCs) for oncology applications are chemotherapeutic agents designed to selectively deliver cytotoxic drug payloads to neoplastic tissue. This book chapter reviews the latest approaches for high drug loaded ADCs. The primary focus of this review is related to ADC drug payload and antibody-drug bioconjugation linker selection strategies resulting in biotherapeutics with improved physicochemical properties, efficacy, and pharmacokinetics. A separate section of this chapter gives a brief overview of antibody targeted nanotherapeutics, a growing and diverse class of anti-cancer agents specifically designed for delivery of significant amounts of drug payload. New strategies to design the highly potent antibody targeted agents discussed in this chapter provide the opportunity to expand the list of drug payloads suitable for ADC applications and introduce agents with new mechanisms of action, which in turn may potentially lead to improvement in therapeutic index of the ADCs for the treatment of cancer.

Keywords Antibody drug conjugates · High DAR ADCs · High drug loaded ADCs · Nanotherapeutics

Abbreviations

ADC	Antibody drug conjugate
ADCM	Antibody/drug-conjugated micelle
AM	Aminomethylene
DAR	Drug antibody ratio
EPR	Enhanced permeability and retention

N. Bodyak (✉)
Mersana Therapeutics, Inc., Cambridge, MA, USA
e-mail: nbodyak@mersana.com

A. V. Yurkovetskiy
Valley Cross Consulting, Inc., North Grafton, MA, USA

M. Damelin (ed.), *Innovations for Next-Generation Antibody-Drug Conjugates*, Cancer Drug Discovery and Development,
https://doi.org/10.1007/978-3-319-78154-9_9

F-HPA	F-hydroxypropylamide
GGFG	Glycine-glycine-phenylalanine-glycine
HPMA	N-(2-hydroxypropyl) methacrylamide
IFN	Interferon
IL	Immunoliposome
MAP-CPT	Mucic acid polymer conjugate of camptothecin
mDPR	Maleimidodiaminopropionic acid
MDR	Multidrug resistance
MMAD	Monomethyl auristatin D
MMAE	Monomethyl auristatin E
MMAF	Monomethyl auristatin F
OC	Ovarian cancer
PBD	pyrrolobenzodiazepine
P-gp	P-glycoprotein
PHF	Poly-1-hydroxymethylethylene hydroxymethylformal
PK	Pharmacokinetics
RES	Reticular endothelial system
SCID	Severe combined immunodeficiency disease
TCEP	Tris-carboxyethylphosphine
TI	Therapeutic index
TNBC	Triple-negative breast cancer
TOPO I	Topoisomerase I
val-cit-PABC	Valine-citrulline-p-aminobenzylcarbamate

Introduction

Antibody drug conjugates (ADCs) for oncology applications are chemotherapeutic agents designed to selectively deliver cytotoxic drug payloads to neoplastic tissue. These agents target cells that are characterized by surface presentation of tumor-associated antigens that are recognized by the antigen specific domains of antibodies. Although a variety of clinically validated chemotherapeutic agents with different biological mechanisms of action have been evaluated as payloads for ADC therapeutics (e.g., vinblastine, methotrexate, doxorubicin) [17, 69, 76], only a few classes of highly potent antitumor agents have shown clinical efficacy in an ADC format. Trial and error over the last two decades of ADC development has led to the conclusion that efficacious ADCs minimally require cytotoxic drug payloads with potency in the sub-nanomolar range. Not surprisingly, the first ADCs approved by the FDA for treatment of cancer utilized highly potent payloads, such as calicheamicin, auristatin, and maytansine derivatives, compounds with anti-proliferative activity in cell-based assays from low picomolar to nanomolar range [11, 43, 70].

This high potency requirement for ADC payloads resulted from the understanding that the pharmacokinetics (PK), biodistribution, and tolerability of ADC therapeutics depend on their physico-chemical properties, which directly relates to drug antibody ratio (DAR). Extensive research by Seattle Genetics and Immunogen on monomethyl auristatin E (MMAE)- and maytansine-based ADCs has shown that for the same payload/linker combination, the ADCs with higher DARs always outperform their lower DAR analogs in vitro, but often show lower efficacy and tolerability in vivo due to more rapid systemic clearance of the highly modified antibody species ([29, 75]). The conclusion drawn from these studies was that DAR is a key parameter in the design of ADCs and that maximum therapeutic index (TI) can be achieved by decreasing antibody drug loading. For auristatin- and maytansine-based ADCs, which dominated clinical development for more than a decade, an average DAR of 3–4 was accepted as an optimal range for achieving maximum TI, and this became a key feature for these ADC classes independent of bioconjugation strategies or linker design. DNA alkylating agents, such as pyrrolobenzodiazepines (PBDs), are another class of highly potent ADC payloads that have shown promising clinical results and are even more potent and show in vitro activity in the low picomolar range [6, 73]. Due to the ultrahigh potency of these payloads, the ADC DAR is typically limited to 2, which is achieved by site-specific bioconjugation methods [53, 54].

The level of cytotoxic activity for the majority of validated small molecule chemotherapeutic agents, including targeted agents used in the clinic to treat a variety of neoplastic malignancies, is significantly lower (10- to 10,000-fold) than the activity of ADC payloads. Can these agents be considered for ADC applications? In addition, a number of conventional ADCs employing auristatin or maytansine derivatives with a DAR of approximately 4 failed in efficacy studies, although toxicity was dose-limiting and target-independent and resulted in thrombocytopenia, neutropenia, and neuropathy underscoring the limitations of these platforms [16]. Over the last few years, continuous improvements in drug linker selection, bioconjugation chemistry, and site-specific antibody engineering have dramatically changed the approaches of ADC design and have created new opportunities for ADCs with high drug load (Table 1). There is a growing body of evidence from both animal oncology models and clinical studies that a new generation of ADCs with high drug load that combine moderately active chemotherapeutic agents with novel hydrophilic linkers may be a means of addressing this problem.

This chapter reviews new approaches for high DAR ADCs primarily focusing on drug linker and payload selection strategies that result in therapeutics with improved physicochemical and PK properties. A separate section of this chapter gives a brief overview of antibody targeted nanotherapeutics, a growing and diverse class of anticancer agents specifically designed for delivery of significant amounts of drug payload. These strategies applied to the next generation of antibody targeted agents could potentially expand the range of drug payloads, introduce new mechanisms of action, and improve the TI of ADCs for the treatment of cancer.

Table 1 High drug load ADC technologies

Technology	Payload Class	DAR	Company	Advantages	Stage	Reference
Hydrophilic CL2A-SN-38 drug linker incorporating PEG_7 unit to improve ADC physicochemical properties. Carbonate drug linker to provide plasma stability necessary for optimal therapeutic activity. Suitable for conjugation via the native cysteine residues.	SN-38, topoisomerase I inhibitor	7–8	Immunomedics	Demonstrated clinical activity and good tolerability.	Phase III	[24–26]
A novel self-immolative linker system permitting drug release on elimination of aminomethylene moiety. ADC hydrophilicity is improved by incorporation of diethylene glycol hydrophilic fragment into the linker. Conventional cysteine conjugation strategy.	Exatecan derivative, topoisomerase I inhibitor	7–8	Daiichi Sankyo	Good physicochemical properties, good linker stability, favorable PK and safety profile, efficacious in low target expressing models.	Phase I	[56, 58, 59]
Amino-containing PEG_6-C2-MMAD linker for transglutaminase catalyzed site-specific antibody conjugation. Applicable to antibodies with engineered glutamine sites selected to improve ADC hydrophilicity and PK profile.	MMAD, tubulin polymerization inhibitor	6, 8	Rinat Laboratories, Pfizer	Good PK profile, high drug linker in vivo stability, efficacy in low target expressing models.	Preclinical	[74]
Side chain PEG/glucuronide-PABC linkers designed to improve hydrophilicity of ADCs by shielding hydrophobic drug exposure to aqueous environment with PEG_{24}. Linkers suitable for conventional cysteine conjugation.	MMAF and MMAE, tubulin polymerization inhibitors	8	Seattle Genetics	Homogeneous DAR8 ADCs with improved hydrophilicity, PK, and efficacy.	Preclinical	[49]
Second generation side chain PEG/glucuronide-PABC linkers for hydrophilic ADCs with improved plasma stability. Thioether linker stability improved by incorporation of self-stabilizing maleimide mDPR. PEG length optimized to PEG_{12}. Suitable for conventional cysteine conjugation.	MMAE, tubulin polymerization inhibitors	8	Seattle Genetics	Homogeneous DAR8 ADCs with improved hydrophilicity, PK, and efficacy compared with first generation linkers.	Preclinical	[13]

PEG_{24}-capped polypeptide drug linkers designed to carry two different drug payloads. Selective drug immobilization on linker scaffold achieved by differential protection and sequential unmasking of two drug-reactive cysteine residues on polypeptide backbone. Delivery of two drug payloads with complementary cytotoxic properties demonstrated for MMAF/MMAE drug combination. Suitable for conventional cysteine and site-specific conjugation.	MMAF/MMAE combination, tubulin polymerization inhibitors	16	Seattle Genetics	Dual-drug payload ADCs demonstrate activity in cells and tumor models that are refractory to treatment with either of the individual component drugs. Good physicochemical properties, PK, and efficacy.	Preclinical	[45, 46]
PEG_{24}-capped bifunctional bis-sulfone linkers. Bis-sulfone bioconjugation unit designed to religate reduced interchain disulfides and stabilize ADC structure. Linker capping with PEG_{24} improves ADC hydrophilicity. Suitable for conventional cysteine conjugation of IgG1 and IgG2 antibody isotypes. Linker variants can support up to two drugs per linker.	MMAE, tubulin polymerization inhibitor	6, 8	Abzena	Homogeneous ADCs, extended systemic exposure, high efficacy.	Preclinical	[61]
A platinum(II)-based linker that can re-bridge the inter-chain cysteines in the antibody, post-reduction.	Camptothecin, topoisomerase I inhibitor used as a proof of concept	8	Invictus Oncology	Superior stability when compared with maleimide-based ADCs.	Preclinical	[28]
Branched cleavable linkers, microbial transglutaminase (MTGase)-mediated conjugation.	MMAF	Up to 8	Texas Therapeutics institute, the Brown Foundation Institute of Molecular Medicine, the University of Texas Health Science Center at Houston	Homogeneous ADCs.	Preclinical	[4]

(continued)

Table 1 (continued)

Technology	Payload Class	DAR	Company	Advantages	Stage	Reference
Fleximer® polyacetal polymer-based platform for high ADC drug load. Fleximer is a highly hydrophilic, fully biodegradable, biocompatible polymer capable of carrying multiple drug payloads. Utility of this platform to produce highly potent ADC based on nanomolar potency drugs was demonstrated using a vinca derivative. Suitable for bioconjugation via lysine amino groups.	Vinca derivative, microtubule inhibitor – Anti-mitotic	20	Mersana Therapeutics	Improved hydrophilicity, good linker stability, and favorable PK and tumor accumulation profile.	Preclinical	[84]
Fleximer polyacetal polymer-based platform for delivery of novel auristatin derivative Auristatin F HPA (Dolaflexin®). Highly potent ADCs with high drug load and improved physicochemical properties. Suitable for conventional cysteine and site-specific conjugation.	Auristatin F HPA, tubulin polymerization inhibitor	12–15	Mersana Therapeutics	Improved hydrophilicity and linker stability, favorable PK and tissue distribution profile, high efficacy in low target expressing tumors.	Phase 1	[82]
HPMA biocompatible polymer-based platform for high drug load. HPMA is a hydrophilic biocompatible polymer incorporating drug payload by copolymerization method. Utility of this platform to produce high DAR ADCs was demonstrated using DNA intercalator epirubicin. HPMA-epirubicin ADC produced by conventional cysteine conjugation.	Epirubicin, DNA intercalator, topoisomerase II inhibitor	About 20	University of Utah	Good physicochemical properties. Good in vivo efficacy and tolerability in mice.	Preclinical	[86]

ADCs with High Drug Antibody Ratio

High DAR ADCs Utilizing PEG-Based Bioconjugation Technology

PEGylation is a well-established, widely employed technology for improving the biomedical efficacy and physicochemical properties of therapeutic agents. The first attempts to PEGylate proteins were undertaken in the 1970s. The first PEGylated product, a PEGylated form of adenosine deaminase (Adagen®, Enzon Pharmaceuticals, USA), was approved by the FDA in 1990 for the treatment of severe combined immunodeficiency disease (SCID). Since then, multiple PEGylated products have received FDA approval including the following blockbuster drugs: PegIntron® (Schering-Plough, USA), a PEGylated form of interferon (IFN)-α2b and Pegasys® (Hoffman-La Roche, Inc., USA), a PEGylated form of IFN-α2a, both for the treatment of hepatitis C. PEG-protein conjugates are regarded as immunologically safe and non-toxic [36]. The highly hydrophilic nature of PEGs makes them very amenable for ADC applications because they reduce the hydrophobicity of linkers and cytotoxic payloads.

In Immunomedics' high-loaded ADC technology, the hydrophobicity of the highly insoluble payload SN-38, a DNA topoisomerase I (Topo I) inhibitor, is reduced with the introduction of a short PEG moiety in the drug-linker. The drug payload is stabilized by attaching the drug-linker to the 20-hydroxy position of SN-38, thereby preventing the lactone ring from opening to the less active carboxylic acid form under physiological conditions. Conjugation was conducted via the native cysteine residues. The conjugate incorporated a maleimide group for fast thiol-maleimide conjugation to mildly reduced antibody and introduced a benzylcarbonate to provide a pH-mediated cleavage site to release the drug from the linker [24]. For best therapeutic activity, a moderately stable linker (designated as CL2A-SN-38) with an intermediate drug release rate in serum was specifically selected over more stable linkers (Fig. 1a) [25]. The resulting anti Trop-2 ADC (IMMU-132) and anti CEACAM5 ADC (IMMU-130) were consistently manufactured, and five clinical lots had average DAR values of 7.6 and 7.51, respectively [24, 26]. Although the range of ADCs with DARs of 6, 7, and 8 were identified by hydrophobic interaction HPLC and confirmed by LC-MS, the largest fraction (about 70%) was represented by DAR8 species [24]. High drug loaded anti Trop-2 ADCs showed better efficacy than lower DAR ADCs in mouse xenograft models and maintained a similar PK profile to unconjugated antibody. ADCs were well tolerated in cynomolgus monkeys, a pharmacologically relevant species, where dose-limiting toxicities were identical to that of irinotecan; namely, intestinal and hematologic [14]. In the clinic, anti Trop-2 ADC sacituzumab govitecan (IMMU-132) was well tolerated and induced early and durable responses in heavily pre-treated patients with metastatic, triple-negative breast cancers (TNBCs) [5]. The confirmed objective response rate was 30% of the median response; the duration was 8.9 months, and the clinical benefit rate was 46%. Adverse events included

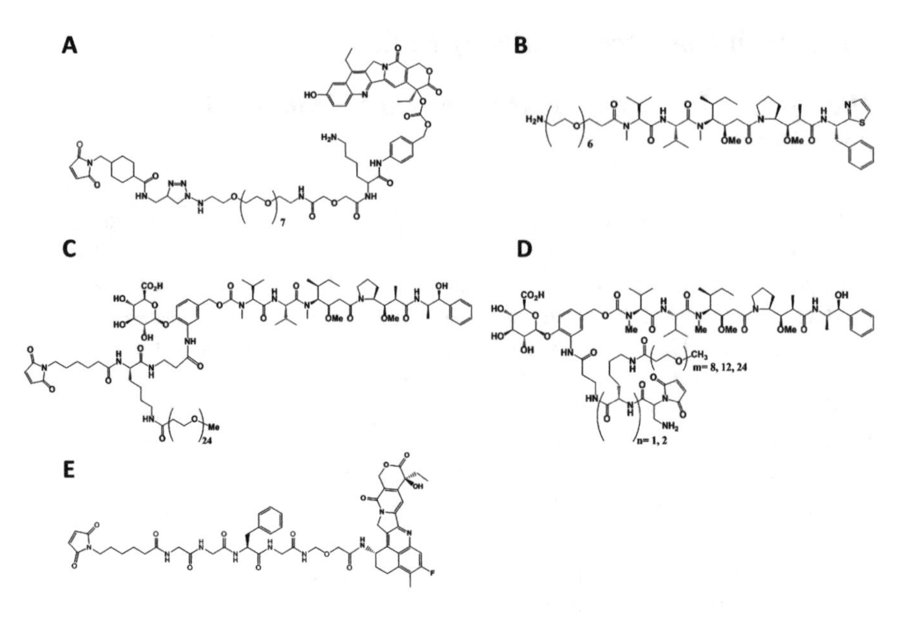

Fig. 1 PEG-based bioconjugation linkers for high DAR ADCs with improved hydrophilicity. (**a**) PEG-based linker for cysteine conjugation: CL2A-SN-38 [24]; (**b**) PEG-based linker for transglutaminase conjugation: PEG_6-C2-MMAD [74]; PEG-based linkers for cysteine conjugation; (**c**) MMAE-glucuronide/PEG/MI [49]; (**d**) MMAE-glucuronide/PEG/mDPR [13]; (**e**) MI-GGFG-DXd [58, 59]

neutropenia (39%), leukopenia (16%), anemia (14%), and diarrhea (13%); the incidence of febrile neutropenia was 7%. Sacituzumab govitecan has received Breakthrough Therapy Designation from the FDA for the treatment of patients with TNBC who failed at least two prior therapies for metastatic disease. The Breakthrough Therapy Designation was supported by a Phase II study in patients with metastatic TNBC who had received a median of five prior therapies. Sacituzumab govitecan has also received U.S. Fast Track designation for TNBC and non-small-cell and small-cell lung cancers, and U.S. Orphan Drug status in small-cell lung and pancreatic cancers.

A high-loaded ADC technology with a DAR of approximately 8 was developed by Daiichi Sankyo and is now in the clinic [56, 58, 59]. It combines a conventional cysteine conjugation strategy with the original stable linker and Topo I isomerase inhibitor exatecan derivative DXd (DX-8951 derivative) as a payload. CPT binds and inhibits the DNA enzyme Topo I causing apoptosis. Exatecan shows stronger Topo I inhibitory activity than the other CPT analogs as well as antitumor activity and bystander killing properties [58, 59]. Furthermore, exatecan is effective against P-glycoprotein (P-gp)-mediated multi-drug resistant cells. Increased linker stability was achieved by developing a novel self-immolative linker system with an amino-methylene (AM) moiety. Enzymatically cleavable peptide linker glycine-glycine-phenylalanine-glycine (GGFG) was attached to the antibody cysteine residues via maleimide. Addition of a hydrophilic group at the C-terminus of the peptide moiety led to a reduction in hydrophobicity and was effective at lowering the aggregation of the resulting ADCs. Anti-HER2 high-loaded ADCs with a DAR of approximately 8 showed potent antitumor activity in low target expressing models where T-DM1 or lower DAR ADCs were less efficacious. The Daiichi Sankyo ADCs had homogeneous reverse-phase chromatography profiles, good PK profiles, and no severe toxicities in cynomolgus monkeys at repeated doses of up to 30 mg/kg administered every 3 weeks. In rats, the maximum tolerated dose was 197 mg/kg [58, 59]. The U3–1402 ADC, based on the same technology, targets HER3 and has a DAR of 7–8. In preclinical efficacy models, U3-1402 antitumor activity correlated with HER3 expression levels [77]. U3-1402 is currently under investigation in a Phase I/II clinical trial [66].

Researchers from Pfizer/Rinat have demonstrated that careful selection of sites for specific transglutaminase-mediated conjugation of amino-PEG_6-C2-monomethyl auristatin D (MMAD) (Fig. 1b) resulted in ADCs with high drug loading (DAR6 and DAR8) that overcame the previously reported limitations of conventional high-loaded ADCs [74]. When compared head to head, the site-specific and conventional high-loaded conjugates had similar potency in vitro, but in vivo, the site-specific, high-loaded ADCs were substantially more efficacious, retained good PK properties, were well tolerated, and as a result, demonstrated an improved TI in mice. In addition, the site-specific, high-loaded ADCs showed superior efficacy in a mouse xenograft model with low target expression. The authors hypothesized that ADCs with many hydrophobic payloads located in close proximity to one another can decrease exposure of ADCs. In order to obtain high-loaded conjugates with optimal properties, it may be necessary to find conjugation sites that individually minimize the density and solvent accessibility of hydrophobic payloads and combine these sites in a way that prevents the close proximity of too many hydrophobic payloads.

Another approach to overcome the shortcomings of conventionally conjugated ADCs with a DAR of 8 was developed by Seattle Genetics [49]. This approach arose following the discovery of the mechanism of accelerated clearance of homogeneous ADCs with a DAR of 8 generated by conjugation via native cysteine residues with a conventional drug linker. To achieve highly homogeneous drug loading, IgG1 antibody was reduced with excess tris-carboxyethylphosphine (TCEP). When monomethyl auristatin F (MMAF) was conjugated to IgG1 antibody via the protease cleavable valine-citrulline-p-aminobenzylcarbamate (val-cit-PABC) linker, the resulting ADC was rapidly taken up by the liver and consequently had accelerated clearance. The underlying cause for accelerated clearance was linked to the hydrophobic nature of the drug linker and not to destabilization of the IgG structure due to an excessive reduction of the interchain disulfides. The val-cit-PABC motif adds considerable hydrophobicity to drug linkers. When compared with ADCs that contain fewer hydrophobic linkers, the noncleavable drug linker mcMMAF exhibited slower plasma clearance. The negative role of hydrophobicity in ADCs was also confirmed by replacing the phenylalanine of MMAF with threonine and linking it directly to a hydrophilic cleavable peptide, thereby eliminating the need for the val-cit-PABC motif. Most cytotoxic drugs require hydrophobic moieties to retain their potency; hence, reducing hydrophobicity by direct engineering may lead to a loss in potency. As an alternative approach, a hydrophilic moiety, such as PEG_{24}, was incorporated to mask the inherent hydrophobicity of the cytotoxic payload. The advantage of this approach was demonstrated with an MMAE payload and a glucuronide cleavable linker (Fig. 1c). In the optimal design, the hydrophobic drug remained close to the antibody, thereby allowing PEG to shield it. These homogeneous ADCs with minimized hydrophobicity and high DAR demonstrated superior antitumor efficacy, enhanced drug accumulation in the tumor, good PK properties, and improved TI.

The Seattle Genetics ADC technology described above was further optimized by stabilization of the maleimide by incorporation of the maleimidodiaminopropionic acid (mDPR) self-stabilizing maleimide and optimization of the length of the PEG side chain (Fig. 1d) [13]. Different PEG chains were explored including PEG_2, PEG_4, PEG_8, PEG_{12}, and PEG_{24}. PEG_8 was shown to be sufficient to shield the hydrophobic moieties of the drug linker and improve ADC circulation, but PEG_{12} was selected over PEG_8 because it had a higher threshold for ADC-accelerated plasma clearance than that observed for shorter PEG chains, accounting for potential interspecies differences when ADCs are tested in higher species. In addition, bone marrow toxicity was mitigated with increasing PEG length [71]. PEG_{24} was deprioritized due to its increased hydrodynamic volume, which may affect tumor penetration. The resulting PEG_{12} ADCs demonstrated enhanced intratumoral drug delivery, minimized non-specific ADC clearance, and subsequent improved tolerability in rats. The greater efficacy exhibited a good correlation with plasma exposure. The therapeutic window was widened by both greater activity and reduced toxicity. This technology is currently applied to create an SGN-CD48A clinical drug candidate.

Seattle Genetics developed a strategy to create ADCs containing complementary multiple drug payloads with a DAR of 16, allowing for increased activity within heterogeneous tumor cell populations and enhanced cancer therapy [46]. To obtain dual drug conjugation, the multiplexing drug carrier with two orthogonally protected cysteine residues was designed: Cys(SiPr), which carries reducible disulfide protecting groups and Cys(Acm), an acetamidomethyl-protected cysteine that can be sequentially unmasked and conjugated with different drug linkers. Conjugation to a native, non-engineered antibody through maleimide chemistry with a self-stabilizing maleimide (mDPR) was employed to minimize in vivo drug linker deconjugation. To reduce hydrophobicity and aggregation, a PEG_{24} stretcher was introduced. Two drugs with complementary activities, MMAE and MMAF, were chosen to create ADCs with enhanced activity on heterogeneous cell populations. Cell permeable MMAE exhibits bystander effects and is a substrate for multidrug resistance (MDR) exporters, whereas MMAF is minimally cell permeable, not susceptible to drug export, and retains activity on MDR(+) cells. The resulting homogeneous dual-drug ADCs had 16 total drugs split evenly (8 + 8) between the two component drugs. In vivo, dual auristatin ADCs were active on tumors that were high in MDR expression, had heterogeneous antigen levels, and were refractory to either of the individual component drugs.

In a recent report, a novel technology employs platinum(II) as a linker to rebridge the antibody chains after conjugation via cysteines [28]. CPT was used as a 'proof of concept' payload to generate novel Pt(II)-based prototype ADCs. A PEG chain, which was included in the linker design to compensate for the hydrophobicity of the drug, decreased the aggregation of the resulting ADCs. The platinum(II) ion was incorporated by the reaction between PEG–CPT and the amine ligand, resulting in the formation of a Pt–PEG–CPT molecule with two labile Pt–Cl bonds that would enable Pt–S bridge formation in the presence of thiol groups. These Pt-based ADCs exhibited superior stability when compared with maleimide-based ADCs and were active in vivo in an A549 lung adenocarcinoma xenograft model.

The utility of branched linkers to create homogeneous ADCs with DAR of up to 8 was reported by scientists from Texas Therapeutics Institute at The Brown Foundation Institute of Molecular Medicine. Branched cleavable linkers were efficiently conjugated to an antibody using enzymatic microbial transglutaminase to create homogeneous ADCs [4].

The benefit of high-loaded ADCs with a DAR of 8 was demonstrated in preclinical studies by the Abzena group of companies [61]. Cysteine conjugation in combination with the bis-sulfone linker technology (24-unit PEG chain and val-cit-PAB-MMAE attached via the same glutamic acid moiety to the bis-sulfone linker) resulted in homogeneous ADCs with well-defined conjugation sites and good PK properties. Incorporation of PEG significantly increased the stability and reduced premature drug loss of the ADC in circulation. The ADCs showed a stepwise increase in potency from 4 to 6 to 8 drugs. DAR8 ADCs with the bis-sulfone linker technology maintained structural integrity better than maleimide DAR8-based constructs that lead to full disruption of interchain disulfides and potential destabilization of the antibody.

High DAR ADCs Utilizing Hydrophilic Polymer-Based Linkers

Water soluble polymer drug conjugates were recognized as an attractive drug delivery platform for active drug targeting by antibodies about three decades ago [67]. Early examples of polymer-containing ADCs with high drug load were related to N-(2-hydroxypropyl) methacrylamide (HPMA) copolymerized with anthracycline derivatives (e.g., doxorubicin and daunomycin). The design of these bioconjugates and their physicochemical and biological properties were extensively reported in the literature [20, 21, 60, 78].

Recent progress in the ADC field and better understanding of the relationships between ADC drug load, drug linker stability, hydrophilicity, size, and in vivo properties, such as PK and tissue disposition, as well as better understanding of the interaction with biological targets and reticular endothelial system (RES) opened up new opportunities to design ADCs with high drug load. Water soluble stealth polymer carriers allow for an increase in ADC drug payload from DARs of 2 to 4 to DARs of 10 to 20 and provide a significant increase in ADC antitumor activity without loss of PK properties. Several examples of these new polymer-based, high DAR ADC platforms are described below.

Biodegradable Polyacetal Drug Carriers for ADC Applications

Fleximer® Platform with Vinca Derivative

Mersana Therapeutics, Inc. has developed a novel, highly differentiated, polymer-based approach to high DAR ADCs. The biodegradable polyacetal polymer carrier poly-1-hydroxymethylethylene hydroxymethylformal (PHF) [81], also known as Fleximer®, was used to create high drug load ADCs. The high hydrophilic nature and polyvalency properties of the Fleximer polymer can be used to reduce the hydrophobicity associated with high DAR ADCs and thus overcome the limitations of direct ADCs by permitting high drug loading with a variety of payloads without compromising the physicochemical and PK properties of the ADC. The polymer backbone has several hydroxy groups suitable for further modification and can be used to accommodate a high drug load. This allows for a significant increase in the ADC drug load even when a limited number of bioconjugation sites are available on the antibody. Therefore, this approach is very appealing for both conventional cysteine and lysine modification strategies and is even more important for site-specific bioconjugation.

To demonstrate the advantage of high drug-loaded ADCs, the Fleximer platform was applied to a moderately potent cytotoxic payload – vinca derivative [84]. An ester-based linker was used to conjugate the vinca derivative payload to the polymer backbone, which in turn was conjugated to the anti-HER2 antibody (trastuzumab) via lysine conjugation. The resultant Fleximer-based ADC with a DAR of 20 maintained excellent physicochemical properties, was highly stable in plasma, and cleared from circulation with a terminal elimination half-life of approximately 3.5 days. Binding affinity for HER2 antigen was maintained along with in vitro cytotoxicity. In vivo, the trastuzumab Fleximer vinca ADC exhibited robust, dose-dependent efficacy in the HER2 high expressing breast cancer xenograft model BT-474. Dosing regimens of 3.5 mg/kg once a week ×3 or 10 mg/kg single dose resulted in 10 of 10 tumor-free survivors on the final day of the study (day 60). Intratumoral accumulation of the drug was confirmed. Trastuzumab Fleximer vinca ADC showed 4-fold greater tumor tissue Cmax and 9-fold greater tumor exposure relative to the non-binding ADC [84].

Dolaflexin® Platform

Mersana Therapeutics' most advanced polymer-based bioconjugation platform, Dolaflexin®, was designed to create high-loaded ADCs with auristatin F-hydroxypropylamide (auristatin F-HPA) (Fig. 2a), a novel, synthetic analogue of the natural product dolastatin 10. Auristatin F-HPA, a primary drug release product of Dolaflexin ADCs, is a potent, tubulin polymerization inhibitor with sub-nanomolar

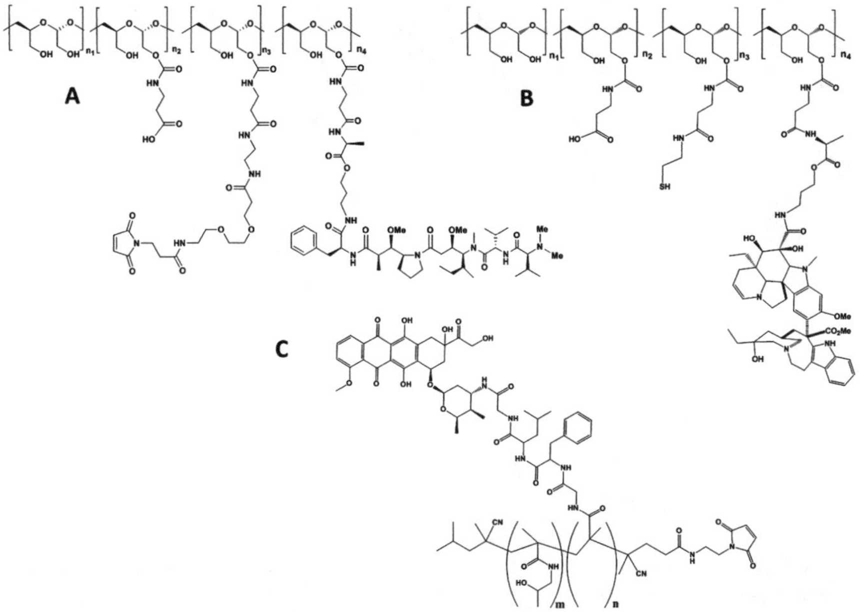

Fig. 2 Polymer-based multi-drug linkers for high DAR ADCs with improved hydrophilicity: (**a**) Dolaflexin® auristatin F-HPA biodegradable polyacetal polymer linker for cysteine conjugation, [85]; (**b**) thiol containing Vinca derivative polyacetal polymer linker for lysine conjugation [84]; (**c**) HPMA-Epirubicin, water soluble HPMA copolymer linker for cysteine conjugation [86]

to low nanomolar activity as a free small molecule in in vitro cytotoxicity assays in several cancer cell lines [82]. Auristatin F-HPA is cell permeable and has bystander cell killing properties. It is further metabolized via deamidation of the C-terminal amino group, resulting in formation of auristatin F. Auristatin F also has specific anti-tubulin activity, but it is not cell permeable, and is less active in vitro, presumably due to impaired cell permeability [7, 8]. Dolaflexin consists of the Fleximer polymer conjugated to 4–5 molecules of auristatin F-HPA. A conventional conjugation approach via cysteine residues was used, achieving a DAR of 12–15 (Fig. 3) [9, 10, 85]. Fleximer creates a highly hydrophilic environment and shields the linker and the payload. The resulting high DAR ADCs are highly efficacious, stable in circulation, and maintain good PK and tolerability profiles. Mersana Therapeutics' lead Dolaflexin ADC, XMT-1522, has entered Phase I clinical studies. It targets HER2 and utilizes a novel, proprietary, anti-HER2 antibody specifically selected for ADC applications that is not competitive with either trastuzumab or pertuzumab.

In vitro, XMT-1522 showed low nanomolar potency in cell lines with HER2 receptor densities as low as 10,000 per cell, and is typically 1–3 logs more potent than ado-trastuzumab emtansine T-DM1 across a panel of 25 tumor cell lines representing a range of tumor indications and HER2 expression levels. In mouse xenograft models, XMT-1522 was active in a range of HER2 expressing models (Fig. 4) [7, 8, 83].

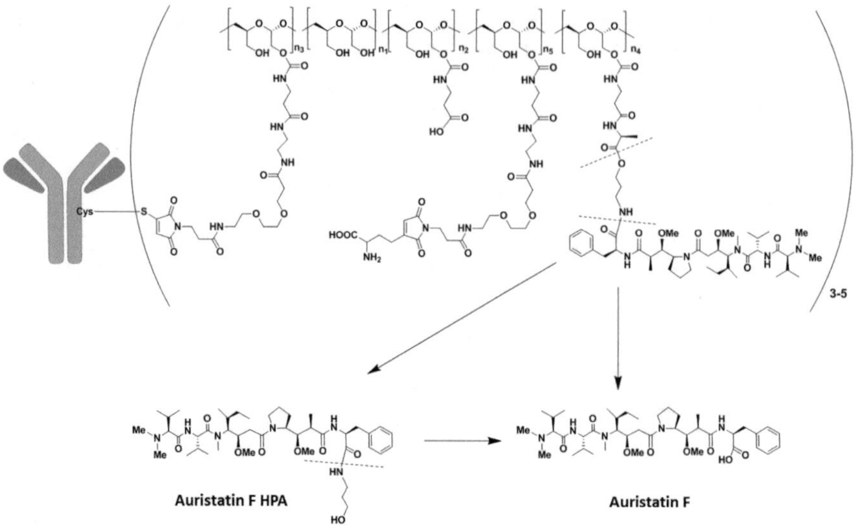

Auristatin F HPA

Auristatin F

Fig. 3 Cellular processing of Dolaflexin® ADCs by antigen expressing tumor cells results in intracellular release of potent cytotoxic compounds: cell permeable drug auristatin F-HPA and cell impermeable active metabolite auristatin F, which lacks bystander capability

In the high HER2-expressing NCI-N87 gastric cancer model (800,000 HER2 receptors/cell, IHC 3+), complete regressions were achieved with a single 1 mg/kg dose of XMT-1522, whereas 10 mg/kg T-DM1 was required for comparable activity. In the medium HER2-expressing JIMT-1 breast cancer (80,000 HER2 receptors/cell, IHC 2+), and the low HER2 expressing SNU5 gastric cancer (22,000 HER2 receptors/cell, IHC 0/1+) models, complete regressions were achieved with a single 1 mg/kg or 0.67 mg/kg dose of XMT-1522, respectively, whereas T-DM1 was inactive at doses ≥10 mg/kg [8]. XMT-1522 tissue analysis in NCI-N87 xenograft tumor-bearing mice demonstrated that both the primary drug release product auristatin F-HPA and its metabolite auristatin F were generated intracellularly from XMT-1522. The carboxylate-containing active metabolite auristatin F was retained in tumor tissue for over 2 weeks, suggesting intracellular trapping, as auristatin F is not cell permeable and cannot reach normal tissues. XMT-1522 demonstrated good stability of the drug conjugate in plasma in mice, rats, and cynomolgus monkeys. In all species, the PK of XMT-1522 was mostly linear, approximately dose proportional, and characterized by extended exposure to conjugated auristatin F-HPA drug payload. Exposure to free auristatin F-HPA and auristatin F was less than 1/1000th the exposure to total auristatin F-HPA. Clearance and volume of distribution were similar for conjugated auristatin F-HPA and anti-HER2 antibody, indicating high stability of the drug polymer linkage in the systemic circulation. In rats, XMT-1522 excretion studies showed that the auristatin F-HPA payload was mainly excreted by the gastrointestinal route. In the first 96 h after administration, 33% of the auristatin F-HPA dose was excreted in feces compared with 3% excretion in urine. The major contributing metabolites both in feces and urine were conjugated auristatin F-HPA, auristatin F, and free

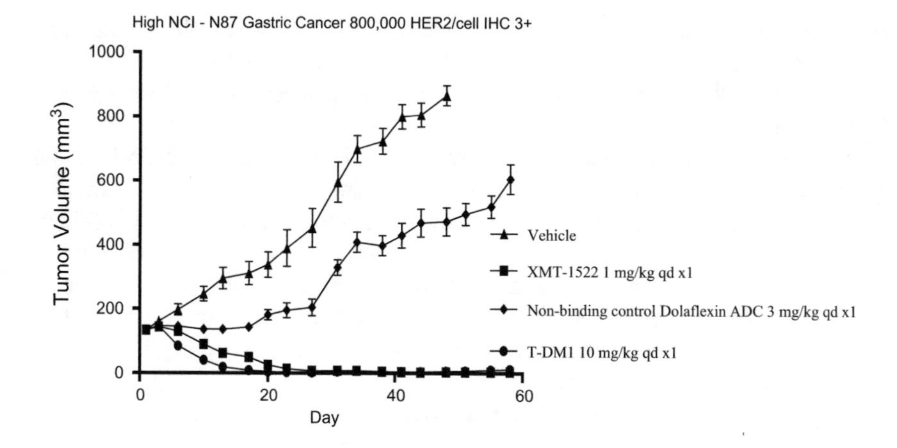

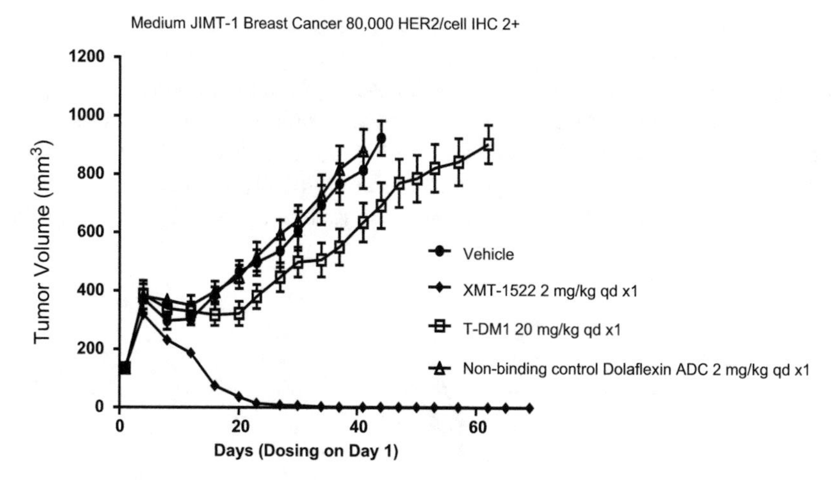

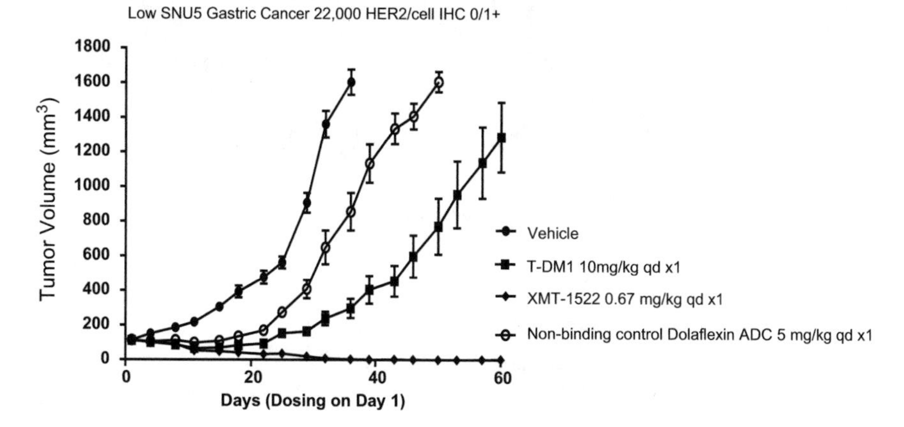

Fig. 4 In vivo efficacy of XMT-1522. XMT-1522 achieved durable complete regressions across models with a range of HER2 expression levels

auristatin F-HPA [85]. In non-human primates, XMT-1522 was well tolerated and there was no XMT-1522-related toxicity observed in critical HER2-expressing tissues, including the heart and lungs, despite the high potency of XMT-1522 in low HER2 tumor models [8].

A second Dolaflexin-based ADC, XMT-1536, targets NaPi2b. NaPi2b is an attractive ADC target, as it is highly expressed in non-squamous NSCLC and non-mucinous ovarian cancer (OC) with restricted normal tissue expression. XMT-1536 induced partial tumor regressions in the OVCAR3 OC model with low receptor density (32,000 NaPi2b/cell) after a single dose of 3 mg/kg and complete tumor regressions after a single dose of 5 mg/kg or 3 weekly doses of 3 mg/kg [10], whereas lifastuzumab vedotin administered as 3 weekly doses of 3 mg/kg failed to achieve tumor regressions. A non-binding Dolaflexin ADC with comparable drug loading was inactive after 3 weekly administrations of 3 mg/kg, consistent with the anti-tumor activity of XMT-1536 being mediated through binding to the NaPi2b target (Fig. 5). XMT-1536 was also tested in patient-derived models of NSCLC where 3 weekly doses of 3 mg/kg led to significant tumor growth delay, and durable tumor regressions were sustained for more than 45 days after treatment was stopped [9]. XMT-1536 had good plasma exposure and was well-tolerated in cynomolgus monkeys after a single 5 mg/kg ADC dose (4294 μg/m^2 auristatin F-HPA payload equivalents) with no evidence of significant toxicity. Notably, no bone marrow toxicity was observed, in contrast to what has been reported generally for cleavable

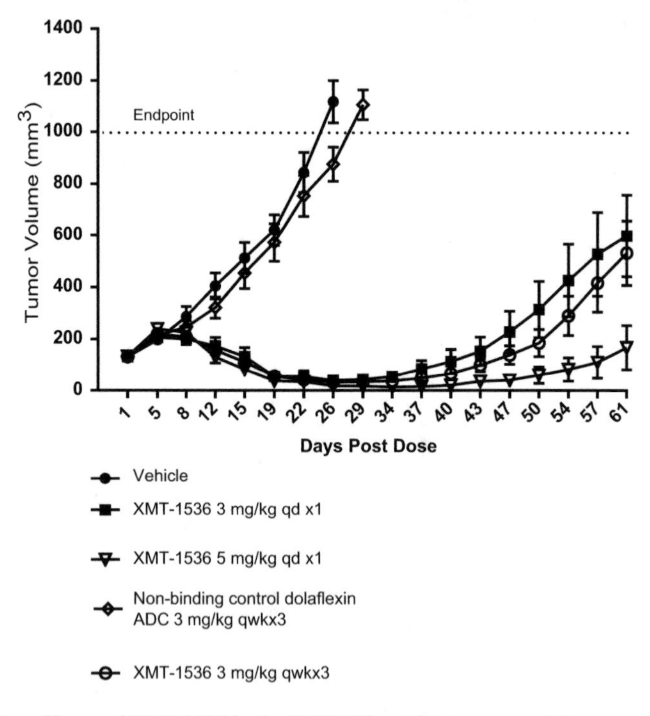

Fig. 5 In vivo efficacy of XMT-1536 in the OVCAR3 ovarian cancer model

auristatin ADCs and specifically for the vcMMAE-based NaPi2b ADCs [47]. XMT-1536 IND-enabling studies are ongoing.

HPMA-Drug Conjugate Based ADCs

HPMA-based ADCs were developed for the treatment of B-cell non-Hodgkin's lymphomas and tested in preclinical models [86]. Epirubicin, a clinically validated chemotherapeutic agent with sub-micromolar potency [27, 37], was incorporated onto HPMA polymer carrier by a controlled living polymerization technique, resulting in a well-defined, high-loaded, polymer-drug conjugate functionalized with terminally maleimido groups for cysteine conjugation (Fig. 2b). This construct was attached to anti-CD20 antibody using the cysteine conjugation approach via reduced disulfide bonds. Depending on the number of polymer chains attached to an antibody, ADC DAR varied from approximately 20 to 40. Conjugates retained water solubility even when the DAR reached over 40 and there was no detectable aggregation. When the number of polymer chains attached to an antibody exceeded 4, the target binding affinity was impacted. ADCs with about 3 polymer chains and 20 drugs per antibody were shown to have the lowest impact and retained over 50% binding affinity compared with unconjugated antibody and were therefore selected. In an in vivo Ramos xenograft mouse model the anti-CD20 HPMA-epirubicin ADC with a DAR of 20 demonstrated superior efficacy compared with HPMA-epirubicin and the non-binding HPMA-epirubicin ADC, was well tolerated, maintained a good PK profile, and showed tumor accumulation [86].

Antibody-Targeted Nanotherapeutics

Antibody-targeted nanotherapeutics are a diverse class of therapeutic agents that combine active tumor targeting with antibodies, antibody fragments, or alternative protein-based recognition scaffolds. These therapies can use a wide range of drug delivery systems or nanocarriers, such as liposomes, water soluble polymer drug conjugates, polymeric nanoparticles, polymeric micelles, carbon nanotubes, and others [65]. Targeted nanocarriers have been developed for delivery of a variety of macromolecular agents, such as proteins, oligonucleotides, siRNA, mRNA, and other emerging gene therapy products. This section will focus on the application of targeted nanotherapeutics for delivery of small molecule cytotoxic drugs. Nanotherapeutics are very attractive carriers for targeted delivery due to their ability to carry significant amounts of payload – a few to dozens of molecules per construct in the case of water soluble polymer drug conjugates [33, 80] and hundreds of thousands of drug molecules per nanoparticle in the case of liposomes [40]. Several non-targeted nanotherapeutics were approved for cancer treatment and include the seven liposomal formulations Doxil® (doxorubicin), DaunoXome®

(daunorubicine), Depocyt® (cytarabine/Ara-C), Myocet® (doxorubicine), Mepact® (mifamurtide), Marqibo® (vincristine), and Onivide® (irinotecan) [12] and one macromolecular drug conjugate Abraxane® (albumin-bound paclitaxel) [34]. Currently, several clinical trials with multiple targeted nanocarriers are ongoing; however, none of the therapeutics in this category have been approved for use.

Immunoliposomes

Immunoliposomes (ILs) are the most represented agents in the nanotherapeutics class, both in preclinical and clinical development. Liposomal drug delivery systems provide a means to alter the biodistribution and PK of small molecule chemotherapeutics and improve their toxicity profiles and therapeutic window. Significant improvements achieved in the design of liposomal formulations over the past two decades have resulted from the careful selection of lipid components to control membrane fluidity, surface charge, hydrophilicity, and drug release, and the introduction of PEG lipids to prevent non-specific interactions with biological milieu and provide long-circulating PK. The liposomes and ILs are typically about 100 nm in diameter. The size of these constructs prevents their extravasation from normal vasculature and results in deposition and retention in areas of functionally porous vasculature, such as the liver and spleen, or leaky vasculature in tumor lesions and areas of inflammation [12, 34, 39]. Accumulation of nanocarriers in tumor lesions is often described as enhanced permeability and retention (EPR) effect. EPR, considered as a non-specific phenomenon, is governed primarily by agent size and surface characteristics [3] and is well characterized in animal models [33, 65]. The capacity of the ILs to carry a significant drug load of up to 20,000–150,000 molecules per unit [40] allows them to be utilized with a broad range of both hydrophilic and hydrophobic small molecule drugs with moderate to high anti-proliferative activity; this clearly differentiates liposomes from ADCs that employ payloads with picomolar to sub-nanomolar potency. Small molecule payloads for liposomal formulations typically do not require chemical modification, thereby providing an opportunity for use in a wide range of clinically validated chemotherapeutic agents, such as Topo I inhibitors irinotecan and topotecan, tubulin agents paclitaxel and vincristine, DNA intercalators doxorubicin and daunorubicin, cisplatin, methotrexate, 5-fluorouridine, bleomycin, rapamycin, and a combination of paclitaxel and rapamycin [3, 15, 18, 19, 39, 42, 72]. Unlike ADCs, in which the antibody functions simultaneously as the recognition ligand and drug carrier, and depending on isotype and modification, it ether retains or abolishes antibody specific immunomodulatory functions (Fc-gamma and FcRn receptor binding and complement binding), IL formulations rely exclusively on target recognition properties to mitigate toxicity and utilize Fab fragments or scFv molecules as targeting moieties to avoid premature Fc receptor-mediated phagocytosis [57]. Depending on design, these ILs can accommodate on average from a few to hundreds of copies of the targeting ligand [40].

In preclinical studies, targeted ILs, such as EGFR [51], HER2 [39, 64], GD2 [62], and CD19 [68], have demonstrated the ability to improve the activity of non-targeted liposomal formulations. Comparative tissue disposition studies of ILs and non-targeted liposomes in tumor xenograft-bearing mice showed similar intratumoral accumulation of drug payload (7–8% ID/g) and no significant differences in PK and biodistribution. However, detailed analysis of tumor samples revealed significant uptake of ILs by tumor cells, whereas non-targeted liposomes accumulated predominantly in tumor resident macrophages [22, 40]. Several IL formulations are currently in clinical development, including HER2-targeted doxorubicin (MM-302), EGFR-targeted doxorubicin (C225-ILs-Dox), and EphA2-targeted doxorubicin (MM-310).

In phase I clinical trials, MM-302 was given to heavily pretreated patients with metastatic HER2-positive breast cancer as a monotherapy and in combination with trastuzumab or trastuzumab and cyclophosphamide. This study demonstrated that MM-302 was safe and there were promising signs of therapeutic activity when administered alone or in combination with trastuzumab [48]. A companion PET/CT 64Cu-MM-302 diagnostic study that was conducted as part of the MM-302 phase I clinical trial (NCT01304797) showed a significant background uptake of ILs in the liver and spleen. Tumor accumulation of 64Cu-MM-302, including deposition in bone and brain lesions, peaked at 24–48 h, varied from 0.52% to 18.5% ID/kg, and was independent of systemic plasma exposure. Clinical data analyses indicated that high 64Cu-MM-302 deposition in tumor lesions was associated with more favorable treatment outcomes [44]. Based on phase I trial results, MM-302 was evaluated at a dose of 30 mg/m^2 q3w in combination with trastuzumab in the randomized phase II HERMIONE trial in anthracycline naïve, HER2-positive, locally advanced or metastatic breast cancer patients (completed in 2016). Another MM-302 phase I study in patients with advanced HER2+ cancer with brain metastases is underway [1].

Doxorubicin-loaded anti-EGFR cetuximab Fab targeted ILs (C225-ILs-Dox) were evaluated in a phase I study in patients with EGFR-overexpressing advanced solid tumors. C225-ILs-Dox was well tolerated up to 50 mg of doxorubicin per m^2 and demonstrated significant clinical benefit as a single agent [52].

A phase I open-label study with MM-310 ILs that encapsulate a novel docetaxel prodrug and target ephrin receptor A2 with anti-EphA2 scFv as targeting moiety [23] was initiated in 2017 in solid tumors [2]. MM-310 will be assessed as a monotherapy until a maximum tolerated dose is established, then MM-310 will be assessed in combination with other therapies [2].

The early preclinical and clinical development of ILs has demonstrated that despite some drawbacks (restricted tumor tissue permeability, significant uptake by RES in the liver and spleen, substantial loss of payload due to diffusion though lipid barrier) these nanotherapeutic carriers remain an attractive drug delivery platform due to the flexibility of their design, versatility in drug and targeting ligand selection, and manufacturability. Continuous improvements in assembly methodology and drug payload immobilization strategies of ILs might lead to further progression of targeted liposomal formulations in the clinic, especially for therapeutic application, such as oligonucleotide, siRNA and mRNA delivery, DNA vaccines, and genomic editing.

Antibody/Drug-Conjugated Micelles

Another modality of highly drug loaded antibody targeted antitumor nanomaterials is represented by antibody/drug-conjugated micelle (ADCM) technology. ADCM therapeutics developed by NanoCarrier Co., Ltd. utilize polyethylene glycol/poly (aminoacid derivative) block copolymers, which can spontaneously form a micellar nanoparticle with a diameter of 20–100 nm in aqueous media. Antibodies are attached to the surface of the nanoparticle, while payloads are encapsulated in the inner core, typically at payload-to-antibody molecular ratio of 100–200. The feasibility of ADCM approach was demonstrated for trastuzumab and cetuximab antibody targeted polymer micelles encapsulating anthracycline antibiotic epirubicin or hemiasterlin analogue, anti-tubulin agent E7974 [38]. Anti-EGFR monoclonal antibody NCAB001 targeted ADCM NC-6201, comprising anti-tubulin agent E7974 is currently in preclinical development by NanoCarrier Co., Ltd. [32].

Another example of antibody targeted nanoparticle delivery system is described by researchers from California Institute of Technology [30, 31]. In their report 30–40 nm diameter nanoparticles consisting of a mucic acid polymer conjugate of camptothecin (MAP-CPT) are targeted by anti-HER2 antibody Herceptin at approximately one antibody per nanoparticle. The specificity of antibody association with nanoparticles is achieved by using boronic acid diol complexation methodology via reaction of boronic acid modified antibody with diol containing nanoparticles [30, 31]. Herceptin targeted MAP-CPT nanoparticles demonstrated prolonged circulation in vivo, tumor accumulation, and complete tumor regression in mice bearing HER2 overexpressing BT-474 human breast cancer tumors.

Antibody Targeted Dendrimers

Dendrimers are highly branched biocompatible polymer scaffolds suitable for covalent surface immobilization of therapeutic agents or entrapment of low soluble drugs in the hydrophobic core of the molecule [63]. Starpharma, a pioneer in not targeted dendrimer technology, has demonstrated high potential for this class of nanotherapeutics by commercializing new dendrimer-based antimicrobial agent VivaGel® and successful completion of Phase I studies with antitumor agent, DEP® docetaxel. Dendrimers, which offer high degree of flexibility in polymer scaffold chemistry, therapeutic agent selection, drug loading capacity, and conjugation strategy, are an attractive platform for antibody drug targeting [79]. Examples of early development of antibody targeted dendrimer agents include several HER2 targeted docetaxel dendrimers from Starpharma and antibody-dendrimer conjugates from other groups [41, 50], and anti-mesothelin antibody K1 targeted paclitaxel containing poly(propylene imine) dendrimer mAbK1-PPI-PTX for treatment of ovarian adenocarcinoma [35].

Conclusion

Emerging technologies and innovative approaches to create a new generation of high drug-loaded ADCs are transforming the current ADC playing field. These innovations allow for a variety of moderately potent drugs as ADC payloads and alter the existing paradigm of a DAR of 4 as optimal for anti-mitotic cytotoxic payloads, which has recently shifted towards site-specific homogeneous ADCs with a DAR of 2. New generation, high-loaded ADCs have demonstrated good physico-chemical properties, excellent PK profiles, superior efficacy in low target expressing tumors, and acceptable tolerability. Several high drug-loaded ADCs based on distinct technologies are currently in clinical development and a few more are in the late stages of preclinical development. There is a high potential for these new generation ADCs to enhance therapeutic response. Antibody targeted nanotherapeutics are a diverse class of agents designed to improve the therapeutic performance of well-understood, clinically established anti-cancer drugs and have a great potential to become a less toxic and more effective treatment option in oncology.

Acknowledgements The authors thank Radha Iyengar for thoughtful and insightful comments on the manuscript. The authors also thank Theresa E. Singleton, PhD of Singleton Science, LLC for editorial support, which was funded by Mersana Therapeutics in accordance with Good Publication Practice (GPP3) guidelines.

References

1. A pilot study of 64-Cu labeled brain PET/MRI for MM-302, a novel HER2 targeting agent, in advanced HER2+ cancer with brain metastases – NCT02735798
2. A study evaluating MM-310 in patients with solid tumors – NCT03076372
3. Ali MF, Salah M, Rafea M, Saleh N (2008) Liposomal methotrexate hydrogel for treatment of localized psoriasis: preparation, characterization and laser targeting. Med Sci Monit 14(12):PI66–PI74
4. Anami Y, Xiong W, Gui X, Deng M, Zhang CC, Zhang N, An Z, Tsuchikama K (2017) Enzymatic conjugation using branched linkers for constructing homogeneous antibody-drugconjugates with high potency. Org Biomol Chem 15(26):5635–5642
5. Bardia A, Mayer IA, Diamond JR, Moroose RL, Isakoff SJ, Starodub AN, Shah NC, O'Shaughnessy J, Kalinsky K, Guarino M, Abramson V, Juric D, Tolaney SM, Berlin J, Messersmith WA, Ocean AJ, Wegener WA, Maliakal P, Sharkey RM, Govindan SV, Goldenberg DM, Vahdat LT (2017) Efficacy and safety of anti-Trop-2 antibody drug conjugate sacituzumab govitecan (IMMU-132) in heavily pretreated patients with metastatic triple-negative breast Cancer. J Clin Oncol 35:2141
6. Bauer TM, Spigel D, Ready N, Morgensztern D, Glisson BS, Byers LA, Burris H, Robert F, Strickland DK, Pietanza MC, Govindan R, Dylla SJ, Peng S, Rudin C (2016) ORAL02.01: safety and efficacy of single-agent Rovalpituzumab Tesirine, a DLL3-targeted ADC, in recurrent or refractory SCLC. Topic Med Oncol J Thorac Oncol 11S(11):S252–S253
7. Bergstrom DA A, Bodyak N, Park PU, Yurkovetskiy A, DeVit M, Yin M, Poling L, Thomas JD, Gumerov D, Xiao D, Ter-Ovanesyan E, Qin L, Uttard A, Johnson A, Lowinger TB (2015) XMT-1522 induces tumor regressions in pre-clinical models representing

HER2-positive and HER2 low-expressing breast cancer. 38th annual SABCS Dec. 8–12, 2015, Publication Number: P4-14-28

8. Bergstrom DA, Bodyak N, Yurkovetskiy A, Park PU, DeVit M, Yin M, Poling L, Thomas JD, Gumerov D, Xiao D, Ter-Ovanesyan E, Qin L, Uttard U, Johnson A, Lowinger TB (2015) A novel, highly potent HER2-targeted antibody-drug conjugate (ADC) for the treatment of low HER2-expressing tumors and combination with trastuzumab-based regimens in HER2-driven tumors. [abstract]. In: Proceedings of the 106th Annual Meeting of the American Association for Cancer Research; 2015; Philadelphia, PA. Philadelphia (PA): AACR; Cancer Res 75(15 Suppl):Abstract nr LB-231
9. Bergstrom D, Bodyak N, Yurkovetskiy A, Poling L, Yin M, Protopopova M, Devit M, Qin L, Gumerov D, Ter-Ovanesyan E, Mosher R, Lowinger T (2016) A NaPi2b antibody-drug conjugate induces durable complete tumor regressions in patient-derived xenograft models of NSCLC. IASLC 17th World Conference on Lung Cancer; Dec 4-7, Vienna, Austria. Abstract nr 5769
10. Bodyak N, Yurkovetskiy A, Yin M, Gumerov G, Bollu R, Conlon P, Gurijala VR, McGillicuddy D, Stevenson C, Ter-Ovanesyan E, Park PU, Poling P, Lee W, DeVit M, Xiao D, Qin L, Lowinger TB, Bergstrom DA (2016) Discovery and preclinical development of a highly potent NaPi2b-targeted antibody-drug conjugate (ADC) with significant activity in patient-derived non-small cell lung cancer (NSCLC) xenograft models. In: Proceedings of the 107th annual meeting of the American Association for Cancer Research; 2016; New Orleans, LA: AACR. Cancer Res 76(14 Suppl):Abstract nr 1194
11. Bross PF, Beitz J, Chen G, Chen XH, Duffy E, Kieffer L, Roy S, Sridhara R, Rahman A, Williams G, Pazdur R (2001) Approval summary: gemtuzumab ozogamicin in relapsed acute myeloid leukemia. Clin Cancer Res 7(6):1490–6. Erratum in: Clin Cancer Res 2002;8(1):300
12. Bulbake U, Doppalapudi S, Kommineni N, Khan W (2017) Liposomal formulations in clinical use: an updated review. Pharmaceutics 9(2):1–33
13. Burke PJ, Hamilton JZ, Jeffrey SC, Hunter JH, Doronina SO, Okeley NM, Miyamoto JB, Anderson ME, Stone IJ, Ulrich ML, Simmons JK, McKinney EE, Senter PD, Lyon RP (2017) Optimization of a PEGylated glucuronide-monomethylauristatin E linker for antibody-drug conjugates. Mol Cancer Ther 16(1):116–123
14. Cardillo TM, Govindan SV, Sharkey RM, Trisal P, Goldenberg DM (2011) Humanized anti-Trop-2 IgG-SN-38 conjugate for effective treatment of diverse epithelial cancers: preclinical studies in human cancer xenograft models and monkeys. Clin Cancer Res 17(10):3157–3169
15. Crosasso P, Brusa P, Dosio F, Arpicco S, Pacchioni D, Schuber F, Cattel L (1997) Antitumoral activity of liposomes and immunoliposomes containing 5-fluorouridine prodrugs. J Pharm Sci 86(7):832–839
16. de Goeij BE, Lambert JM (2016) New developments for antibody-drug conjugate-based therapeutic approaches. Curr Opin Immunol 40:14–23
17. Elias DJ, Hirschowitz L, Kline LE, Kroener JF, Dillman RO, Walker LE, Robb JA, Timms RM (1990) Phase I clinical comparative study of monoclonal antibody KS1/4 and KS1/4-methotrexate immunconjugate in patients with non-small cell lung carcinoma. Cancer Res 50(13):4154–4159
18. Eloy JO, Petrilli R, Chesca DL, Saggioro FP, Lee RJ, Marchetti JM (2017) Anti-HER2 immunoliposomes for co-delivery of paclitaxel and rapamycin for breast cancer therapy. Eur J Pharm Biopharm 115:159
19. Eloy JO, Petrilli R, Brueggemeier RW, Marchetti JM, Lee RJ (2017) Rapamycin-loaded immunoliposomes functionalized with trastuzumab: a strategy to enhance cytotoxicity to HER2-positive breast cancer cells. Anti Cancer Agents Med Chem 17(1):48–56
20. Etrych T, Mrkvan T, Říhová B, Ulbrich K (2007) Star-shaped immunoglobulin-containing HPMA-based conjugates with doxorubicin for cancer therapy. J Control Release 122(1):31–38
21. Etrych T, Strohalm J, Kovár L, Kabesová M, Říhová B, Ulbrich K (2009) HPMA copolymer conjugates with reduced anti-CD20 antibody for cell-specific drug targeting. I. Synthesis and in vitro evaluation of binding efficacy and cytostatic activity. J Control Release 140(1):18–26

22. Gaddy DF, Lee H, Zheng J, Jaffray DA, Wickham TJ, Hendriks BS (2015) Whole-body organ-level and kidney microdosimetric evaluations of 64Cu-loaded HER2/ErbB2- targeted liposomal doxorubicin (64Cu-MM-302) in rodents and primates. EJNMMI Res 5:24
23. Geddie ML, Kohli N, Kirpotin DB, Razlog M, Jiao Y, Kornaga T, Rennard R, Xu L, Schoerberl B, Marks JD, Drummond DC, Lugovskoy AA (2017) Improving the developability of an anti-EphA2 single-chain variable fragment for nanoparticle targeting. MAbs 9(1):58–67. Epub 2016 Nov 17
24. Goldenberg DM, Cardillo TM, Govindan SV, Rossi EA, Sharkey RM (2015) Trop-2 is a novel target for solid cancer therapy with sacituzumab govitecan (IMMU-132), an antibody-drug conjugate (ADC). Oncotarget 6(26):22496–22512
25. Govindan SV, Cardillo TM, Sharkey RM, Tat F, Gold DV, Goldenberg DM (2013) Milatuzumab-SN-38 conjugates for the treatment of CD74+ cancers. Mol Cancer Ther 12(6):968–978
26. Govindan SV, Cardillo TM, Rossi EA, Trisal P, McBride WJ, Sharkey RM, Goldenberg DM (2015) Improving the therapeutic index in cancer therapy by using antibody-drug conjugates designed with a moderately cytotoxic drug. Mol Pharm 12(6):1836–1847
27. Gray J, Cubitt CL, Zhang S, Chiappori A (2012) Combination of HDAC and topoisomerase inhibitors in small cell lung cancer. Cancer Biol Ther 13(8):614–622
28. Gupta N, Kancharla J, Kaushik S, Ansari A, Hossain S, Goyal R, Pandey M, Sivaccumar J, Hussain S, Sarkar A, Sengupta A, Mandal SK, Roy M, Sengupta S (2017) Development of a facile antibody–drug conjugate platform for increased stability and homogeneity. Chem Sci 8:2387
29. Hamblett KJ, Senter PD, Chace DF, Sun MM, Lenox J, Cerveny CG, Kissler KM, Bernhardt SX, Kopcha AK, Zabinski RF, Meyer DL, Francisco JA (2004) Effects of drug loading on the antitumor activity of a monoclonal antibody drug conjugate. Clin Cancer Res 10:7063–7070
30. Han H, Davis ME (2013) Single-antibody, targeted nanoparticle delivery of camptothecin. Mol Pharm 10(7):2558–2567
31. Han H, Davis ME (2013) Targeted nanoparticles assembled via complexation of boronic-acid-containing targeting moieties to diol-containing polymers. Bioconjug Chem 24(4):669–677
32. Harada M, Tsuchiya M, Miyazaki R, Inoue T, Tanaka R, Yanagisawa Y, Ito M, Yu I, Naito K (2016) Preclinical evaluation of NC-6201, an antibody/drug-conjugated micelle incorporating novel hemiasterlin analogue E7974. AACR 107th annual meeting 2016; April 16–20, 2016; New Orleans. Abstract 1368
33. Hoch U, Staschen CM, Johnson RK, Eldon MA (2014) Nonclinical pharmacokinetics and activity of etirinotecan pegol (NKTR-102), a long-acting topoisomerase 1 inhibitor, in multiple cancer models. Cancer Chemother Pharmacol 74(6):1125–1137
34. Ibrahim NK, Desai N, Legha S, Soon-Shiong P, Theriault RL, Rivera E, Esmaeli B, Ring SE, Bedikian A, Hortobagyi GN, Ellerhorst JA (2002) Phase I and pharmacokinetic study of ABI-007, a Cremophor-free, protein-stabilized, nanoparticle formulation of paclitaxel. Clin Cancer Res 8(5):1038–1044
35. Jain NK, Tare MS, Mishra V, Tripathi PK (2015) The development, characterization and in vivo anti-ovarian cancer activity of poly(propylene imine) (PPI)-antibody conjugates containing encapsulated paclitaxel. Nanomedicine 11(1):207–218
36. Jevsevar S, Kunstelj M, Porekar VG (2010) PEGylation of therapeutic proteins. Biotechnol J 5(1):113–128
37. Jiang P, Mukthavaram R, Chao Y, Bharati IS, Fogal V, Pastorino S, Cong X, Nomura N, Gallagher M, Abbasi T, Vali S, Pingle SC, Makale M, Kesari S (2014) Novel anti-glioblastoma agents and therapeutic combinations identified from a collection of FDA approved drugs. J Transl Med 12:13
38. Kato Y, Harada M, Saito H, Hayashi T. Active targeting polymer micelle encapsulating drug, and pharmaceutical composition. US Patent Application 20100221320
39. Kirpotin DB, Drummond DC, Shao Y, Shalaby MR, Hong K, Nielsen UB, Marks JD, Benz CC, Park JW (2006) Antibody targeting of long-circulating lipidic nanoparticles does

not increase tumor localization but does increase internalization in animal models. Cancer Res 66(13):6732–6740
40. Kirpotin DB, Noble CO, Hayes ME, Huang Z, Kornaga T, Zhou Y, Nielsen UB, Marks JD, Building DDC (2012) Characterizing antibody-targeted lipidic nanotherapeutics. Methods Enzymol 502:139–166
41. Kulhari H, Pooja D, Shrivastava S, Kuncha M, Naidu VG, Bansal V, Sistla R, Adams DJ (2016) Trastuzumab-grafted PAMAM dendrimers for the selective delivery of anticancer drugs to HER2-positive breast cancer. Sci Rep 6:23179
42. Kullberg M, Mann K, Anchordoquy TJ (2012) Targeting Her-2+ breast cancer cells with bleomycin immunoliposomes linked to LLO. Mol Pharm 9(7):2000–2008
43. Lambert JM, Chari RVJ (2014) Ado-trastuzumab emtansine (T-DM1): an antibody-drug conjugate (ADC) for HER2-positive breast cancer. J Med Chem 57:6949–6964
44. Lee H, Shields AF, Siegel BA, Miller KD, Krop I, Ma CX, LoRusso PM, Munster PN, Campbell K, Gaddy DF, Leonard SC, Geretti E, Blocker SJ, Kirpotin DB, Moyo V, Wickham TJ, Hendriks BS (2017) 64Cu-MM-302 positron emission tomography quantifies variability of enhanced permeability and retention of nanoparticles in relation to treatment response in patients with metastatic breast cancer. Clin Cancer Res. https://doi.org/10.1158/1078-0432.CCR-16-3193
45. Levengood MR, Zhang X, Emmerton KK, Hunter JH, Peter D Senter PD (2017) Development of homogeneous dual-drug ADCs: application to the co-delivery of auristatin payloads with complementary antitumor activities. Proceedings of the American Association for Cancer Research, vol 58. April 2017, Abstract# 982, p 250
46. Levengood MR, Zhang X, Hunter JH, Emmerton KK, Miyamoto JB, Lewis TS, Senter PD (2017) Orthogonal cysteine protection enables homogeneous multi-drug antibody-drug conjugates. Angew Chem Int Ed Engl 56(3):733–737
47. Lin K, Rubinfeld B, Zhang C, Firestein R, Harstad E, Roth L, Tsai SP, Schutten M, Xu K, Hristopoulos M, Polakis P (2015) Preclinical Development of an Anti-NaPi2b (SLC34A2) Antibody-Drug Conjugate as a Therapeutic for Non-Small Cell Lung and Ovarian Cancers. Clin Cancer Res 21(22):5139–5150
48. LoRusso P, Krop I, Miller K et al (2015) A Phase 1 study of MM-302, a HER2-targeted PEGylated liposomal doxorubicin, in patients with HER2+ metastatic breast cancer (mBC). Presented at: 2015 AACR Annual Meeting; April 18–22, 2015; Philadelphia. Abstract CT234
49. Lyon RP, Bovee TD, Doronina SO, Burke PJ, Hunter JH, Neff-LaFord HD, Jonas M, Anderson ME, Setter JR, Senter PD (2015) Reducing hydrophobicity of homogeneous antibody-drug conjugates improves pharmacokinetics and therapeutic index. Nat Biotechnol 33(7):733–735
50. Ma P, Zhang X, Ni L, Li J, Zhang F, Wang Z, Lian S, Sun K (2015) Targeted delivery of polyamidoamine-paclitaxel conjugate functionalized with anti-human epidermal growth factor receptor 2 trastuzumab. Int J Nanomedicine 10:2173–2190
51. Mamot C, Drummond DC, Noble CO, Kallab V, Guo Z, Hong K, Kirpotin DB, Park JW (2005) Epidermal growth factor receptor-targeted immunoliposomes significantly enhance the efficacy of multiple anticancer drugs in vivo. Cancer Res 65(24):11631–11638
52. Mamot C, Ritschard R, Wicki A, Stehle G, Dieterle T, Bubendorf L, Hilker C, Deuster S, Herrmann R, Rochlitz C (2012) Tolerability, safety, pharmacokinetics, and efficacy of doxorubicin-loaded anti-EGFR immunoliposomes in advanced solid tumours: a phase 1 dose-escalation study. Lancet Oncol 3(12):1234–1241
53. Mantaj J, Jackson PJ, Rahman KM, Thurston DE (2017) From Anthramycin to Pyrrolobenzodiazepine (PBD)-containing antibody-drug conjugates (ADCs). Angew Chem Int Ed Engl 56(2):462–488
54. Miller ML, Fishkin NE, Li W, Whiteman KR, Kovtun Y, Reid EE, Archer KE, Maloney EK, Audette CA, Mayo MF, Wilhelm A, Modafferi HA, Singh R, Pinkas J, Goldmacher V, Lambert JM, Chari RV (2016) A new class of antibody-drug conjugates with potent DNA alkylating activity. Mol Cancer Ther 15(8):1870–1878

55. MM-302 plus trastuzumab vs. chemotherapy of physician's choice plus trastuzumab in HER2-positive locally advanced/metastatic breast cancer patients (HERMIONE)–NCT02213744
56. Nakada T, Masuda T, Naito H, Yoshida M, Ashida S, Morita K, Miyazaki H, Kasuya Y, Ogitani Y, Yamaguchi J, Abe Y, Honda T (2016) Novel antibody drug conjugates containing exatecan derivative-based cytotoxic payloads. Bioorg Med Chem Lett 26(6):1542–1545
57. Noble CO, Kirpotin DB, Hayes ME, Mamot C, Hong K, Park JW, Benz CC, Marks JD, Drummond DC (2004) Development of ligand-targeted liposomes for cancer therapy. Expert Opin Ther Targets 8(4):335–353
58. Ogitani Y, Aida T, Hagihara K, Yamaguchi J, Ishii C, Harada N, Soma M, Okamoto H, Oitate M, Arakawa S, Hirai T, Atsumi R, Nakada T, Hayakawa I, Abe Y, Agatsuma T (2016) DS-8201a, a novel HER2-targeting ADC with a novel DNA topoisomerase I inhibitor, demonstrates a promising antitumor efficacy with differentiation from T-DM1. Clin Cancer Res 22(20):5097–5108
59. Ogitani Y, Hagihara K, Oitate M, Naito H, Agatsuma T (2016) Bystander killing effect of DS-8201a, a novel anti-human epidermal growth factor receptor 2 antibody-drug conjugate, in tumors with human epidermal growth factor receptor 2 heterogeneity. Cancer Sci 107(7):1039–1046
60. Omelyanenko V, Kopecková P, Gentry C, Shiah JG, Kopecek J (1996) HPMA copolymer-anticancer drug-OV-TL16 antibody conjugates. 1. Influence of the method of synthesis on the binding affinity to OVCAR-3 ovarian carcinoma cells in vitro. J Drug Target 3(5):357–373
61. Pabst M, McDowell W, Manin A, Kyle A, Camper N, De Juan E, Parekh V, Rudge F, Makwana H, Kantner T, Parekh H, Michelet A, Sheng X, Popa G, Tucker C, Khayrzad F, Pollard D, Kozakowska K, Resende R, Jenkins A, Simoes F, Morris D, Williams P, Badescu G, Baker MP, Bird M, Frigerio M, Godwin A (2017) 18. Modulation of drug-linker design to enhance in vivo potency of homogeneous antibody-drug conjugates. J Control Release 253:160–164
62. Pagnan G, Stuart DD, Pastorino F, Raffaghello L, Montaldo PG, Allen TM, Calabretta B, Ponzoni M (2000) Delivery of c-myb antisense oligodeoxynucleotides to human neuroblastoma cells via disialoganglioside GD2-targeted immunoliposomes: antitumor effects. J Natl Cancer Inst 92(3):253–261
63. Palmerston Mendes L, Pan J, Torchilin VP (2017) Dendrimers as nanocarriers for nucleic acid and drug delivery in cancer therapy. Molecules 22(9):1401
64. Park JW, Hong K, Kirpotin DB, Meyer O, Papahadjopoulos D, Benz CC (1997) Anti-HER2 immunoliposomes for targeted therapy of human tumors. Cancer Lett 118(2):153–160
65. Pérez-Herrero E, Fernández-Medarde A (2015) Advanced targeted therapies in cancer: drug nanocarriers, the future of chemotherapy. Eur J Pharm Biopharm 93:52–79
66. Phase I/II study of U3-1402 in subjects with human epidermal growth factor receptor 3 (HER3) positive metastatic breast cancer – NCT02980341
67. Řihová B, Kopeček J (1985) Biological properties of targetable poly[N-(2-hydroxypropyl)-methacrylamide]-antibody conjugates. J Control Release 2:289–310
68. Sapra P, Allen TM (2002) Internalizing antibodies are necessary for improved therapeutic efficacy of antibody-targeted liposomal drugs. Cancer Res 62(24):7190–7194
69. Schneck D, Butler F, Dugan W, Littrell D, Petersen B, Bowsher R, DeLong A, Dorrbecker S (1990) Disposition of a murine monoclonal antibody vinca conjugate (KS1/4-DAVLB) in patients with adenocarcinomas. Clin Pharmacol Ther 47(1):36–41
70. Senter PD, Sievers EL (2012) The discovery and development of brentuximab vedotin for use in relapsed Hodgkin lymphoma and systemic anaplastic large cell lymphoma. Nature Biotech 30:631–637
71. Simmons J, Zapata F, Neff-Laford H, Hunter J, Cochran J, Burke P, Lyon RP. Reducing toxicity of antibody-drug conjugates through modulation of pharmacokinetics. Proceedings of the American Association for Cancer Research. Vol 58. April 2017, Abstract# 60. p 15
72. Stathopoulos GP, Antoniou D, Dimitroulis J, Stathopoulos J, Marosis K, Michalopoulou P (2011) Comparison of liposomal cisplatin versus cisplatin in non-squamous cell non-small-cell lung cancer. Cancer Chemother Pharmacol 68(4):945–950

73. Stein EM, Stein A, Walter RB et al (2014) Interim analysis of a phase 1 trial of SGN-CD33A in patients with CD33-positive acute myeloid leukemia (AML) [abstract]. Blood 124(21). Abstract 623
74. Strop P, Delaria K, Foletti D, Witt JM, Hasa-Moreno A, Poulsen K, Casas MG, Dorywalska M, Farias S, Pios A, Lui V, Dushin R, Zhou D, Navaratnam T, Tran TT, Sutton J, Lindquist KC, Han B, Liu SH, Shelton DL, Pons J, Rajpal A (2015) Site-specific conjugation improves therapeutic index of antibody drug conjugates with high drug loading. Nat Biotechnol 33(7):694–696
75. Sun X, Ponte JF, Yoder NC, Laleau R, Coccia J, Lanieri L, Qiu Q, Wu R, Hong E, Bogalhas M, Wang L, Dong L, Setiady Y, Maloney EK, Ab O, Zhang X, Pinkas J, Keating TA, Chari R, Erickson HK, Lambert JM (2017) Effects of drug-antibody ratio on pharmacokinetics, biodistribution, efficacy, and tolerability of antibody-maytansinoid conjugates. Bioconjug Chem 28(5):1371–1381
76. Tolcher AW, Sugarman S, Gelmon KA, Cohen R, Saleh M, Isaacs C, Young L, Healey D, Onetto N, Slichenmyer W (1999) Randomized phase II study of BR96-doxorubicin conjugate in patients with metastatic breast cancer. J Clin Oncol 17(2):478–484
77. Ueno S, Hirotani K, Abraham R, Blum S, Frankenberger B, Redondo-Muller M, Bange J, Ogitani Y, Zembutsu A, Morita K, Nakada T, Majima S, Abe Y, Agatsuma T (2017) U3-1402a, a novel HER3-targeting ADC with a novel DNA topoisomerase I inhibitor, demonstrates a potent antitumor efficacy. In: Proceedings of the 108th Annual Meeting of the American Association for Cancer Research; 2017; Washington, DC: AACR; Cancer Res 76(14 Suppl):Abstract nr 3092
78. Ulbrich K, Etrych T, Chytil P, Jelínková M, Ríhová B (2004) Antibody-targeted polymer-doxorubicin conjugates with pH-controlled activation. J Drug Target 12(8):477–489
79. Yang H (2016) Targeted nanosystems: advances in targeted dendrimers for cancer therapy. Nanomedicine 12(2):309–316
80. Yurkovetskiy AV, Fram RJ (2009) XMT-1001, a novel polymeric camptothecin pro-drug in clinical development for patients with advanced cancer. Adv Drug Deliv Rev 61(13):1193–1202
81. Yurkovetskiy A, Choi S, Hiller A, Yin M, McCusker C, Syed S, Fischman AJ, Papisov MI (2005) Fully degradable hydrophilic polyals for protein modification. Biomacromolecules 6(5):2648–2658
82. Yurkovetskiy A, Bodyak N, Yin M, Thomas J, Conlon P, Stevenson C, Uttard U, Qin L, Gumerov D, Ter-Ovaneysan E, DeVit M, Lowinger TB (2013) Advantages of polyacetal polymer-based antibody drug conjugates employing cysteine bioconjugation. In: Proceedings of the 104th annual meeting of the American Association for Cancer Research; 2013; Washington, DC: AACR; Cancer Res 73(8 Suppl):Abstract nr 4331
83. Yurkovetskiy A, Bodyak N, Yin M, Thomas JD, Conlon PR, Stevenson CA, Uttard A, Qin LL, Gumerov DR, Ter-Ovanesyan E, Gurijala VR, McGillicuddy D, Glynn RE, DeVit M, Poling LL, Park PU, Lowinger TB (2014) Antibody drug conjugate (ADC) designed with Fleximer® platform enables high drug-loading of payloads and potent anti-tumor activities in tumor cells with low target expression. The Antibody Biology & Engineering Gordon Research Conference. Lucca (Barga), March 23–28
84. Yurkovetskiy AV, Yin M, Bodyak N, Stevenson CA, Thomas JD, Hammond CE, Qin L, Zhu B, Gumerov DR, Ter-Ovanesyan E, Uttard A, Lowinger TB (2015) A polymer-based antibody-vinca drug conjugate platform: characterization and preclinical efficacy. Cancer Res 75(16):3365–3372
85. Yurkovetskiy A, Gumerov D, Ter-Ovanesyan E, Conlon P, Devit M, Bu C, Bodyak N, Lowinger T, Bergstrom D (2017) Non-clinical pharmacokinetics of XMT-1522, a HER2 targeting auristatin-based antibody drug conjugate. In: Proceedings of the 108th annual meeting of the American Association for Cancer Research; 2017; Washington, DC: AACR; Cancer Res 76(14 Suppl):Abstract nr 48
86. Zhang L, Fang Y, Kopeček J, Yang J (2017) A new construct of antibody-drug conjugates for treatment of B-cell non-Hodgkin's lymphomas. Eur J Pharm Sci. Accepted manuscript 103:36–46

Site-Specific Antibody-Drug Conjugates

Feng Tian, Dowdy Jackson, and Yun Bai

Abstract Site-specific antibody drug conjugates are the next stage in the evolution of antibody drug conjugates. The enhanced in vivo stability, potent anti-tumor efficacy and favorable toxicology profiles make site-specific ADCs an attractive option for treating cancer patients. The well-defined structure provides a base for further optimization through structure-property-relationship. We provide a comprehensive review of site-specific ADC technologies and offer insights into the future direction of ADCs.

Keywords Site-specific · Antibody drug conjugate · ADC · Bioconjugation

Overview

Monoclonal antibodies are an important modality in the treatment of various diseases including cancer. Monoclonal antibodies selectively bind to specific proteins and can be used for the diagnosis and treatment of cancer patients. The first therapeutic monoclonal antibody, Muromonab-CD3 (Orthoclone OKT 3) was approved in 1986 to reduce organ rejection in organ transplant patients [1]. Eleven years later the first therapeutic monoclonal antibody for an oncology indication, Rituximab (Rituxin/Mabthera), was approved in 1997 to treat non-Hodgkin's lymphoma patients [1]. To date approximately 24 monoclonal antibodies have been approved to treat cancer patients (Table 1).

Monoclonal antibodies can be used to treat cancer patients by utilizing several mechanisms of action. Monoclonal antibodies can bind to the extra cellular domain of tyrosine kinase receptors and inhibit vital signal transduction pathways, which inhibit tumor growth [2]. They can bind to receptors or ligands involved in tumor angiogenesis and inhibit the formation of blood vessels thus starving the tumor [3,

F. Tian (✉) · D. Jackson · Y. Bai
Ambrx, Inc., La Jolla, CA, USA
e-mail: feng.tian@ambrx.com

M. Damelin (ed.), *Innovations for Next-Generation Antibody-Drug Conjugates*, Cancer Drug Discovery and Development,
https://doi.org/10.1007/978-3-319-78154-9_10

Table 1 Approved monoclonal antibodies for cancer treatment

Generic name	Proprietary name	Target	Technology	Isotype	Additional manipulations	Year FDA approved	Approved clinical indication
Rituximab	Rituxin/ Mabthera	CD20	Mouse Hybridoma	IgG1-kappa	Chimeric	1997	NHL; later CD20 + CLL, FL, RA
Transtuzumab	Herceptin	HER-2	Mouse Hybridoma	IgG1-kappa	Humanized	1998	HER-2+ MBC
Gemtuzumab ozogamicin	Mylotarg	CD33	Mouse Hybridoma	IgG4-kappa	Humanized-ADC	2000	AML
Alemtuzumab	Campath/ Mabcampath	CD52	Rat Hybridoma	IgG1-kappa	Humanized	2001	CL L, T-cell lymphoma
Ibritomomab tiuxitan	Zevalin	CD20	Mouse monoclonal	IgG1-kappa	Conjugated to Yittrium-90	2002	NHL
Tositumomab	Bexxar	CD20	Mouse monoclonal	IgG2a-lambda	Conjugated to I-131	2003	NHL
Cetuximab	Erbitux	EGRF, HER-1	Mouse monoclonal	IgG1-kappa	Chimeric	2004	EGRF+ MCC
Bevacizumab	Avastin	VEGF	Mouse monoclonal	IgG1-kappa	Humanized	2004	MCC
Panitumumab	Vectibix	EGRF, HER-1	Human monoclonal	IgG2-kappa	Human	2006	MCC
Ofatumumab	Arzerra	CD20	Human monoclonal	IgG1-kappa	Human	2009	Refractory CLL
Ipilimumab	Yervoy	CTLA-4	Human monoclonal	IgG1-kappa	Human	2011	MMel
Brentuximab vedotin	Adcetris	CD30	Mouse Hybridoma	IgG1-kappa	Chimeric - ADC	2011	Hodgkin lymphoma and ALCL
Pertuzumab	Perjeta	EGFR2, HER-2	Mouse monoclonal	IgG1-kappa	Humanized	2012	Breast

Generic name	Proprietary name	Target	Technology	Isotype	Additional manipulations	Year FDA approved	Approved clinical indication
Obinutuzumab	Gazyva	CD20	Mouse Hybridoma	IgG1-kappa	Humanized	2013	CLL
Ado-trastuzumab emtansine	Kadcyla	Her2	Mouse Hybridoma	IgG1-kappa	Humanized - ADC	2013	Breast
Ramucirumab	Cyramza	VEGFR-2	Human monoclonal	IgG1-kappa	Human	2014	Colorectal
Blinatumomab	Blincyto	CD3-CD19	Human monoclonal		Bispecific (BiTe)	2014	ALL
Pembrolizumab	Keytruda	PD-1	Mouse Hybridoma	IgG4-kappa	Humanized	2014	Head and neck
Nivolumab	Opdivo	PD-1	Mouse Hybridoma (Hu-Mab)	IgG4-kappa	Humanized	2014	Locally advanced or metastatic urothelial carcinoma
Elotuzumab	Empliciti	SLAMF7	Mouse Hybridoma	IgG1-kappa	Humanized	2015	Multiple myeloma
Necitumumab	Portrazza	EGFR	Human monoclonal	IgG1-kappa	Human	2015	Non small cell lung cancer
Dinutuximab	Unituxin	Glycolipid-GD2	Mouse Hybridoma	IgG1-kappa	Chimeric	2015	Neuroblastoma
Olaratumab	Lartuvo	PDGFR-α	Human monoclonal	IgG1-kappa	Human	2016	Soft tissue sarcoma
Atezolizumab	Tecentriq	PD-L1	Human monoclonal	IgG1-kappa	Human (deglycosylated)	2016	Urothelial carcinoma

4]. They can be used to recruit the immune system, using their ADCC and CDC functionality, to kill antigen expressing tumor cells. More recently, they can be used to block the immune check points to break the tolerance of our immune system toward cancer [5, 6]. Finally, cytotoxic payloads can be conjugated to antibodies to create antibody drug conjugates (ADCs), which can selectively deliver cytotoxic payloads to tumors to inhibit tumor growth.

Cytotoxic small molecule chemotherapeutic drugs are commonly used to treat a variety of cancers. However, small molecule chemotherapeutic drugs are toxic to both cancerous and normal cells, which results in unwanted and often debilitating side effects. To maximize the effectiveness of these chemotherapeutic drugs and minimize the unwanted side effects, the drugs should be selectively delivered to tumors. Paul Ehrlich, a German physician/scientist, in 1906 first described the concept of a "Magic Bullet", where a toxin is selectively delivered to tumors [7], which is transformed into today's antibody drug conjugates (ADCs) [8–10].

ADCs are tumor targeting monoclonal antibodies that are covalently attached to cytotoxic chemotherapeutic drugs, using conventional conjugation methodologies, which utilizes cysteines from reduced inter-chain disulfide bonds or surface exposed lysines [11]. Once the ADCs bind to the antigen expressing tumor cells, they are internalized and transported into the lysosomes where the ADCs are degraded and/or the peptide linker is enzymatically cleaved. The cytotoxic payload is released in the intracellular compartment of the cell. The cytotoxic payload binds to the appropriate intracellular target and induces apoptotic cell death. Unlike small molecule chemotherapeutic agents, generally ADCs are not transported across cell membrane into cells in the absence of a cell surface antigen. Upon administration to patients, the ADC will deliver the cytotoxic drugs to the antigen expressing tumors and spare the normal non-antigen expressing tissues.

One of the first ADCs to be evaluated in humans was a mouse IgG2 monoclonal antibody against the KS1/4 protein, which is a 40–42 kD glycoprotein expressed by human lung adenocarcimonas [12]. The anti-KS1/4 antibody was conjugated using methotrexate or vinblastine on surface exposed lysines using hemisuccinate linkers. This resulted in a heterogeneous distribution of drugs per antibody with an average of 4–6 drugs per antibody. Patients treated with this ADC developed antibodies against the mouse antibody/ADC, which resulted in the neutralization and rapid clearance of the ADC thus making the ADC ineffective. To overcome the immunogenicity issue of mouse antibody, Bristol-Myers Squibb and Seattle Genetics utilized a chimeric anti-Lewis Y protein antibody, BR96 (SGN15), which was conjugated with doxorubicin on reduced inter-chain cysteines using a hydrazine linker [13]. The clinical development of BR96 was terminated due to lack of antitumor efficacy, which was attributed to the lack of potency of doxorubicin and the instability of the hydrazine linker. Subsequently another ADC against Lewis Y, CMD-193, was developed using a humanized antibody conjugated to calicheamicin on lysines [14]. Although the payload potency was significantly improved, the linker, which includes a trisulfide and an acid labile hydrazone moieties, was not stable. The linker instability resulted in myelosuppression and impaired liver function due to premature release of the payload, which lead to the discontinuation of CMD-193.

Currently, there are more than 50 ADCs at various stages of clinical development. Most of the ADCs in clinical development use conventional conjugation of the cytotoxic drugs to cysteines or lysines, which results in the heterogeneous distribution of drugs. The majority of the ADCs in clinical development are either in phase I or phase II, while only three have progressed to phase III [15]. The clinical development of more than 20 ADCs have been terminated and only four ADCs have gained regulatory approval for use in acute myelogenous leukemia (Mylotarg®), Her2 positive breast cancer (Kadcyla®), Hodgkin lymphoma (Adcetris®) and most recently, acute lymphoblastic leukemia (Besponsa®) [9].

The low rate of ADCs progressing into later stage clinical trials suggests that further improvements in ADC technology may be required to improve the clinical success rates. The predominate reason why ADCs fail in clinical development is due to a lack of significant anti-tumor activity and significant dose-limiting toxicities which leads to a poor therapeutic index [15, 16]. Efforts are underway to improve the anti-tumor efficacy and reduce the toxicities to widen the therapeutic index.

Several companies have adopted a strategy where they are producing ADCs with high DARs, (i.e. eight or more drugs/antibody) and improved *in-vivo* serum stability in the hopes that delivering more drug to the tumor, while improving the ADC's serum stability, will result in improved tumor efficacy and an improved safety profile. Seattle Genetics recently reported that the use of a hydrophilic linker and the addition of PEG reduces the hydrophobicity of an ADC which enables the production of ADCs with high homogeneous DARs and improved *in vivo* pharmacokinetic properties [17]. Mersana's ADC, XMT-1522, which targets Her2 and uses a biodegradable and hydrophilic Fleximer polymer, has 12–15 drugs/antibody with improved pharmacokinetic properties over the first generation ADCs [18]. Daiichi Sankyo's ADC, DS-8201, which also targets Her2, has eight drugs/antibody and also reports to have improved pharmacokinetic properties [19].

Among these efforts, a new approach utilizing site-specific conjugation of cytotoxic drugs to antibodies, appeared in 2008 and largely has become the consensus approach recently in the ADC community [20]. The preclinical data for site-specific ADCs suggests that site-specific ADCs should be superior to conventional ADCs in improving the therapeutic index. Today, there are seven site-specific ADCs in clinical development and all of them are currently in Phase I. The clinical development of two site specific ADCs, SGN-CD70A and SGN-CD33A were discontinued (Table 2).

Site-Specific ADCs

Site-specific ADCs are created through conjugation of cytotoxic drugs to specific sites on antibodies, which result in a homogenous population of ADCs with a well-defined drug antibody ratio (DAR) and site of conjugation. Conventional ADCs have an average DAR of 4 and are created through conjugation to solvent exposed lysines and cysteines after reduction of the inter-chain disulfide bonds. For a commonly used IgG1 antibody, there are over 70 solvent exposed lysines and 8 cysteines for inter-chain disulfide bonds. This results in a large population of heterogeneous ADCs, with a distribution of drugs that range from 0 to 8 drugs

Table 2 Clinical development of site-specific ADC programs

ADC	Target	Payload	Site	Indication(s)	Phase
SGN-CD19B	CD19	PBD	Engineered cysteine	Non-Hodgkin lymphoma, diffuse large B-cell lymphoma, follicular lymphoma (high grade)	Phase I
SGN-CD70A	CD70	PBD	Engineered cysteine	Renal cell carcinoma, diffuse large B-cell lymphoma, mantle cell lymphoma (high grade), mantle cell lymphoma (low grade), grade III follicular lymphoma	Discontinued (phase I)
SGN-CD33A	CD33	PBD	Engineered cysteine	Acute myeloid leukemia (AML)	Discontinued (phase III)
SGN-CD123A	CD123	PBD	Engineered cysteine	Acute myeloid leukemia (AML)	Phase I
ADCT-301	CD25	PBD	Engineered cysteine	Acute myelogenous/myeloid leukemia (AML), Hodgkin lymphoma, non-Hodgkin lymphoma	Phase I
ADCT-402	CD19	PBD	Engineered cysteine	Non-Hodgkin lymphoma, diffuse large B-cell lymphoma, follicular lymphoma (high grade), acute lymphoblastic leukemia (ALL)	Phase I
ADCT-401 (MEDI3726)	PSMA	PBD	Engineered cysteine	Prostate	Suspended (Phase I)
ARX788	Her2	Auristatin	Non-natural amino acid (*p*AF)	Breast, gastric	Phase I
AGS62P1	FLT3	Auristatin	Non-natural amino acid (*p*AF)	Acute myeloid leukemia (AML)	Phase I

per antibody and undefined sites of conjugation. Compared to conventional ADCs, site-specific ADCs have several advantages. First, site-specific conjugation provides a molecule with well-defined structure, which is a starting point for optimization of any molecule through structure-property-relationship (SPR). A similar concept, structure-activity-relationship (SAR) has been routinely used in medicinal chemistry for small molecule drug optimization. A truly meaningful SPR capability brought in by site-specific ADCs will accelerate the evolution of ADC technology toward more desirable therapeutic properties. Second, site-specific ADCs tend to be more stable than conventional ADCs *in vivo*. The number of drugs conjugated to an antibody has an impact on the rate of *in vivo* clearance. ADCs with higher drug loading are cleared faster from circulation than ADCs with lower drug loads [21]. In addition, the selection of the conjugation site is also critical to cleavable linker stability. Tian et al. showed that an enzymatic labile cleavable linker can be highly stabilized in plasma and in animal models by changing the conjugation side to its neighboring site [22]. Third, based on preclinical research, site-specific ADCs have better or equivalent *in vivo* anti-tumor efficacy and lower toxicity than conventionally conjugated ADCs, thus potentially resulting in a widened therapeutic index [20]. Fourth, site-specific ADCs have a homogeneous and well-defined DAR. The typical DAR is 2 and higher DARs are achievable. The homogeneous DAR simplifies the production process and characterization of the ADCs for manufacturing.

Here, we will review the development of site-specific ADC technologies with a focus on their conjugation methodologies. Site-specific conjugation technology can be categorized into four groups: (1) genetic engineered cysteine or selenocysteine residues, (2) incorporation of non-natural amino acids containing reactive functional groups, (3) enzymatic modification and (4) other emerging technologies such as re-bridging inter-chain disulfide bonds and photoactive protein z. All of these methods results in site-specific conjugation, but there are several differences between the methods, including the requirement for genetic modification of antibodies, the use of enzymes for conjugation, and the conjugation site number and locations. A comparison of the site-specific methods is summarized in Table 3.

Conjugation Using Natural Amino Acids

Engineered Cysteines

The amino acid cysteine contains a reactive thiol group that serves an essential function in the structure and function of many proteins. Conjugation of thio-reactive probes to proteins through cysteine residues has long been used in protein labeling, and it has also been applied to ADC generation [23]. The use of native cysteines for conjugation resulted in DARs ranging from 0 to 8 and increased ADC instability at the higher DARs. The systemic replacement of solvent exposed cysteine for inter-chain disulfide bond formation with serine resulted in a more homogenous ADC [24].

Inspired by the first generation or conventional conjugation via inter-chain cysteine residues, the engineered cysteine conjugation technology is based on introduction of the extra cysteine residues using site-directed mutagenesis onto pre-determined sites to allow site-specific conjugation without interrupting antibody structure and function (Fig. 1a). This technology for ADC development, named Thiomab, was demonstrated by scientists at Genentech [25].The engineered unpaired cysteines on Thiomab are capped, by cysteine and glutathione etc. after antibodies are produced from CHO cell culture process. A reduction process is required to de-cap the engineered cysteines for conjugation. During the reduction process, not only are the engineered cysteines de-capped but the native inter-chain disulfide bonds are reduced. Subsequently, a re-oxidation step using a gentle oxidant such as $CuSO_4$ or dehydro-ascorbic acid is implemented to reform proper

Table 3 Site specific ADC technologies

Technology	Conjugation chemistry	DAR	Conjugation site	Companies or institutes	Advantage	Disadvantage	Phase of development
Cysteine	Maleimide, Bromoacetamide	2–4	Any	Genentech, Medimmune, Seattle genetics etc.	Defined DAR, homogeneity	Multiple steps (de-cap, re-oxidize),	Clinical (phase III)
Selenocysteine	Maleimide, iodoacetamide	2	C-terminus	NCI	Defined DAR Homogeneity	Multiple step (de-cap, re-oxidize), need C-his for purification	Preclinical
EuCODE™ (CHO cell, non-natural amino acids)	Oxime and click	2–4	Any	Ambrx	Defined DAR, homogeneity	Special platform cell line	Clinical (phase I)
OCFS (cell free, non-natural amino acid)	Click	1–2	Any	Sutro	Defined DAR, homogeneity	Special techniques, biological agents and manufacturing facility	Preclinical
Glycotransferase	Oxime and click	2–4	Glycan at Asn-297	SynAffix	Defined DAR, homogeneity	Multiple steps (deglycosylation, glycosylation, conjugation)	Preclinical
Glycotransferase	Oxime	@1.6	Sialic acid	Sanofi, Genzyme	Defined DAR, homogeneity	Multiple steps	Research
BTG	Gln with primary amino group	2–4	Any	Rinat-Pfizer, innate pharma	Defined DAR, homogeneity	Removal of N-glycan on N297 or incorporate enzyme substrate motif (LLQGA)	Preclinical
Sortase A	Hydrolysis of Thr-Gly in LPxTG motif	2–4	N and C-termini	NBE therapeutics	Known conjugate site	Incorporation of LPETG motif and reversible reaction	Preclinical
FGE	Hydrazino-iso-Pictet-Spengler ligation	2–4	Multiple	Catalent	Defined DAR, homogeneity	Incorporation of CXPXR motif	Preclinical

Technology	Conjugation chemistry	DAR	Conjugation site	Companies or institutes	Advantage	Disadvantage	Phase of development
Rebridge inter-chain disulfide bonds	Disulfide bond (Bis-alkylating reagents)	4	Interchain cysteine	UCL Cancer Institute, Abzena	Defined DAR, homogeneity, high structural stability	Potential disulfide scrambling	Preclinical
Photoactive protein z	4-benzoyl-L-phenylalanine photo cross-linking	2	Fc region	N/A	Defined DAR, homogeneity	Multiple steps required, exposure to UV light, reversible reaction	Research

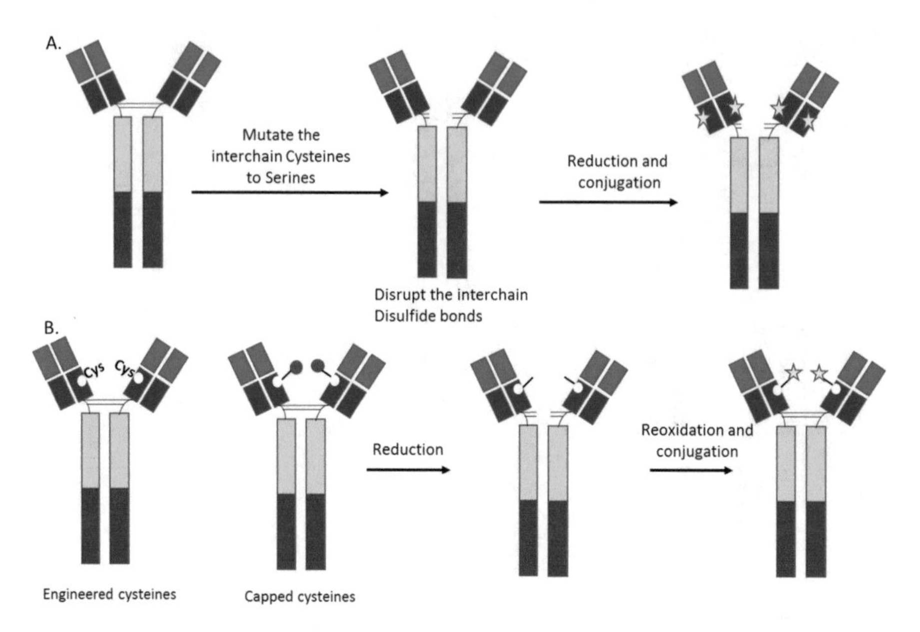

Fig. 1 Random cysteine conjugation compared to site specific conjugation. (**a**) The conversion of the inter-chain cysteines to serines results in ADCs with more homogeneous DARs. (**b**) The incorporation of cysteines at specific sites results in a homogeneous ADC with a DAR of 2

inter-chain disulfide bonds. The antibody is then, ready for conjugation with a cytotoxic drug linked to a thio-reactive maleimide moiety to provide site-specific antibody conjugates (Fig. 1b).

The common challenges with the engineered cysteine conjugation technology are (1) engineered free cysteines on the protein surface can pair with cysteines intermolecularly, on other molecules to form protein dimers [26]; (2) the introduced-cysteines can pair intra-molecularly with native cysteines to create improper disulfide bonds, resulting in disulfide bond shuffling and possibly protein inactivation [27]; (3) cytotoxic payloads conjugated on cysteines can lose their payloads via a retro-Michael reaction [28]. The retro-Michael reaction results in the transfer of the cytotoxic drug to albumin which reduces the ADC's serum exposure and anti-tumor effect. This can potentially result in non-target mediated toxicities and reduce the therapeutic index of the ADC [28–30]; (4) the control of the reduction and re-oxidation steps at manufacturing scale to ensure process robustness and efficiency can be quite challenging.

To overcome the challenges of disulfide shuffling, Phage Elisa for Selection of Reactive Thiols (PHESELECTOR) was developed to identify proper sites on antibodies in which the cysteine-substitution is unlikely to react with other intra-antibody cysteines, so that mAb structure and its function will be maintained [20, 25]. Using PHESELECTOR method, ten residues are identified as suitable for cysteine substitution and site-specific conjugation.

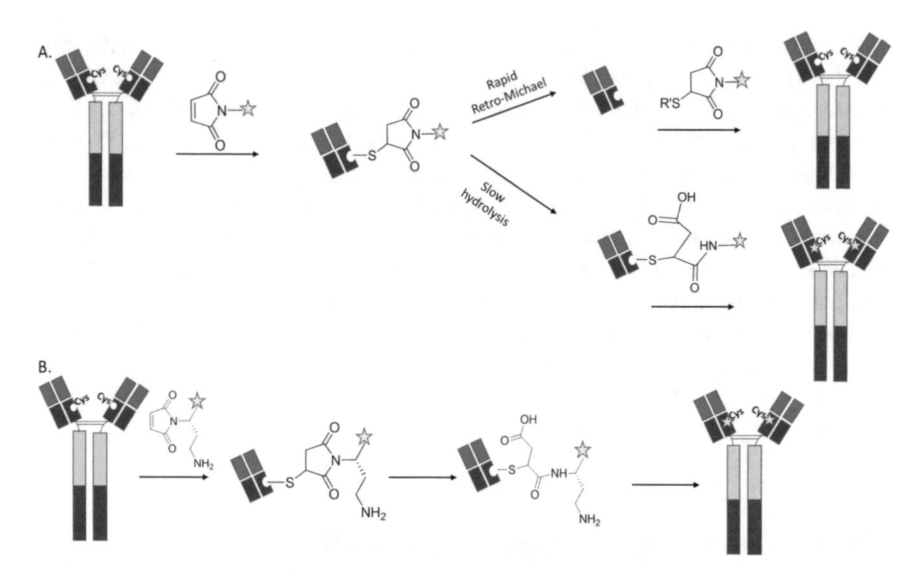

Fig. 2 Blocking the retro-Michael reaction. (**a**) The retro-Michael reaction results in premature release of the ADC payload and ADC instability. The thiosuccinimide ring can also undergo a slow hydrolysis. (**b**) The placement of a basic amino group next to the thiosuccinimide ring results in the rapid hydrolysis of the thiosuccinimide ring

Chemically, the retro-Michael reaction can be prevented by the hydrolysis of the thiosuccinimide ring (Fig. 2a). The ring opening can be achieved through either screening of the conjugation sites or the incorporation of a basic group on the linker adjacent to the maleimide, which induces the thiosuccinimide ring to rapidly hydrolyze at neutral pH and room temperature (Fig. 2b) [31]. Currently, there are several clinical trials with ADCs created using this approach (Table 2).

Selenocysteine

Selenocysteine is a naturally existing proteinogenic amino acid which presents in a wide number of species as a component of selenoproteins [32]. There are approximately 25 known selenoproteins in mammals, including proteins such as glutathione peroxidases and thioreductases. Selenocysteine is very similar to the classical cysteine amino acid, but contains a selenium atom in place of the sulfur atom. The selenolate group makes selenocysteine more reactive to electrophilic moieties (maleimide, maleimide-like or iodoacetamide) in acidic conditions (~ pH 5.2) than its classic counterpart cysteine. This chemical property of selenocysteine is therefore used to selectively conjugate maleimide or iodoacetamide containing agents to the antibodies with genetically engineered selenocysteine [33–35].

Incorporation of selenocysteine requires genetic engineering of the target antibodies. The opal stop codon (UGA) which is a stop codon for translational termination is used to signal the selenocysteine incorporation in the presence of a Sec insertion sequence (SECIS), which is a stem-loop structure located in the 3′ untranslated regions (UTR) of Sec-containing proteins in mammilian cells. A selenocysteine specific $tRNA^{Sec}$ is required on which selenocysteine is synthesized. As the initial step of the incorporation process, the selenocysteine specific $tRNA^{Sec}$ is charged with a serine by seryl-tRNA synthetase. The tRNA bond serine is then, converted to selenocysteine by two enzymes: O-phosphoseryl-$tRNA^{Sec}$ kinase (PSTK) and selenocysteine synthase. Finally, selenocysteine-tRNA is recognized and delivered to ribosome by an alternative enlongation factor, eEFSec for selenocysteine incorporation to site on mRNA with the UGA codon and the SECIS at the 3′ end of gene of interest [36]. Due the low suppression efficiency of UGA codon, a histag 3′ to UGA codon, is required to facilitate the purification of full length antibody from the truncated fragment .

Conjugation Using Non-natural Amino Acids

Site-specific incorporation of non-natural amino acids into proteins provide invaluable tools for biomedical research as well as promising solutions for creating effective therapeutics. Over 71 non-natural amino acids have been incorporated into proteins in different strain of *E. Coli*, yeast, mammalian cells and animals [37, 38]. Non-natural amino acids, by design, can bring a spectrum of chemical functionality, such as keto and azido groups, that enable chemical reactions orthogonal to the functionalities found on natural amino acids [39]. The incorporation of non-natural amino acid residues with a reactive handle, is a strategy that allows for site-specific chemical conjugation, leading to ADC products with strictly controlled DAR values and substantially improved serum stability compared to the conventional conjugation technologies. The option to select "designer" reactions which are not limited by the functionalities of 20 natural amino acids, makes this approach immune to the challenges encountered in the engineered cysteine approach. This also expands the repertoire of the conjugate site selection over engineered cysteines. The freedom it brought into protein engineering allows us to create highly optimized site-specific protein conjugates.

Non-natural amino acids, *para*-acetylphenylalanine (*p*-AcF) and *para*-azidophenylalanine (*p*-AzF) are the two most commonly used for site-specific conjugation [22, 40, 41]. *p*-AcF contains a ketone group that is not found in any of the 20 natural amino acid side chains, therefore it can be used to selectively conjugate to a drug containing an alkoxy-amine through an oxime ligation without interference from other amino acids under acidic conditions in aqueous solution. While, *p*-AzF contains an azido group, which can enable "Click Chemistry" under any pH condition in aqueous solution [41].

The expression of recombinant antibodies with non-natural amino acids can be accomplished using an orthogonal tRNA/aminoacyl-tRNA synthetase (aaRS) pair [9, 15]. The orthogonal aaRS is engineered to only recognize a specific non-natural amino acid and charges it to the orthogonal tRNA which is not recognized by 20 canonical tRNA synthetases. The orthogonal tRNA is engineered to recognize a stop codon such as the amber codon (TAG). The codon on the DNA sequence of the gene of interest, where the non-natural amino acid is designated for incorporation, is mutated to the amber codon. During translation, the charged orthogonal tRNA will be brought to ribosome by EF-Tu, where the non-natural amino acid is incorporated into the target antibody sequence. Ambrx developed the technology using living cells which includes *E. Coli* (ReCODE™) [40], yeast and mammalian (EuCODE™) [22, 40] for product development. Sutro Biopharma, Inc. translated the concept and technology into a cell free system for product development [42]. The main challenge for the non-natural amino acid approach is the lower antibody expression yields relative to wildtype antibodies. The incorporation efficiency of the non-natural amino acid is less than that of natural amino acids due to the competition of orthogonal tRNA with amber codon recognizing release factors during protein synthesis. However, this challenge seems to have been overcome by Ambrx, Inc., with recent technology improvements evidenced by the initiation of the clinical development of two ADCs [9, 15]. In addition, even though no observations or data on the potential immunogenicity of non-natural amino acids and their bioorthogonal linages have been reported, this question needs to be further evaluated during the clinical development of these ADCs.

EuCODE™ Technology

In order to develop an efficient system for the production of non-natural amino acid containing proteins in mammalian cells, Ambrx created a platform cell line, in which the genes of orthogonal tRNA and tRNA synthetase pair are integrated in to CHO cells (Fig. 3a). Their expressions are optimized to achieve a balance between the non-natural amino acid incorporation efficiency and cell viability to maximize antibody production. From this platform cell line, stable antibody or protein producing cell lines were created by following current industry standard methodologies, which includes introducing antibody encoding vectors into the cells and selection with appropriate conditions according to the selection marker used on the vectors [22]. The equipment and medium used for antibody production is similar to wild type antibody production. Current antibody manufacturing facilities used for clinical studies and commercial manufacturing can be used for an antibody containing non-natural amino acids without any modification. Recent improvements in the EuCODE™ technology has increased the antibody production titers up to 1.5 g/L, which has alleviated some concerns for the manufacturability of the EuCODE technology for antibody production (unpublished results).

In the following conjugation step, the ketone functional group in *p*-AcF reacts with the alkoxy-amine linked to the cytotoxic drug to form a stable oxime bond (Fig. 3b). This results in the cytotoxic drug being covalently attached to the antibody at a specific site where the *p*-AcF is incorporated. This oxime formation

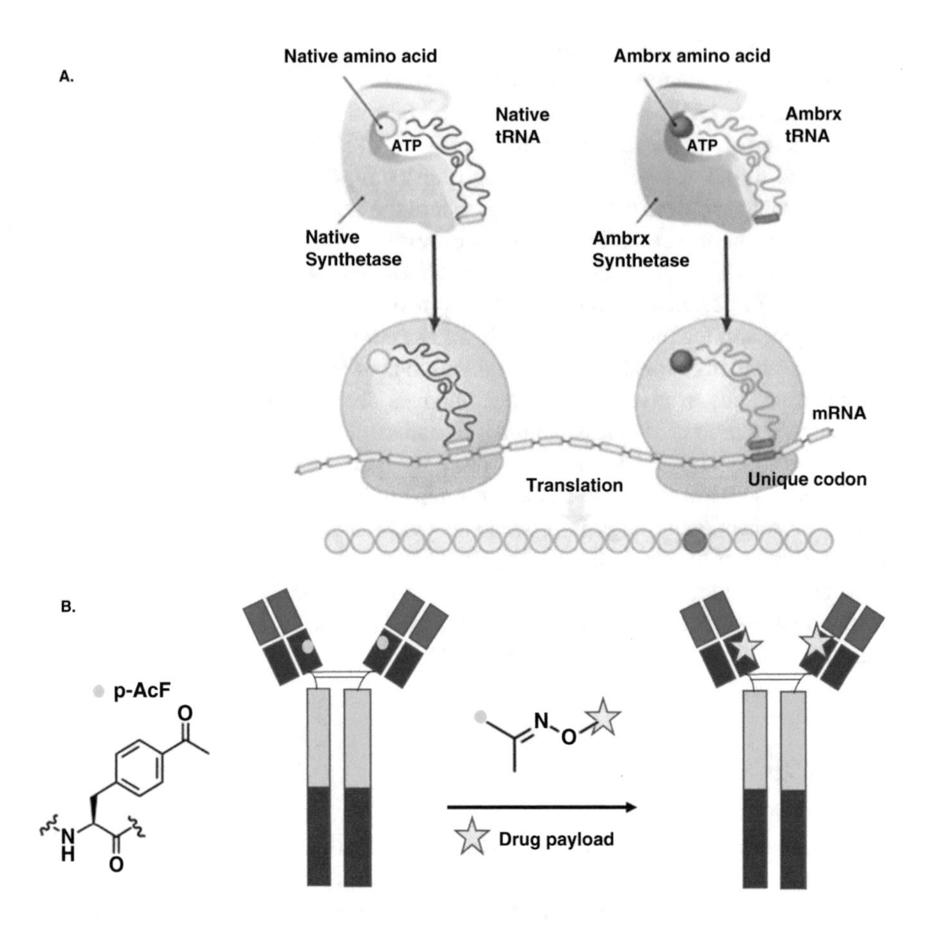

Fig. 3 EuCODE™ technology. (**a**) tRNA synthase, which has been modified to recognize an amber stop codon, is stably expressed in CHO cells, and incorporates the non-natural amino acid, p-acetyl phenyalanine (*p*-AcF), into the antibody at the site of the amber stop codon. (**b**) The linker/payload is conjugated to the *p*-AcF via an oxime bond

reaction generally requires acidic pH conditions. The reaction kinetics are fast, and the use of a catalyst can drive the reaction to a near complete state within a few hours [43]. Azido group could also be introduced onto antibodies through the incorporation of either *p*-AzF or *N*6-((2-azidoethoxy)carbonyl)-l-lysine for site-specific ADC generation with "Click Chemistry" [44, 45].

Through various *in vitro* and *in vivo* testing for multiple ADC molecules, Ambrx and its collaborators have shown that site-specific ADCs, using the incorporation of non-natural amino acids, generally have comparable efficacy but improved pharmacokinetics (PK) and safety than both engineered and conventional cysteine-conjugated ADCs. This is most likely due to the improved stability of the aryl oximes relative to maleimide thioethers in cysteines-conjugated ADCs. In a rat safety study comparing a conventionally cysteine conjugated anti-Her2 ADC and a *p*-AcF version of the anti-Her2-ADC, the *p*-AcF version of the ADC had a superior pharmacokinetic and safety profile compared to the conventionally cysteine conjugated anti-Her2 ADC [46]. Two ADC programs, AGS62P1 (anti-FLT3) and ARX788 (anti-Her2/ERBB2), based on this technology are undergoing phase I clinical evaluation.

OCFS Technology

At Sutro Biopharma, Inc., an open cell free synthesis system (OCFS) technology has been developed to express antibodies and proteins containing non-natural amino acids. In OCFS system, proteins are synthesized by mixing *E. Coli* cell extracts with essential chemical substrates (nucleoside triphosphates, amino acids, salts and cofactors etc.), an energy regeneration system and the corresponding DNA template encoding genes of interest [42, 47, 48]. Without the constraints of living cells, OCFS can be developed to increase the amber suppression efficiency by, for example, deleting release factor (RF1) which competes for Amber codon recognition with orthogonal tRNA. Correctly folded full length antibodies are produced in the cell free system. The non-natural amino acid *para*-azidomethyl-L-phenylalanine is incorporated and is used for conjugation with cyclic alkyne-functionalized linkers through a copper-free cycloaddition (also called "Click Chemistry") to produce site-specific ADCs [42, 45]. Sutro has developed a GMP manufacturing facility, which specially fits this process, however, the production of *E. Coli* cell extract with well controlled quality could be a challenge. The antibodies produced in cell free system are not glycosylated in the Fc region.

Deglycosylation in the Fc region will have impacts on antibody effector functions and their development as biotherapeutics. The deglycosylation of antibodies is commonly associated with the loss of effector function, such as ADCC, which is mediated through the binding of the Fcγ IIIa receptor on immune cells [49, 50]. Deglycosylated antibodies do not bind to the Fcγ IIIa receptor while afucosylated antibodies show strong binding to the Fcγ IIIa receptor and induces ADCC [50]. It has been suspected that some ADCs, such as Kadcyla, which is glycosylated, bind to Fcγ receptors on immune cells which may be responsible for some of the non-target mediated side effects. The thrombocytopenia observed for Kadcyla (T-DM1) has been attributed to FcγRIIa receptor binding on megakaryocytes, which results in the death of megakaryocytes and the reduction of platelets [51]. Furthermore, a recent study suggests that non-specific anti-tumor efficacy displayed by a non-binding isotype control ADC in some preclinical tumor models may be the result of ADCs binding to the Fcγ receptors on tumor associated macrophages (TAMs), which results in the release of the cytotoxic payload in these tumors [52]. While the deglycosylation of antibodies may reduce the non-target mediated activities of the ADC, which is associated with binding to the Fcγ receptors, it may also result in increased antibody instability and increased aggregation. It was observed that deglycosylated antibodies are less thermally stable in their CH2 domains, which renders the antibodies more susceptibility to proteolytic cleavage [53]. These observations show the potential strengths and challenges of the OCFC technology, which is currently in preclinical development.

Enzymatic Ligations

The use of enzymes to catalyze the ligation of a drug to an antibody is another strategy being explored for use in site-specific conjugation. In this approach, one of the enzyme ligation substrates, either a short peptide sequence or a carbohydrate moiety is engineered to a specific site on an antibody. In the presence of respective enzyme and antibody, the second enzyme substrate linked to cytotoxic drug is ligated to the antibody. Multiple enzymatic platforms such as glycotransferase, transglutaminase and sortase are actively explored and appear to have promising results. We will also review formylglycine generating enzyme (FGE) in this section, where the cysteine within the recognition peptide is converted to formylglycine for conjugation.

Glycotransferase

Human IgG antibodies contain an N-glycosylation site at the conserved heavy chain Asn-297 of the Fc fragment. The glycans attached to this site are generally complex and are commonly referred to as G0, G1 and G2 based on the number of the terminal galactoses. Glycotransferases are a large family of enzymes involved in the synthesis of oligosaccharides and are responsible for the transfer of a sugar residue from an activated sugar nucleotide to a sugar acceptor or glycoprotein/lipid.

Qasba and coworkers had developed β1, 4-glycotransferase mutant that can transfer a galactose derivative containing a ketone reactive group to carbohydrate on antibody [54, 55]. An IgG1 antibody is first degalactosylated with *Streptococcus pneumoniae* β1,4-glycotransferase to release galactose from antibody to form a homogeneous antibody with only G0 glycoforms. After degalactosylation, a galactose UDP derivative with a chemically reactive ketone group, UDP-C2-keto-Gal, was added back onto the degalactosylated glycans using the mutant β1,4-glycotransferase-T1-Y289L with high efficiency [56]. This is followed with the conjugation of alkoxy-amine linker-derivatized auristatin F by reacting with the ketone group on the modified galactose to produce a site-specific DAR 4 ADC.

Similar to conjugation to galactose, sialic acid residues on the native glycans have also been used as a chemical handle to allow for site-specific conjugation. In this method, sialic acid units are first incorporated onto the glycans using a mixture of β1,4-glycotransferase and α2,6-sialyltransferase. Periodate oxidation of these sialic acids yielded aldehyde groups which were then reacted with the aminooxyl-funcationized toxin-linker via oxime ligation to provide site-specific ADC [57].

Bacterial Transglutaminase (BTG)

This technique uses a microbial transglutaminase to couple an amine-containing toxin payload to an engineered glutamine residue on the antibody. A transglutaminase from *Streptoverticillium mobaraense* is a commercially available enzyme that catalyzes amide bond formation between the acyl group of a glutamine side chain and a primary amine-containing drug linker. The bacterial transglutaminase interacts with the glutamine "tag" sequence (LLQG) that can be incorporated into the mAb via genetic engineering technology [58].

In order to explore more conjugation sites, a short glutamine tag (LLQG) can be incorporated into the location of choice on the antibody during genetic engineering and served as a BTG substrate for conjugation [59, 60] After evaluating 90 surface-accessible locations across the antibody backbone, 12 sites are identified by the Rinat group with efficient conjugation. ADCs made using BTG methods were compared to the conventional ADCs and demonstrated comparable efficacy to the conventional ADCs but had better PK, safety and tolerability than the conventional ADCs.

The BTG-based method can also utilize the native sequence on antibodies at position 295 (Q295) for site-specific conjugation. For this approach, the conjugation process generally involves two steps: (1) removal of the glycan attached to N297 site using peptide-N-glycosidase F (PGNase F) to reveal the adjacent conjugation site – Q295; (2) site-specifically conjugation of the cytotoxic payload with a primary amine group onto the glutamine at 295 position catalyzed by BTG to produce the site-specific ADC with a DAR of 2. The Q295 site can also be revealed for conjugation by the removal of glycosylation through N297Q mutation [56, 58, 61] (Fig. 4).

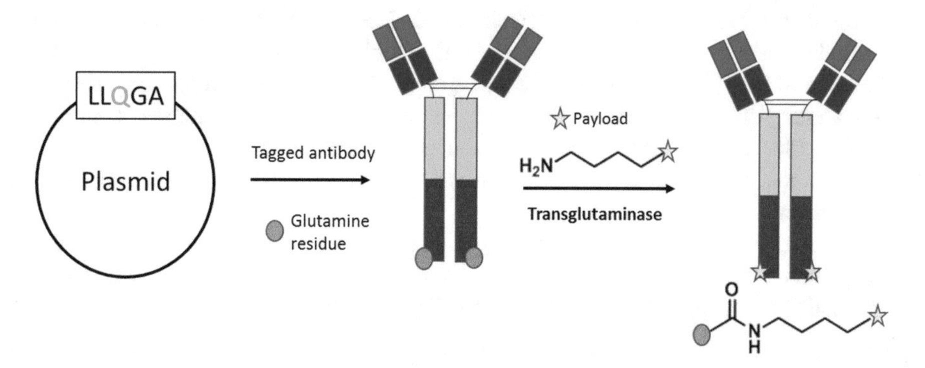

Fig. 4 Using Bacterial Transglutaminase (BTG) for site-specific conjugation. BTG couples an amine-containing toxin payload to an engineered glutamine residue (LLQA) on an antibody. This will allow for the site-specific incorporation of a toxin on an antibody using oxime conjugation

Sortase A

The transpeptidase Sortase A from *Staphylococcus aureus* has been explored for site-specific modification either at the N or C terminus of proteins. The thiol group of the enzyme at C148 recognizes the LPXTG motif, where X can be any amino acid, cleaves the threonine-glycine (T-G) bond to release the terminal glycine and form a thioacyl intermediate. This intermediate can react with an oligoglycine-containing molecule such as GGGY to form a new T-G bond, where Y can be any payload. Various molecules can be fused to the oligoglycine for Sortase A-mediated conjugation such as peptides, proteins, cytotoxic drugs and nucleic acids [60, 62, 63]. The reversibility of transpeptidase mediated reactions is a major drawback for this technology and a large excess of substrate and sortase are needed to drive the reaction to high yield. This issue has been partially addressed by using depsipeptide substrates and enhanced Sortase A variants [63].

Formylglycine-Generating Enzyme (FGE)

Redwood Bioscience, Inc., now part of Catalent, developed a novel chemoenzymatic approach that uses the naturally occurring FGE to introduce a formyl glycine (fGly) residue into protein backbones which serves as a handle for site-specific conjugation. This technique is also referred to as SMARTag technology [64]. The formylglycine-generating enzyme recognizes cysteines in the aldehyde tags (CxPxR), where x is usually serine, threonine, alanine or glycine, and oxidizes the cysteine residues to an aldehyde-bearing formylglycine, thus generating a protein with an aldehyde tag. The aldehyde group can then be conjugated to cytotoxic payloads through Hydrazino-iso-Pictet-Spengler (HIPS) ligation chemistry which forms a stable carbon-carbon bond between antibody and payload linker [64, 65].

The fGly tag is incorporated into a desired location of the antibody heavy or light chain using genetic engineering techniques. The tagged antibody is produced recombinantly in cells that co-express FGE, which converts the thiol group of the cysteine in the fGly tag into an aldehyde group which can be used for conjugation. Apparently, unlike the BTG method, the enzyme FGE is used to create the conjugation handle for conjugation in the following step, rather than catalyze the conjugation process. The chemoenzymatic reaction is integrated into the process of antibody expression.

Through a series of animal studies, FGE conjugation at the C-terminus of the heavy chain was shown to be the optimal site in terms of ADC plasma stability, *in vivo* half-life and anti-tumor efficacy [66] (Fig. 5) (FGE Method)

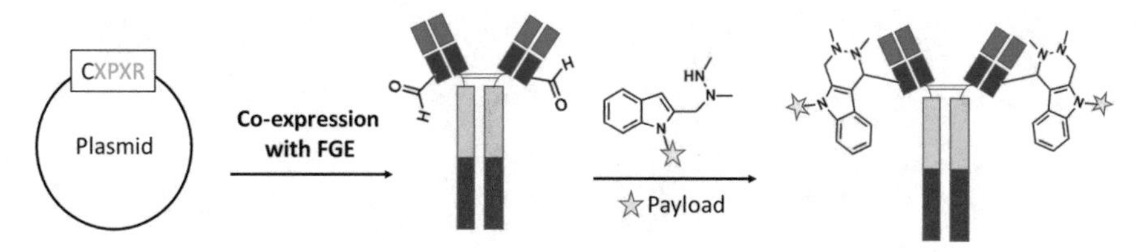

Fig. 5 Using Formylglycine-Generating Enzyme (FGE) for site-specific conjugation. FGE recognizes cysteines in the aldehyde tags (CxPxR) and oxidizes the cysteine residues to an aldehyde-bearing formylglycine, thus generating a protein with an aldehyde tag. The aldehyde group can then be used to attach a cytotoxic payload

Tub-Tag Labeling

Tub-tag labeling for site-specific conjugation combines the use of UAA incorporation with a highly efficient chemoenzymatic system [67]. The technique is based on the enzyme tubulin tyrosine ligase (TLL) which recognizes a 14-amino acid recognition motif at the C-terminus of alpha-tubulin and post-translationally attaches a terminal tyrosine residue [68]. When recombinantly fused to an antibody, the recognition motif (Tub-tag) allows the TTL-mediated attachment of non-natural tyrosine derivatives that carry uniquely reactive groups for chemoselective conjugation such as strain-promoted alkyne azide cycloadditions (SPAAC). One potential benefit is that the human-derived peptide on the C-terminus is glutamate-rich and strongly hydrophilic, it potentially can help to improve the ADC instability due to strong hydrophobicity nature.

Other Technologies

Re-bridge of Reduced Inter-chain Disulfide Bonds of a Native Antibody

Cysteine re-bridging is a recently developed strategy to improve the control of the DAR and reduce the heterogeneity of ADCs. This method takes advantage of bis-sulfone reagents that undergo bis-alkylation to conjugate both thiols of the two cysteine residues that were obtained through the reduction of native disulfide bonds. Dibromomaleimide [69, 70], dibromopyridazinediones [71] and a 1,3-bis(p-toluenesulfonyl)propane-based core [72] can link two reduced cysteines derived from inter-chain disulfide bonds to form a re-bridged and homogenous ADC (Fig. 6).

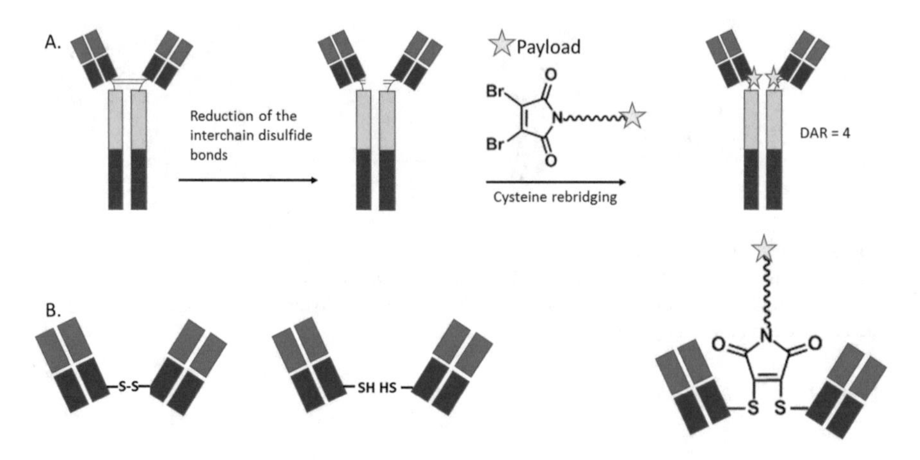

Fig. 6 Cysteine re-bridging. (**a**) Cysteine re-bridging can link two reduced cysteines derived from inter-chain disulfide bonds to form a re-bridged and homogenous ADC. (**b**) A detailed view of the reduction of the inter-chain disulfides followed by the cysteine re-bridging, which results in the conjugation of the payload

Photoactive Protein Z

Conjugation of a photoactive protein Z to antibodies has recently emerged as an unconventional approach to make homogeneous ADCs. Protein Z is a small helical protein, consisting of 58 amino acids, derived from the IgG-binding B domain of Protein A. Protein Z binds to the antibody's Fc domain, but the binding is non-covalent, thus reversible. In order to form a stable linkage to create a site-specific ADC, Tsourks's group developed a photo cross-linking methodology [73]. The photo reactive non-natural amino acid, 4-benzoyl-L-phenylalanine (BPA) are introduced at various locations on protein Z. A payload linked to a peptide is then introduced into C terminal of protein Z through either intein-mediated expressed peptide ligation (EPL) or more recently sortase-tag expressed protein ligation (STEPL). Protein Z-BPA variants with payload bound antibody Fc domain is exposed to long wavelength UV light (365 nm) and forms a covalent linkage to the target antibody. The site of BPA incorporation on protein Z is critical for photo-linking efficiency. Protein Z variants, L17BPA and K35BPA, are the best sites capable of crosslinking many commonly used IgG isotypes with efficiencies ranging from 60% to 95% after only 1 h of UV exposure [73, 74].

Conclusion and Future Direction

Antibody drug conjugates are the manifestation of a nearly century old vision conceived by Dr. Paul Ehrlich to simply deliver drugs to the corresponding disease site, such as cancer. Today, only four ADCs are approved for cancer treatment. This result speaks to the challenges the ADC field is facing. To design ADC therapeutics, we need to address five aspects simultaneously, namely target selection, antibody technology, cytotoxic drug optimization, linker design and antibody conjugation methodology development. The development of ADC therapeutics continues to evolve and improve. The recent wave of technology development has increased the number of site-specific conjugation methodologies and ADCs. With the improved precision in ADC drug design, we are able to conduct medicinal chemistry-like research on protein conjugates. Site-specific ADCs will serve as a new starting point for the future rounds of ADC technology evolution to further improve anti-tumor efficacy and increase safety.

The preclinical toxicology and anti-tumor efficacy studies suggest that site-specific ADCs will have an improved therapeutic index compared to conventional ADCs. This is the rationle and motivation for the recent surge of site-specific ADCs in clinical development. There are seven site-specific ADCs in clinical development. Although there are several options available to produce site-specific ADCs, the site-specific ADCs currently in clinical development utilize either engineered cysteines or non-natural amino acids in combination with PBDs or Auristatin payloads.

Looking forward, increasing the therapeutic index remains a major challenge for ADC therapeutics. While the anti-tumor efficacy can be improved by employing more potent cytotoxic payloads or by increasing the DAR, these changes also appear to elevate unwanted toxicities. Understanding the mechanisms for on-target and off-target toxicities are challenges for ADCs. On-target toxicity is caused by tumor antigen expression in normal tissues where, the ADC is internalized, the cytotoxic payload is released intracellularly, which causes normal tissue damage. The number of receptors required to internalize enough cytotoxic payload to kill antigen expressing cells is unclear and may vary depending on the biology of the targeted cell surface antigen. Off-target toxicity is caused by the non-target antigen mediated uptake of the ADC via pinocytosis or the premature release of the cytotoxic payload due to the linker instability. Various studies have been initiated to address these issues. For example, the on-target toxicity issue could potentially be addressed as we learn more about the solid tumor's microenviroment and how different it is from the normal tissue's microenvironment. The lower pH of the tumor's extracellular environment and/or increased expression and activity of certain proteases, may help to differentiate the tumor from normal tissues and allow an ADC, which can take advantage of these conditions, to selectively deliver the payload to the tumor.

CytomX Therapeutics has developed a Probody platform in which the antibody binding sites are masked during circulation. Upon reaching the tumor, where specific proteases, such as urokinase type plasminogen activator, membrane-type serine protease and legumain, are over expressed and active, the antibody binding sites are unmasked through protealytic cleavage of an enzyme specific peptide linker connecting the mask and antibody. This allows the ADC/Probody drug conjugate (PDC) to bind selectively to the tumor cells and not to the antigen expressing normal cells [75]. The PDC, is in the preclinical evaluation phase and will hopefully begin clinical evaluation in the near future.

The mechanism of action of ADCs may synergize with immunotherapies, which rely on the either recruiting or enhancing immune response toward the tumor. The tumor and the tumor microenviroment can be immuno-suppressive, which can render the immunotherapy ineffective for solid tumors. ADCs could serve as the first wave of attack to damage the solid tumor and alter the tumor's immune suppressive microenviroment. This could potentially enhance the sensitivity of solid tumors to immunotherapies, such as checkpoint inhibitors (anti-PD-1 antibody) which are effective in 20–30% of lung cancer patients. With the approval of the immune checkpoint inhibitors Avelumab, Atezolizumab (αPD-L1 antibody), Pembrolizumab and Nivolumab (αPD-1 antibody), and the bispecific T-cell engager (BiTE) Blinatumomab (CD3-CD19 BiTE), the role of ADCs in combination with anti-cancer immunotherapy are being explored.

The future of ADCs is very promising. The number of ADCs entering into clinical development has seen a steady increase over the years. As more information emergs during the clinical development of ADCs, this new round of learning will help improve the preclinical development of ADC linkers, payloads and conjugation technology. Site-specific ADCs addressed some of the off-target toxicity issues through improved in vivo stability of ADC, which eliminates the premature release of the cytotoxc payload. Future ADC technologies will emerge to further improve the therapeutic index by addressing ways to limit or eliminate on-target activity in normal tissues as well as the off-target toxicities. This will hopefully increase the number of ADCs in clinical development transitioning from early stage to later stage clinical development and approval. As more novel therapeutics, such as immune checkpoint inhibitors, CD3 bispecific antibodies, etc. are approved, the use of ADCs in combination with these therapies will hopefully provided added benefit to the cancer patients.

References

1. Ecker DM, Jones SD, Levine HL (2015) The therapeutic monoclonal antibody market. MAbs 7(1):9–14
2. Scott AM, Wolchok JD, Old LJ (2012) Antibody therapy of cancer. Nat Rev Cancer 12(4):278–287
3. Sanz L, Alvarez-Vallina L (2005) Antibody-based antiangiogenic cancer therapy. Expert Opin Ther Targets 9(6):1235–1245
4. Roviello G et al (2017) The role of bevacizumab in solid tumours: a literature based meta-analysis of randomised trials. Eur J Cancer 75:245–258
5. Azoury SC, Straughan DM, Shukla V (2015) Immune checkpoint inhibitors for cancer therapy: clinical efficacy and safety. Curr Cancer Drug Targets 15(6):452–462
6. Chen DS, Mellman I (2017) Elements of cancer immunity and the cancer-immune set point. Nature 541(7637):321–330
7. Ho RJ, Chien J (2014) Trends in translational medicine and drug targeting and delivery: new insights on an old concept-targeted drug delivery with antibody-drug conjugates for cancers. J Pharm Sci 103(1):71–77
8. Polakis P (2016) Antibody drug conjugates for Cancer therapy. Pharmacol Rev 68(1):3–19

9. Beck A et al (2017) Strategies and challenges for the next generation of antibody-drug conjugates. Nat Rev Drug Discov 16(5):315–337
10. Schrama D, Reisfeld RA, Becker JC (2006) Antibody targeted drugs as cancer therapeutics. Nat Rev Drug Discov 5(2):147–159
11. Peters C, Brown S (2015) Antibody-drug conjugates as novel anti-cancer chemotherapeutics. Biosci Rep 35(4):e00225
12. Varki NM, Reisfeld RA, Walker LE (1984) Antigens associated with a human lung adenocarcinoma defined by monoclonal antibodies. Cancer Res 44(2):681–687
13. Trail PA et al (1993) Cure of xenografted human carcinomas by BR96-doxorubicin immunoconjugates. Science 261(5118):212–215
14. Herbertson RA et al (2009) Phase I biodistribution and pharmacokinetic study of Lewis Y-targeting immunoconjugate CMD-193 in patients with advanced epithelial cancers. Clin Cancer Res 15(21):6709–6715
15. Jackson D, Stover D (2015) Using the lessons learned from the clinic to improve the preclinical development of antibody drug conjugates. Pharm Res 32(11):3458–3469
16. Donaghy H (2016) Effects of antibody, drug and linker on the preclinical and clinical toxicities of antibody-drug conjugates. MAbs 8(4):659–671
17. Lyon RP et al (2015) Reducing hydrophobicity of homogeneous antibody-drug conjugates improves pharmacokinetics and therapeutic index. Nat Biotechnol 33(7):733–735
18. Yurkovetskiy AV et al (2015) A polymer-based antibody-Vinca drug conjugate platform: characterization and preclinical efficacy. Cancer Res 75(16):3365–3372
19. Ogitani Y et al (2016) DS-8201a, a novel HER2-targeting ADC with a novel DNA topoisomerase I inhibitor, demonstrates a promising antitumor efficacy with differentiation from T-DM1. Clin Cancer Res 22(20):5097–5108
20. Junutula JR et al (2008) Site-specific conjugation of a cytotoxic drug to an antibody improves the therapeutic index. Nat Biotechnol 26(8):925–932
21. Hamblett KJ et al (2004) Effects of drug loading on the antitumor activity of a monoclonal antibody drug conjugate. Clin Cancer Res 10(20):7063–7070
22. Tian F et al (2014) A general approach to site-specific antibody drug conjugates. Proc Natl Acad Sci U S A 111(5):1766–1771
23. Peng H et al (2012) Thiol reactive probes and chemosensors. Sensors (Basel) 12(11):15907–15946
24. McDonagh CF et al (2006) Engineered antibody-drug conjugates with defined sites and stoichiometries of drug attachment. Protein Eng Des Sel 19(7):299–307
25. Junutula JR et al (2008) Rapid identification of reactive cysteine residues for site-specific labeling of antibody-Fabs. J Immunol Methods 332(1–2):41–52
26. Woo HJ et al (1991) Carbohydrate-binding protein 35 (mac-2), a laminin-binding lectin, forms functional dimers using cysteine 186. J Biol Chem 266(28):18419–18422
27. Wootton SK, Yoo D (2003) Homo-oligomerization of the porcine reproductive and respiratory syndrome virus nucleocapsid protein and the role of disulfide linkages. J Virol 77(8):4546–4557
28. Alley SC et al (2008) Contribution of linker stability to the activities of anticancer immunoconjugates. Bioconjug Chem 19(3):759–765
29. Baldwin AD, Kiick KL (2011) Tunable degradation of maleimide-thiol adducts in reducing environments. Bioconjug Chem 22(10):1946–1953
30. Shen BQ et al (2012) Conjugation site modulates the in vivo stability and therapeutic activity of antibody-drug conjugates. Nat Biotechnol 30(2):184–189
31. Lyon RP et al (2014) Self-hydrolyzing maleimides improve the stability and pharmacological properties of antibody-drug conjugates. Nat Biotechnol 32(10):1059–1062
32. Lu J, Holmgren A (2009) Selenoproteins. J Biol Chem 284(2):723–727
33. Hofer T et al (2009) Molecularly defined antibody conjugation through a selenocysteine interface. Biochemistry 48(50):12047–12057
34. Hofer T et al (2008) An engineered selenocysteine defines a unique class of antibody derivatives. Proc Natl Acad Sci U S A 105(34):12451–12456

35. Li X, Yang J, Rader C (2014) Antibody conjugation via one and two C-terminal selenocysteines. Methods 65(1):133–138
36. Yuan J et al (2006) RNA-dependent conversion of phosphoserine forms selenocysteine in eukaryotes and archaea. Proc Natl Acad Sci U S A 103(50):18923–18927
37. Hohsaka T, Sisido M (2002) Incorporation of non-natural amino acids into proteins. Curr Opin Chem Biol 6(6):809–815
38. Chin JW (2014) Expanding and reprogramming the genetic code of cells and animals. Annu Rev Biochem 83:379–408
39. Hallam TJ, Smider VV (2014) Unnatural amino acids in novel antibody conjugates. Future Med Chem 6(11):1309–1324
40. Cho H et al (2011) Optimized clinical performance of growth hormone with an expanded genetic code. Proc Natl Acad Sci U S A 108(22):9060–9065
41. Kern JC et al (2016) Novel phosphate modified Cathepsin B linkers: improving aqueous solubility and enhancing payload scope of ADCs. Bioconjug Chem 27(9):2081–2088
42. Zimmerman ES et al (2014) Production of site-specific antibody-drug conjugates using optimized non-natural amino acids in a cell-free expression system. Bioconjug Chem 25(2):351–361
43. Axup JY et al (2012) Synthesis of site-specific antibody-drug conjugates using unnatural amino acids. Proc Natl Acad Sci U S A 109(40):16101–16106
44. Kern JC et al (2016) Discovery of pyrophosphate Diesters as tunable, soluble, and bioorthogonal linkers for site-specific antibody-drug conjugates. J Am Chem Soc 138(4):1430–1445
45. VanBrunt MP et al (2015) Genetically encoded Azide containing amino acid in mammalian cells enables site-specific antibody-drug conjugates using click cycloaddition chemistry. Bioconjug Chem 26(11):2249–2260
46. Jackson D et al (2014) In vitro and in vivo evaluation of cysteine and site specific conjugated herceptin antibody-drug conjugates. PLoS One 9(1):e83865
47. Ozawa K et al (2012) High-yield cell-free protein synthesis for site-specific incorporation of unnatural amino acids at two sites. Biochem Biophys Res Commun 418(4):652–656
48. Hong SH, Kwon YC, Jewett MC (2014) Non-standard amino acid incorporation into proteins using Escherichia coli cell-free protein synthesis. Front Chem 2:34
49. Thomann M et al (2015) In vitro glycoengineering of IgG1 and its effect on fc receptor binding and ADCC activity. PLoS One 10(8):e0134949
50. Liu SD et al (2015) Afucosylated antibodies increase activation of FcgammaRIIIa-dependent signaling components to intensify processes promoting ADCC. Cancer Immunol Res 3(2):173–183
51. Uppal H et al (2015) Potential mechanisms for thrombocytopenia development with trastuzumab emtansine (T-DM1). Clin Cancer Res 21(1):123–133
52. Li F et al (2017) Tumor associated macrophages can contribute to antitumor activity through FcgammaRmediated processing of antibody-drug conjugates. Mol Cancer Ther
53. Zheng K, Bantog C, Bayer R (2011) The impact of glycosylation on monoclonal antibody conformation and stability. MAbs 3(6):568–576
54. Ramakrishnan B, Qasba PK (2002) Structure-based design of beta 1,4-galactosyltransferase I (beta 4Gal-T1) with equally efficient N-acetylgalactosaminyltransferase activity: point mutation broadens beta 4Gal-T1 donor specificity. J Biol Chem 277(23):20833–20839
55. Boeggeman E et al (2009) Site specific conjugation of fluoroprobes to the remodeled fc N-glycans of monoclonal antibodies using mutant glycosyltransferases: application for cell surface antigen detection. Bioconjug Chem 20(6):1228–1236
56. Sochaj AM, Swiderska KW, Otlewski J (2015) Current methods for the synthesis of homogeneous antibody-drug conjugates. Biotechnol Adv 33(6 Pt 1):775–784
57. Zhou Q et al (2014) Site-specific antibody-drug conjugation through glycoengineering. Bioconjug Chem 25(3):510–520
58. Jeger S et al (2010) Site-specific and stoichiometric modification of antibodies by bacterial transglutaminase. Angew Chem Int Ed Engl 49(51):9995–9997

59. Strop P et al (2013) Location matters: site of conjugation modulates stability and pharmacokinetics of antibody drug conjugates. Chem Biol 20(2):161–167
60. Popp MW, Antos JM, Ploegh HL (2009) Site-specific protein labeling via sortase-mediated transpeptidation. Curr Protoc Protein Sci. Chapter 15: p. Unit 15.3
61. Jefferis R (2009) Glycosylation as a strategy to improve antibody-based therapeutics. Nat Rev Drug Discov 8(3):226–234
62. Swee LK et al (2013) Sortase-mediated modification of alphaDEC205 affords optimization of antigen presentation and immunization against a set of viral epitopes. Proc Natl Acad Sci U S A 110(4):1428–1433
63. Beerli RR et al (2015) Sortase enzyme-mediated generation of site-specifically conjugated antibody drug conjugates with high in vitro and in vivo potency. PLoS One 10(7):e0131177
64. Rabuka D et al (2012) Site-specific chemical protein conjugation using genetically encoded aldehyde tags. Nat Protoc 7(6):1052–1067
65. Agarwal P et al (2013) Hydrazino-Pictet-Spengler ligation as a biocompatible method for the generation of stable protein conjugates. Bioconjug Chem 24(6):846–851
66. Drake PM et al (2014) Aldehyde tag coupled with HIPS chemistry enables the production of ADCs conjugated site-specifically to different antibody regions with distinct in vivo efficacy and PK outcomes. Bioconjug Chem 25(7):1331–1341
67. Schumacher D et al (2015) Versatile and efficient site-specific protein functionalization by tubulin tyrosine ligase. Angew Chem Int Ed Engl 54(46):13787–13791
68. Prota AE et al (2013) Structural basis of tubulin tyrosination by tubulin tyrosine ligase. J Cell Biol 200(3):259–270
69. Behrens CR et al (2015) Antibody-drug conjugates (ADCs) derived from Interchain cysteine cross-linking demonstrate improved homogeneity and other pharmacological properties over conventional heterogeneous ADCs. Mol Pharm 12(11):3986–3998
70. Bryden F et al (2014) Regioselective and stoichiometrically controlled conjugation of photodynamic sensitizers to a HER2 targeting antibody fragment. Bioconjug Chem 25(3):611–617
71. Maruani A et al (2015) A plug-and-play approach to antibody-based therapeutics via a chemoselective dual click strategy. Nat Commun 6:6645
72. Bryant P et al (2015) In vitro and in vivo evaluation of cysteine Rebridged Trastuzumab-MMAE antibody drug conjugates with defined drug-to-antibody ratios. Mol Pharm 12(6):1872–1879
73. Hui JZ, Tsourkas A (2014) Optimization of photoactive protein Z for fast and efficient site-specific conjugation of native IgG. Bioconjug Chem 25(9):1709–1719
74. Sakamoto T et al (2010) Enzyme-mediated site-specific antibody-protein modification using a ZZ domain as a linker. Bioconjug Chem 21(12):2227–2233
75. Polu KR, Lowman HB (2014) Probody therapeutics for targeting antibodies to diseased tissue. Expert Opin Biol Ther 14(8):1049–1053

Bispecific and Biparatopic Antibody Drug Conjugates

Frank Comer, Changshou Gao, and Steve Coats

Abstract The conceptual framework for antibody drug conjugates (ADC's) emerged contemporaneously with the discovery of antibodies, with Paul Ehrlich proposing in the early 1900's the concept of a "magic bullet", an ideal therapeutic that would specifically target a disease-causing agent without causing harm to the body. This concept still underpins the overarching goal of biopharmaceutical development today: to produce drugs that have a broad therapeutic index by effectively targeting the disease while causing minimal damage to normal tissue. Although the concept of ADC's is simple, achieving the ideal combination of properties has proven challenging, as reflected by the limited number of ADC's that have demonstrated success in the clinic to date. Recent years have witnessed a burgeoning field, with the number of clinical stage ADC's more than doubling in just the last two years to more than 70 candidates currently in clinical development. Despite the successes to date and the prospect of new ADC's reaching patients in the coming years, many challenges remain and there is substantial room for improvement, most notably in improving the therapeutic index. The key challenge in developing an ADC is balancing its efficacy and safety. This review will focus on ways to capitalize on bispecific antibody technology to improve the therapeutic index of ADC's, in pursuit of the magic bullet ideal. The nature of bispecific antibodies allows for fine tuning of the interactions between each target to impact the overall properties of the molecule. Here, we discuss some of the cutting edge bispecific antibody strategies that are currently under investigation to address both the efficacy and safety aspects of ADC's.

F. Comer (✉)
Biosuperiors, MedImmune LLC, Gaithersburg, MD, USA
e-mail: comerf@medimmune.com

C. Gao
Antibody Discovery and Protein Engineering, MedImmune LLC, Gaithersburg, MD, USA

S. Coats
Oncology Development, MedImmune LLC, Gaithersburg, MD, USA

M. Damelin (ed.), *Innovations for Next-Generation Antibody-Drug Conjugates*,
Cancer Drug Discovery and Development,
https://doi.org/10.1007/978-3-319-78154-9_11

Keywords Bispecific · Antibody drug conjugate · ADC · Bispecific format · Therapeutic index

Introduction

There are four key elements comprising an antibody drug conjugate (ADC) strategy: the target, the antibody, the cytotoxic warhead, and the linker connecting the warhead to the antibody. Consideration of all of these parameters is crucial for the successful development of an ADC [1, 2]. There has been a great deal of progress made in understanding the relationship between these various components, however several challenges remain, most notably improving the therapeutic index [3, 4]. Over the past few years numerous improvements have been made in the chemical properties of the warheads, the linkers, and the means of conjugation to the antibody. These essential advancements, which have greatly expanded the ADC toolbox, have been reviewed elsewhere in this volume. This chapter will focus on the antibody and the target, with a specific emphasis on how to capitalize on bispecific technology to optimize ADC's. To date, the majority of the bispecific antibody approaches to treat cancer have fallen into one of two broad functional categories: (i) simultaneous blockade of two cancer associated targets (e.g., oncogenic receptors, growth factor ligands, or cytokines) or (ii) redirection of a therapeutic effector (e.g., engaging immune effector cells or molecules, pre-targeting of therapeutic toxin or radionuclide) [5–8]. While many of these prior approaches do not translate directly to ADC's, recent efforts have sought to exploit the unique features of bispecific antibodies to produce ADC's that are more efficacious and better tolerated. Ultimately, the key challenge in developing any ADC is balancing its efficacy and safety [1, 2, 4]. The ability of bispecific antibodies to simultaneously engage two targets affords some creative possibilities to address both the efficacy and safety aspects of ADC's. Several strategies currently in development employ bispecific targeting to enhance ADC internalization and lysosomal delivery, with the goal of improving efficacy [9–11]. Another emerging area of research seeks to use the dual targeting capability of bispecific antibodies to improve selectivity toward the tumor relative to normal tissue, an approach that could impact both the safety and efficacy of ADC's [12–14].

With the approval of catumaxomab (Removab) in 2009 and Blinatumomab in 2015, pharmaceutical companies have started to use bispecific antibodies (BsAbs) more frequently for therapeutic applications. The proof of concept for bispecific antibodies was first demonstrated more than half a century ago, initially by chemical conjugation of two antibodies to form bispecific F(ab')2 molecules [15] and later by fusing two different hybridoma cells [16] which was enabled by the hybridoma technology established in 1975 [17]. The hybridoma approach to produce bispecific antibodies is time consuming, requires multiple purification steps, suffers from low purification yields, and faces potential immunogenicity issues. Advances in protein engineering technologies have enabled the generation of recombinant bispecific antibodies with defined architecture and the desired biochemical, functional, and pharmacological properties. The ability to select among different bispecific formats to tailor these properties for the specific application provides opportunities to extend the potential of therapeutic antibodies. The enhanced capacity for fine tuning of bispecific antibodies is particularly relevant for ADC approaches to improve both their efficacy and safety.

Molecular Formats of Bispecific Antibodies

Bispecific antibodies (BsAbs) provide the ability to recognize two different antigens or two distinct epitopes (a subset of bispecifc antibodies designated biparatopic antibodies) simultaneously as a single molecule and offer the potential to maximize the benefits of therapeutic antibodies by a number of mechanisms, including, but not limited to: (1) simultaneously blocking two different targets or mediators that have a primary role in the disease pathogenesis; (2) retargeting to mediate effector functions, such as antibody-dependent cell-mediated cytotoxicity (ADCC); (3) avoiding or delaying the development of resistance; (4) inducing more potent anti-proliferative effects, and (5) activating cytotoxic T and NK cells to induce tumor lysis (e.g., bispecific T-cell engagers (BiTE) and bispecific killer cell engagers (BiKE)). There are now more than 100 different bispecific formats [18] enabling researchers to select the ideal parameters (e.g., size, half-life, stability, flexibility, orientation, and developability) to achieve the desired therapeutic outcome. Bispecific antibody formats can be classified into five distinct structural groups [18, 19]: (1) monovalent bispecific IgG (IgG-like architecture with a single binding moiety for each specificity); (2) appended IgG (IgG backbone with a second antigen targeting domain fused at specific locations); (3) BsAb fragments; (4) bispecific fusion proteins, and (5) BsAbs generated by chemical conjugations. In this chapter we will focus on recombinant approaches to generate bispecific antibodies and will highlight their potential in ADC applications.

While conventional IgG antibodies are bivalent and monospecific, bispecific IgG-like antibodies that are monovalent for each antigen are most often used (referred to as monovalent bispecific IgG herein). These monovalent bispecific IgG's typically contain an asymmetric Fc region for heterodimerization to avoid heavy chain (HC) mispairing [18–22]. Some approaches for IgG-based bispecifics use a wild-type homodimeric Fc regions. Examples of this approach include two-in-one antibody [23], κλ-body with a common heavy chain [24] and iMab with all four different chains tethered by flexible linkers [25]. However, two-in-one antibodies and κλ-body technologies require extensive antibody engineering and screening and cannot be generated with preexisting mAbs without reengineering the binding sites. To address the HC mispairing problem, heterodimeric Fc technologies have been developed to allow the correct assembly of two different HCs [26–38] into BsAbs (Fig. 1a). The most common Fc heterodimeric technologies are (1) knobs-into-holes (KIH) [36]; (2) electrostatic steering [33, 34]; (3) Fab-arm exchange (Duobody) [37]; and (4) SEED body [30]. Monovalent bispecific IgG's with heterodimeric Fc have been generated using a number of strategies to avoid light and heavy chain

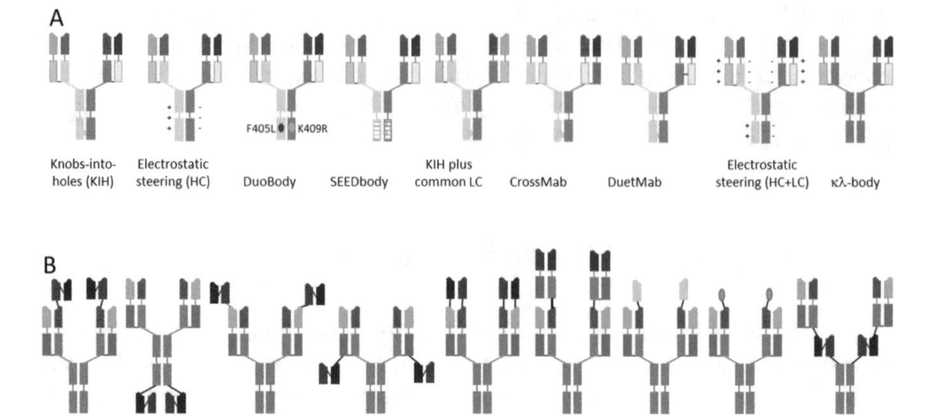

Fig. 1 Schematic bispecific antibody formats, which are grouped to (**a**) monovalent bispecific IgG's and (**b**) Appended IgG's

mispairing including combination with a common light chain (LC) approach [24] or with two distinct LCs, using the CrossMab [39], DuetMab [40] with a reengineered HC-LC disulfide bond, electrostatic steering [41], and κλ-body with a common heavy chain [24].

In contrast to the monovalent bispecific IgG format, bivalent bispecific antibodies can also be generated by engineering additional antigen binding units into different locations on IgG's [18, 19], including appended IgG fused to the heavy chain [42, 43]. Besides the N- and C-terminal fusion of scFvs to heavy chain, scFvs have been successfully inserted into the heavy chain hinge [43, 44] (Some examples are listed in Fig. 1b) and Fc regions (manuscript in preparation) to generate fully functional BsAbs.

Selection of Bispecific Formats and Binding Modalities for ADC's

Identification of bispecific antibody formats with the desired functionality is critical to develop bispecific antibody drug conjugates. Selection of the correct bispecific format for drug development is a challenge, with many different bispecific formats to choose from [18]. The choice of molecular format can impart key features, such as binding modality (ex. monovalent or bivalent binding to each target, biparatopic binding, etc.). Typically, the bispecific format is chosen to match the proposed mechanisms of action and the specific clinical application. Ideally, several alternative bispecific formats are constructed and the final lead candidate is chosen after in vitro and in vivo functional characterization. The conventional IgG-like monovalent bispecific format is usually selected for good developability properties, prolonged in vivo half-life, and desired antibody effector functions such as ADCC and CDC. Although the mechanisms of ADC toxicity are complex, target expression in normal tissue can lead to on-target toxicity [45, 46]. Thus, strategies for increasing tumor selectivity, and thus the therapeutic index, of ADC's are needed to limit toxicity resulting from target engagement in normal tissue. Monovalent bispecific IgG's are the preferred format for increasing target selectivity by altering antibody affinity to maximize killing of cancer cells while sparing normal cells [12, 47]. One potential major advantage of appended IgG's is that they preserve the natural antibody avidity to cell surface receptors and can enable the simultaneous binding of antigen to all variable domains and hence provide a higher specific binding capacity [48]. This may be useful in targeting cells with low abundance receptors for enhanced potency. Biparatopic antibodies (a subset of bispecific antibodies in which each antigen binding domain recognizes unique, non-overlapping epitopes on the same target antigen) have demonstrated the superior ability to promote receptor clustering for improved receptor internalization, lysosomal trafficking, and receptor down regulation, therefore increasing drug potency [11, 49]. Capitalizing on this ability of biparatopic antibodies to increase lysosomal trafficking is a promising strategy to enhance delivery of ADC's to target cells and is discussed in detail below. Ultimately, the selection of the appropriate bispecific antibody format will be dictated by the specific biology of the targets, the clinical need, and the features offered by a given format to address those requirements.

Bispecific ADC Strategies: Maximizing Internalization and Trafficking to Lysosomes

The first consideration in developing an ADC is identifying an appropriate target that will serve to deliver the cytotoxic drug into the tumor. Generally, ADC target selection has focused primarily on its expression pattern, with the ideal target showing high, uniform expression in the tumor and little to no expression in normal tissues. Such a clean expression profile affords the best opportunity to achieve a broad therapeutic index. Nevertheless, the expression profile is only one factor that contributes to the success of an ADC target. Virtually all of the ADC payloads to date require not only binding of the target at the tumor cell surface, but also uptake into the cell and subsequent delivery to the lysosome in order to effectively release the active cytotoxic warhead [50, 51]. Many potential ADC targets either internalize poorly or undergo a high rate of endocytic recycling, which causes the ADC to return to the cell surface intact without delivering the payload to the lysosome [50, 52]. Several bispecific ADC approaches have emerged recently that seek to enhance internalization and trafficking to the lysosome, thus maximizing the amount of drug that is effectively delivered to tumor cells at a given dose.

Early work suggested that targeting a single receptor with bispecific antibodies that recognize distinct epitopes could lead to increased avidity/overall affinity toward the target and greater potency [53]. Subsequent studies demonstrated that non-overlapping antibody pairs and biparatopic antibodies or non-antibody scaffolds could drive receptor clustering and cross-linking, which promotes enhanced internalization, trafficking to the lysosome and degradation of the target [54–56]. Importantly, not all non-overlapping antibody pairs are equally effective at promoting receptor down regulation, and there is evidence that the specific epitopes and spatial orientation induced by their combination has an impact on their ability to synergistically drive enhanced lysosomal trafficking [55]. Symphogen applied this principle to achieve targeted degradation of EGFR using a pair of monoclonal antibodies, termed Sym-004, which is currently in PhII clinical testing in multiple solid tumor indications [57, 58]. Similarly, Covagen developed a bispecific, biparatopic HER2 targeted Fynomab, COVA208, which recognizes two distinct epitopes and induces degradation of the receptor, as well as other HER family members, EGFR and HER3 [59]. These investigators noted that simply targeting two distinct epitopes does not ensure functional activity, and they proposed that the molecular architecture and spatial orientation of the different binding arms influences the ability to efficiently induce receptor clusters that are targeted for lysosomal degradation. While these examples demonstrated how biparatopic targeting can promote receptor trafficking to the lysosome and subsequent down modulation of signaling through receptor degradation, the MOA is also well suited to an ADC approach that seeks to maximize delivery of a cytotoxic drug to tumor cells.

As noted above, there are a number of targets that show promising tumor expression profiles, but poor lysosomal trafficking limits their full potential as effective ADC targets. HER2 is an example of a recycling receptor that exhibits a dynamic equilibrium between the cell surface and recycling endosomes [52]. As a result, when anti-HER2 antibodies, such as trastuzumab, bind to HER2 at the cell surface, the majority of the antibody-receptor complex is internalized and rapidly recycled back to the cell surface intact, with only a small fraction trafficking to lysosomes. Consequently, the Her2 targeted ADC, T-DM1 (Kadcyla®), which consists of trastuzumab conjugated to the microtubule toxin maytansinoid DM1, exhibits only limited delivery to lysosomes [52]. While it is currently the only ADC approved for solid tumors, and provides clinical benefit for a subset of HER2 positive breast cancer patients, its clinical utility is restricted to patients whose tumors express a high level of HER2. Disappointingly, T-DM1 failed to show a treatment benefit in gastric cancer (GATSBY trial, NCT01641939 [60]), an indication for which the unarmed trastuzumab is approved. Similarly, it has been slow to move up to earlier lines of therapy in breast cancer, as multiple Phase II and III clinical trials have been terminated or have failed to demonstrate superiority compared to other standard of care therapies, including trastuzumab plus taxane (e.g., MARIANNE trial, NCT01120184 [61]). Several investigators have suggested that the limited clinical benefit of T-DM1 can be attributed in part to its poor lysosomal trafficking and have developed bispecific ADC strategies to overcome this limitation ([11] Zymeworks ZW33). Li et al. recently demonstrated that a biparatopic antibody produced by combining two binding arms from each of two non-competing HER2 antibodies (for a total of four HER2 binding moieties per molecule) was capable of efficiently inducing large cross-linked antibody-receptor clusters, causing internalization

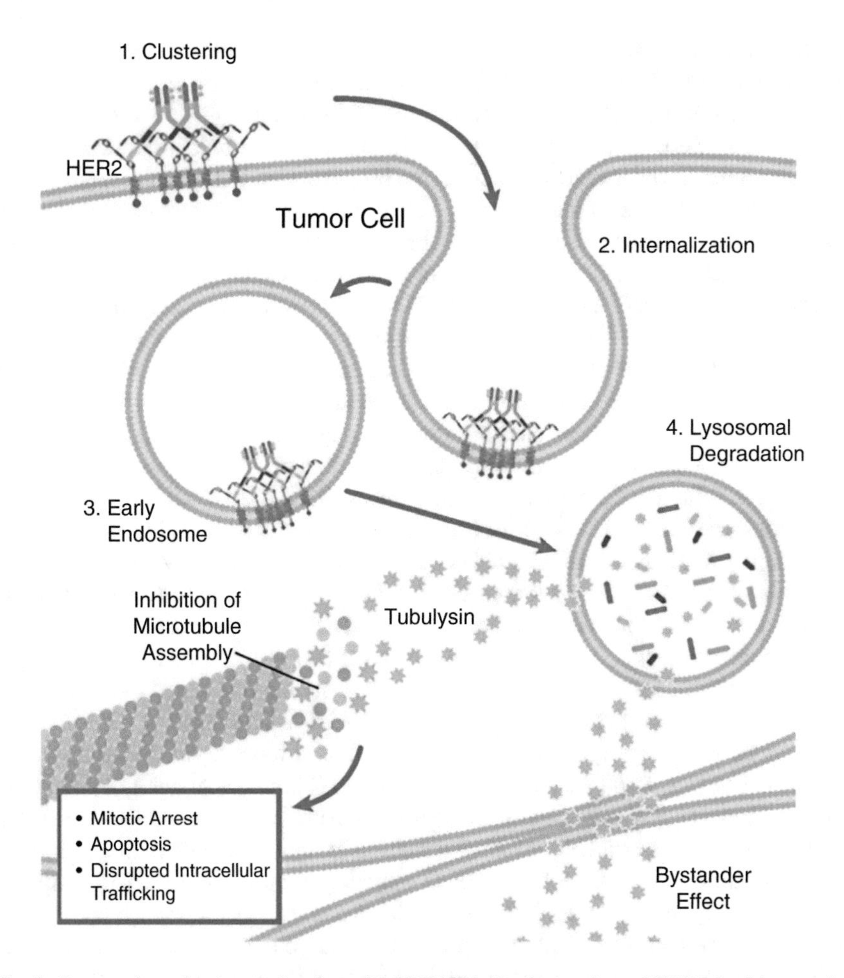

Fig. 2 Proposed mechanisms of action of MEDI4276. Dual targeting of HER2 by biparatopic ADC maximizes toxin delivery into tumor cells by inducing receptor clustering, enhanced internalization, and trafficking to lysosomes. The released cytotoxin acts directly on target cells by inhibition of microtubule assembly, leading to mitotic arrest and apoptosis. In addition, the cytotoxin is membrane permeable, allowing it to passively diffuse out of target cells into the tumor microenvironment, where it can kill neighboring tumor cells. This enhances the ability of the ADC to kill tumor cells that exhibit heterogeneous expression of the target (reviewed in [69]). (From Li et al. [11]. Used with permission from Cell Press)

and lysosomal degradation that resulted in greater than 90% depletion of HER2 from the cell surface within 1 h (Fig. 2). Over the same time period, trastuzumab induced a negligible degree of HER2 internalization and lysosomal degradation. The authors took advantage of this enhanced lysosomal trafficking to produce an ADC that could more effectively deliver a cytotoxic payload to tumor cells and direct it to lysosomes, where the toxin could be released. The resulting biparatopic ADC, conjugated to the microtubule toxin, tubulysin (AZD13599185) and designated MEDI4276, showed superior *in vitro* and *in vivo* activity compared to the trastuzumab based ADC, T-DM1. In patient derived tumor xenograft (PDX) models of human breast cancer representing both T-DM1 ineligible HER2 low tumors and T-DM1 relapsed/refractory HER2 positive tumors, the biparatopic HER2 ADC caused tumor stasis or regression in a large proportion of the models. While it may seem counterintuitive to invoke a mechanism that involves target downregulation, several considerations make this a tractable ADC strategy. First, the enhanced lysosomal trafficking results in more effective tumor cell killing in the first instance. Second, the authors demonstrate that the tubulysin warhead employed in the ADC possesses bystander killing activity, which means that, once liberated from target expressing tumor cells, the cytotoxic warhead can enter and kill nearby non-target expressing tumor cells [11]. Finally, downregulation of HER2 is in itself a potentially viable mechanism of shutting down oncogenic signaling in HER2 driven tumors [62]. MEDI4276 is currently under investigation in a Phase I clinical trial in patients with HER2 expressing solid tumors (NCT02576548). The enhanced lysosomal trafficking and superior preclinical activity of MEDI4276 represents an opportunity to fill an unmet medical need in patients that are T-DM1 resistant or are ineligible for T-DM1 due to low levels of HER2 tumor expression. More recently, Zymeworks has initiated development of ZW33, a biparatopic HER2 targeted ADC built on their IgG-like Azymetric™ platform [35]. The proposed MOA's of ZW33 include cross-linked *trans* HER2 binding and clustering, enhanced toxin-mediated cytotoxicity due to increased HER2-mediated ADC internalization, HER2 downregulation, as well as signaling blockade and effector function-mediated cytotoxicity [10]. The U.S. Food and Drug Administration (FDA) has granted Orphan Drug Designation for ZW33 for the treatment of ovarian cancer and an IND filing is anticipated in the second half of 2017 for multiple indications, including breast and gastric cancer. These examples of HER2 targeting biparatopic ADC's demonstrate that enhancing lysosomal trafficking is a viable strategy for improving the efficacy of ADC's, and could be similarly used for other targets. Enhanced lysosomal trafficking has also been shown with multiple biparatopic molecule formats, including mAb combinations, bispecific antibodies, non-antibody scaffolds, and Ig domain formats. Accordingly, Crescendo Biologics has applied their Humabody® human V_H domain platform to the biparatopic ADC approach [9]. They report that the small size of the molecular format combined with biparatopic targeting leads to an ADC with superior internalization, rapid tumor uptake and penetration, and potent *in vivo* tumor killing.

While induction of receptor clustering and cross linking has emerged as a general strategy for enhancing ADC internalization and trafficking to lysosomes, another strategy that several groups have begun to explore is a passive cargo, or "drag and degrade" mechanism. In this bispecific approach, a poorly internalizing target that provides tumor specificity is paired up with a target that efficiently internalizes and traffics to lysosomes. Lee, J.M., et al. demonstrated this concept in a non-ADC context by constructing bispecific antibodies consisting of a strongly internalizing anti-cMET antibody, SAIT301, paired with anti-HER2 or anti-EGFR antibodies [63]. The authors demonstrated that these bispecific antibodies induce efficient EGFR or HER2 internalization and degradation when cMet was present, a process that they termed “drag and degrade”. They further show that the bispecific antibodies cause HSP90, a chaperone that is known to protect proteins from lysosomal degradation, to dissociate from the target receptors. Although these authors did not use the approach to deliver a cytotoxic drug, their work demonstrates that it is possible to use bispecific antibodies to induce increased lysosomal trafficking of poorly internalizing or highly recycling targets by pairing them with a strongly internalizing target. More recently, de Goeij, et al. demonstrated that one could use a similar approach to deliver an ADC to target tumors [13]. They created a bispecific ADC in which one binding arm specifically targets CD63 (also known as LAMP-3), a protein that shuttles between the plasma membrane and endosomal compartments, including lysosomes, and combined it with a HER2 binding arm, which was selected to provide tumor specific binding. CD63 is a ubiquitously expressed protein in the tetraspanin superfamily. Although the bulk of the cellular pool exists intracellularly in late endosomes and lysosomes, a small fraction is present on the cell surface. While the functions of CD63 are not completely understood, it appears to regulate intracellular transport of interacting proteins via endocytosis, with lysosomal targeting as a major fate of the internalized cargo [64]. The authors selected a low affinity anti-CD63 arm so that efficient binding and internalization preferentially occurred only when the tumor associated HER2 target was present along with the CD63. They demonstrated that bispecific targeting of CD63 and HER2 resulted in enhanced internalization and co-localization with lysosomes on target expressing tumor cells, whereas the monospecific parental antibodies did not internalize appreciably. In contrast, the bispecific antibody showed minimal binding and intracellular accumulation in peripheral blood thrombocytes and granulocytes, which express CD63 but not HER2. Such a strategy has the potential to provide both enhanced lysosomal delivery, thereby improving efficacy, as well as enhanced tumor selectivity, thereby improving safety. In a similar fashion, investigators at Regeneron have recently generated a bispecific ADC targeting HER2 and prolactin receptor (PRLR) and tested its activity *in vitro* [14]. PRLR is a tumor associated target, but in contrast to HER2, it is constitutively internalized, trafficked to lysosomes, and degraded. The HER2xPRLR bispecific antibody dramatically enhanced the degradation of HER2 *in vitro*, and, when conjugated to the toxin, DM1, the resulting ADC kills double positive breast cancer cells more effectively than the corresponding monospecific HER2 ADC. Although these molecules have yet to be proven in the clinic, they show that it is possible to redirect a poorly internalizing target for lysosomal degradation by employing a bispecific antibody that targets a second antigen with enhanced lysosomal trafficking. This strategy has the potential to significantly expand the number of viable ADC targets to include those that do not readily traffic to lysosomes.

A key question going forward is whether these enhanced lysosomal targeting strategies will improve the therapeutic index. While these strategies could, in principle, introduce an increased risk for on-target toxicity, the majority of ADC toxicities observed in the clinic are target independent [45, 46]. Considerations such as proliferative index and regenerative potential of the target organ will also play a role in the toxicity profile of an ADC. For example, the mechanism of many ADC warheads are designed to differentially affect rapidly dividing cells (ex. disruption of the microtubule network required for cell division). Thus, if a normal tissue expresses the target antigen but proliferates slowly, it likely to be less sensitive to the ADC compared to a rapidly dividing tumor that expresses the target [45, 46]. Ongoing and pending clinical trials will provide the key proof of concept for biparatopic ADC's, but preclinical evidence suggests that they represent a promising strategy to enhance lysosomal trafficking and delivery, thus turning poorly internalizing tumor associated antigens into tractable ADC targets.

Bispecific ADC Strategies: Enhancing Selectivity

The examples above demonstrate that bispecific antibodies can improve the efficacy of ADC's by enhancing targeting to lysosomes. Recent work has sought to further capitalize on bispecific technology to improve ADC targeting and selectivity. In its simplest form, bispecific antibodies can employ dual targeting to extend the reach of an ADC, namely to create a two in one ADC. In this scenario, either target is sufficient to deliver the ADC into the tumor cell, which can be useful to broaden the therapeutic benefit when the targets are heterogeneously expressed within the tumor. Waldron, et al. demonstrated the feasibility of such an approach with a bispecific EpCAM-CD133 toxin conjugate [65]. Other more recent efforts are aimed at fine tuning the properties of each binding arm to suit the particular targets and to improve tumor selectivity. As noted above, the HER2-CD63 used a reduced affinity anti-CD63 arm to favor selective binding and ADC delivery to tumor cells expressing both the tumor associated target, HER2, and the lysosomal associated protein, CD63 [13]. This same principle could be applied to two tumor associated targets in order to achieve improved tumor selectivity. That said, an important lesson can be taken from the experience with some immunocytokines, as Tzeng, et al. exemplified with IL2-IgG bispecific fusions [66]. These investigators found that fusion of IL-2 to an antibody against a tumor associated antigen (TAA) caused a dramatic redistribution away from the tumor and toward IL-2 receptor expressing immune cells. These results show that simply creating a bispecific molecule does not ensure that both targets will contribute equally to the behavior of the final molecule. One arm can dominate, and care must be taken to select complementary targets. Likewise, Mazor, et al. have demonstrated that dual targeting alone is not sufficient to achieve tumor selectivity, and that the affinity of the individual arms, the density of the target, the overall avidity and the valency of the bispecific format all play significant roles in producing a bispecific mAb that can discriminate between tumors that express both targets from normal tissue/non-transformed cells that express only one of the targets [12, 47]. The authors systematically evaluated a series of bispecific HER2/EGFR variants with different EGFR affinities and showed that a reduced affinity monovalent bispecific could discriminate dual target expressing tumors, *in vivo*, from those expressing a single target, while the higher affinity variants lacked this selectivity. They further show that incorporating the same antibody arms into a bivalent bispecific format abolished the gains in selectivity, suggesting that achieving optimal tumor selectivity requires a delicate balance of multiple factors, including both affinity and valency. Similarly, Sellmann, et al. generated EGFRxcMET bispecific ADC's with different EGFR affinities and showed that an affinity attenuated variant had greater selectivity *in vitro* for tumor cells overexpressing both antigens [67]. The authors showed that reducing the EGFR affinity led to decreased cytotoxicity toward human keratinocytes, which express moderate levels of EGFR and low cMET. They propose that selecting the appropriate combination of affinity optimized bispecific ADC variants could lead to higher selectivity for tumor versus normal tissue, which could broaden the therapeutic index.

The strategies presented here represent sophisticated applications of bispecific technology that are designed to derive the maximal potential of dual targeting with a single molecular entity, which goes well beyond simply binding and neutralizing two targets. The principle of avidity, defined as the accumulated strength of multiple individual interactions, is likely key to the success of these strategies [68]. Bispecific antibodies may tolerate low affinity interactions toward each individual target because dual targeting drives the overall strength of binding through avidity effects. This property can be advantageous when one or both of the targets has some expression in normal tissues, but are only substantially co-expressed in tumors. The ability to independently fine tune each arm of a bispecific ADC to suit the expression and safety profiles of each target may enable mitigation of potential toxicities in normal tissue while maintaining potency against tumors.

As we move forward, the types of bispecific and biparatopic technologies described in this chapter will likely start to be used more frequently for poorly internalizing tumor antigens where optimization of cytotoxic warhead delivery requires greater tumor selectivity, increased ADC uptake and enhanced lysosomal trafficking. The strides made in antibody engineering technologies coupled with advances made in the development of ADC's make this an ideal time to develop bispecific and biparatopic ADC's with improved activity and a better therapeutic index.

References

1. Beck A et al (2017) Strategies and challenges for the next generation of antibody-drug conjugates. Nat Rev Drug Discov 16:315
2. Thomas A, Teicher BA, Hassan R (2016) Antibody–drug conjugates for cancer therapy. Lancet Oncol 17(6):e254-e262
3. Lambert JM, Morris CQ (2017) Antibody-drug conjugates (ADCs) for personalized treatment of solid tumors: a review. Adv Ther 34:1015
4. Tolcher AW (2016) Antibody drug conjugates: lessons from 20 years of clinical experience. Ann Oncol 27(12):2168–2172
5. Kontermann RE (2012) Dual targeting strategies with bispecific antibodies. MAbs 4(2):182–197
6. May C, Sapra P, Gerber H-P (2012) Advances in bispecific biotherapeutics for the treatment of cancer. Biochem Pharmacol 84(9):1105–1112

7. Yang F, Wen W, Qin W (2016) Bispecific antibodies as a development platform for new concepts and treatment strategies. Int J Mol Sci 18(1)
8. Fan GW et al (2015) Bispecific antibodies and their applications. J Hematol Oncol:8
9. Boku N (2014) HER2-positive gastric cancer. Gastric Cancer 17(1):1–12
10. ZW33, Anti-HER2 x HER2 ADC Overview, Zymeworks Company Website. July 2017.; Available from: https://www.zymeworks.com/our-pipeline/zw33
11. Li JY et al (2016) A Biparatopic HER2-targeting antibody-drug conjugate induces tumor regression in primary models refractory to or ineligible for HER2-targeted therapy. Cancer Cell 29(1):117–129
12. Mazor Y et al (2017) Enhanced tumor-targeting selectivity by modulating bispecific antibody binding affinity and format valence. Sci Rep 7:40098
13. de Goeij BE et al (2016) Efficient payload delivery by a bispecific antibody-drug conjugate targeting HER2 and CD63. Mol Cancer Ther 15(11):2688–2697
14. Andreev J et al (2017) Bispecific antibodies and antibody-drug conjugates (ADCs) bridging HER2 and prolactin receptor improve efficacy of HER2 ADCs. Mol Cancer Ther 16:681
15. Nisonoff A, Rivers MM (1961) Recombination of a mixture of univalent antibody fragments of different specificity. Arch Biochem Biophys 93(2):460
16. Brennan M, Davison PF, Paulus H (1985) Preparation of bispecific antibodies by chemical recombination of monoclonal immunoglobulin G1 fragments. Science 229(4708):81–83
17. Kohler G, Milstein C (1975) Continuous cultures of fused cells secreting antibody of predefined specificity. Nature 256(5517):495–497
18. Brinkmann U, Kontermann RE (2017) The making of bispecific antibodies. MAbs 9(2):182–212
19. Spiess C, Zhai Q, Carter PJ (2015) Alternative molecular formats and therapeutic applications for bispecific antibodies. Therapeutic antibodies: discovery, design and deployment. Mol Immunol 67(2, Part A):95–106
20. Ha JH, Kim JE, Kim YS (2016) Immunoglobulin Fc heterodimer platform technology: from design to applications in therapeutic antibodies and proteins. Front Immunol 7:394
21. Liu H et al (2017) Fc engineering for developing therapeutic bispecific antibodies and novel scaffolds. Front Immunol 8:38
22. Krah S et al (2017) Engineering bispecific antibodies with defined chain pairing. New Biotechnol 39:167
23. Bostrom J et al (2009) Variants of the antibody herceptin that interact with HER2 and VEGF at the antigen binding site. Science 323(5921):1610–1614
24. Fischer N et al (2015) Exploiting light chains for the scalable generation and platform purification of native human bispecific IgG. Nat Commun 6:6113
25. Dimasi N et al (2017) Guiding bispecific monovalent antibody formation through proteolysis of IgG1 single-chain. MAbs 9(3):438–454
26. Choi HJ et al (2015) Engineering of immunoglobulin fc heterodimers using yeast surface-displayed combinatorial fc library screening. PLoS One 10(12):e0145349
27. Wranik BJ et al (2012) LUZ-Y, a novel platform for the mammalian cell production of full-length IgG-bispecific antibodies. J Biol Chem 287(52):43331–43339
28. Leaver-Fay A et al (2016) Computationally designed bispecific antibodies using negative state repertoires. Structure 24(4):641–651
29. Moretti P et al (2013) BEAT® the bispecific challenge: a novel and efficient platform for the expression of bispecific IgGs. BMC Proc 7(6):O9
30. Davis JH et al (2010) SEEDbodies: fusion proteins based on strand-exchange engineered domain (SEED) CH3 heterodimers in an Fc analogue platform for asymmetric binders or immunofusions and bispecific antibodies. Protein Eng Des Sel 23(4):195–202
31. de Kruif C.A., Hendriks L.J.A., Logtenberg T. (2016) Methods and means for the production of Ig-like molecules. Google Patents
32. Choi HJ et al (2013) A heterodimeric Fc-based bispecific antibody simultaneously targeting VEGFR-2 and met exhibits potent antitumor activity. Mol Cancer Ther 12(12):2748–2759

33. Strop P et al (2012) Generating bispecific human IgG1 and IgG2 antibodies from any antibody pair. J Mol Biol 420(3):204–219
34. Gunasekaran K et al (2010) Enhancing antibody fc heterodimer formation through electrostatic steering effects applications to bispecific molecules and monovalent IgG. J Biol Chem 285(25):19637–19646
35. Von Kreudenstein TS et al (2013) Improving biophysical properties of a bispecific antibody scaffold to aid developability: quality by molecular design. MAbs 5(5):646–654
36. Merchant AM et al (1998) An efficient route to human bispecific IgG. Nat Biotechnol 16(7):677–681
37. Labrijn AF et al (2013) Efficient generation of stable bispecific IgG1 by controlled Fab-arm exchange. Proc Natl Acad Sci 110(13):5145–5150
38. Moore GL et al (2011) A novel bispecific antibody format enables simultaneous bivalent and monovalent co-engagement of distinct target antigens. MAbs 3(6):546–557
39. Schaefer W et al (2011) Immunoglobulin domain crossover as a generic approach for the production of bispecific IgG antibodies. Proc Natl Acad Sci U S A 108(27):11187–11192
40. Mazor Y et al (2015) Improving target cell specificity using a novel monovalent bispecific IgG design. MAbs 7(2):377–389
41. Liu Z et al (2015) A novel antibody engineering strategy for making monovalent bispecific heterodimeric IgG antibodies by electrostatic steering mechanism. J Biol Chem 290(12):7535–7562
42. Coloma MJ, Morrison SL (1997) Design and production of novel tetravalent bispecific antibodies. Nat Biotechnol 15(2):159–163
43. DiGiandomenico A et al (2014) A multifunctional bispecific antibody protects against Pseudomonas aeruginosa. Sci Transl Med 6(262):262ra155
44. Bezabeh B et al (2017) Insertion of scFv into the hinge domain of full-length IgG1 monoclonal antibody results in tetravalent bispecific molecule with robust properties. MAbs 9(2):240–256
45. Hinrichs MJ, Dixit R (2015) Antibody drug conjugates: nonclinical safety considerations. AAPS J 17(5):1055–1064
46. Donaghy H (2016) Effects of antibody, drug and linker on the preclinical and clinical toxicities of antibody-drug conjugates. MAbs 8(4):659–671
47. Mazor Y et al (2015) Insights into the molecular basis of a bispecific antibody's target selectivity. MAbs 7(3):461–469
48. Jakob CG et al (2013) Structure reveals function of the dual variable domain immunoglobulin (DVD-Ig (TM)) molecule. MAbs 5(3):358–363
49. Godar M et al (2016) Dual anti-idiotypic purification of a novel, native-format biparatopic anti-MET antibody with improved in vitro and in vivo efficacy. Sci Rep 6
50. Ritchie M, Tchistiakova L, Scott N (2013) Implications of receptor-mediated endocytosis and intracellular trafficking dynamics in the development of antibody drug conjugates. MAbs 5(1):13–21
51. Xu S (2015) Internalization, trafficking, intracellular processing and actions of antibody-drug conjugates. Pharm Res 32(11):3577–3583
52. Austin CD et al (2004) Endocytosis and sorting of ErbB2 and the site of action of cancer therapeutics trastuzumab and geldanamycin. Mol Biol Cell 15(12):5268–5282
53. Robert B et al (1999) Tumor targeting with newly designed biparatopic antibodies directed against two different epitopes of the carcinoembryonic antigen (CEA). Int J Cancer 81(2):285–291
54. Friedman LM et al (2005) Synergistic down-regulation of receptor tyrosine kinases by combinations of mAbs: implications for cancer immunotherapy. Proc Natl Acad Sci U S A 102(6):1915–1920
55. Spangler JB et al (2010) Combination antibody treatment down-regulates epidermal growth factor receptor by inhibiting endosomal recycling. Proc Natl Acad Sci U S A 107(30):13252–13257
56. Hackel BJ et al (2012) Epidermal growth factor receptor downregulation by small heterodimeric binding proteins. Protein Eng Des Sel 25(2):47–57

57. Dienstmann R et al (2015) Safety and activity of the first-in-class Sym004 anti-EGFR antibody mixture in patients with refractory colorectal cancer. Cancer Discov 5(6):598–609
58. Pedersen MW et al (2010) Sym004: a novel synergistic anti-epidermal growth factor receptor antibody mixture with superior anticancer efficacy. Cancer Res 70(2):588–597
59. Brack S et al (2014) A bispecific HER2-targeting FynomAb with superior antitumor activity and novel mode of action. Mol Cancer Ther 13(8):2030–2039
60. Thuss-Patience PC et al (2017) Trastuzumab emtansine versus taxane use for previously treated HER2-positive locally advanced or metastatic gastric or gastro-oesophageal junction adenocarcinoma (GATSBY): an international randomised, open-label, adaptive, phase 2/3 study. Lancet Oncol 18:640
61. Perez EA et al (2017) Trastuzumab emtansine with or without pertuzumab versus trastuzumab plus taxane for human epidermal growth factor receptor 2-positive, advanced breast cancer: primary results from the phase III MARIANNE study. J Clin Oncol 35(2):141–148
62. Burstein HJ (2005) The distinctive nature of HER2-positive breast cancers. N Engl J Med 353(16):1652–1654
63. Lee JM et al (2016) Novel strategy for a bispecific antibody: induction of dual target internalization and degradation. Oncogene 35:4437
64. Pols MS, Klumperman J (2009) Trafficking and function of the tetraspanin CD63. Exp Cell Res 315(9):1584–1592
65. Waldron NN et al (2014) A bispecific EpCAM/CD133-targeted toxin is effective against carcinoma. Target Oncol 9(3):239–249
66. Tzeng A et al (2015) Antigen specificity can be irrelevant to immunocytokine efficacy and biodistribution. Proc Natl Acad Sci 112(11):3320–3325
67. Sellmann C et al (2016) Balancing selectivity and efficacy of bispecific EGFR x c-MET antibodies and antibody-drug conjugates. J Biol Chem 291:25106
68. Rudnick SI, Adams GP (2009) Affinity and avidity in antibody-based tumor targeting. Cancer Biother Radiopharm 24(2):155–161
69. Kovtun YV, Goldmacher VS (2007) Cell killing by antibody-drug conjugates. Cancer Lett 255(2):232–240

Targeting Drug Conjugates to the Tumor Microenvironment: Probody Drug Conjugates

Jack Lin and Jason Sagert

Abstract The tolerability and ultimately efficacy of ADCs are limited by 2 major issues: (1) antigen expression that is too low on tumors, resulting in insufficient toxin delivery to the tumor, especially within the confines of the clinical MTD established by linker/payload-driven off-target toxicity and (2) too much antigen expression on normal healthy tissues, resulting in on-target but off-tumor toxicity. In this chapter, we will review strategies for making antibody prodrugs that have been or could be used to selectively deliver drug to a tumor compared to normal tissues. These technologies have the potential to lower on-target, off-tumor toxicities and enable better efficacy of ADCs due to better target selection and the delivery of higher concentrations of drug to tumors.

Keywords Ab drug conjugate (ADC) · Linker/payload · Linker/toxin · Toxicity · Mask · MMP9 · pH · Probody · Protease · Tumor microenvironment

Introduction

Antibody drug conjugates (ADCs) harness the specificity of antibodies to deliver potent cytotoxic drugs to malignant cells. Conceptually, ADCs widen the therapeutic window of potent cytotoxic drugs that would have been too toxic to deliver on their own without the targeting provided by the antibody. The promise of ADCs has been validated by the FDA approvals of gemtuzumab ozogamicin (Mylotarg) for acute myelogenous leukemia in 2000 [1], brentuximab vedotin (Adcetris) for Hodgkin lymphoma in 2011 [2], ado-trastuzumab emtansine (T-DM1, Kadcyla) for Her2+ metastatic breast cancer in 2013 [3], and more recently, inotuzumab

PROBODY is a trademark of CytomX Therapeutics, Inc. All other brands and trademarks referenced herein are the property of their respective owners.

J. Lin (✉) · J. Sagert
CytomX Therapeutics, Inc., South San Francisco, CA, USA
e-mail: mkavanaugh@cytomx.com

M. Damelin (ed.), *Innovations for Next-Generation Antibody-Drug Conjugates*, Cancer Drug Discovery and Development,
https://doi.org/10.1007/978-3-319-78154-9_12

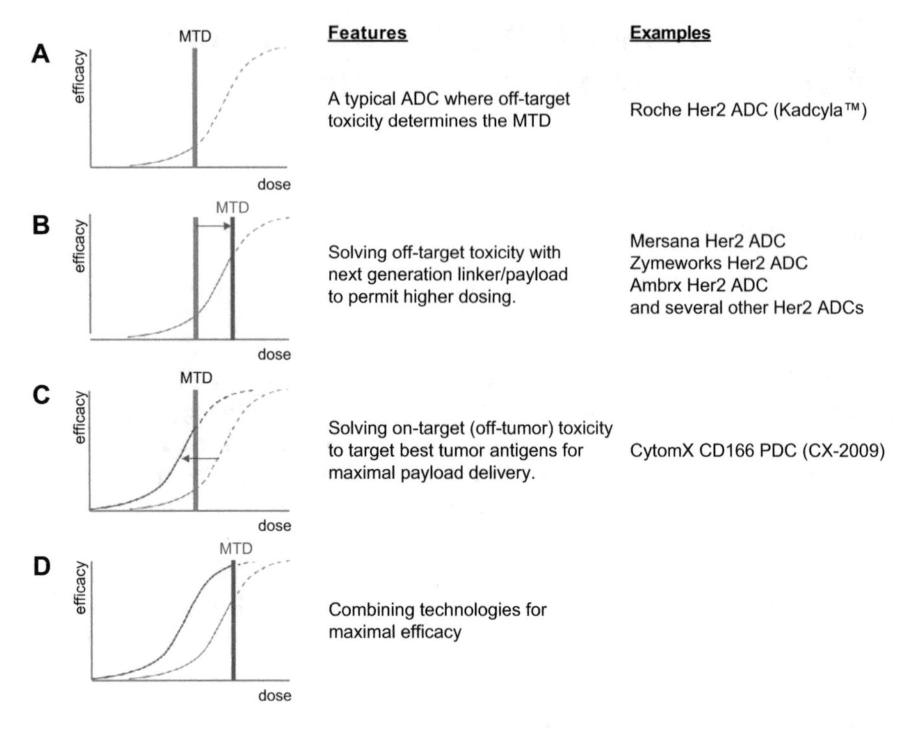

Fig. 1 Conceptual framework for the state of current and future ADCs. The horizontal axis denotes ADC dose and the vertical axis denotes the corresponding antitumor response. MTD, or the maximum tolerated dose, is the highest dose where the probability of encountering a dose-limiting toxicity equals the pre-specified target level (usually less than 30%). Solid lines depict dose-efficacy curves below the MTD and dashed lines depict dose-efficacy curves above the MTD. The intersect of the MTD line and the dose-efficacy curve represents the magnitude of the theoretical antitumor efficacy, which could be improved by increasing the MTD (panel **b**), shifting the dose-efficacy curve to the left (panel **c**), or a combination of both (panel **d**). See text for details

ozogamicin for B-cell precursor ALL in 2017. However, the enthusiasm and optimism for ADCs has been tamed by a string of setbacks in the clinic. Gemtuzumab ozogamicin was withdrawn from the market voluntarily in 2010 [4], only to be re-introduced in 2017. A number of ADCs in clinical development were halted due to excessive toxicity or the inability to dose to sufficient levels to impart strong efficacy signals ([5, 6]). There are now abundant data that identify two main causes of ADC failures in the clinic: (1) antigen expression that is too low on tumors, resulting in insufficient toxin delivery to the tumor, especially within the confines of the clinical MTD established by linker/payload-driven off-target toxicity and (2) too much antigen expression on normal healthy tissues, resulting in on-target but off-tumor toxicity.

Solving the issue of off-target toxicity, which are toxicities resulting from the linker/payload irrespective of the antibody target, has been one of the most active areas of ADC research (Fig. 1a, b). The strongest data that suggest off-target toxicities are a major obstacle in ADC development comes from surveys of auristatin-based and maytansine-based ADCs in clinical development [5–7]. Despite the diversity of targets investigated in the clinic, the maximum tolerated dose (MTD) of ADCs with the two commonly used payloads, the auristatin MMAE and the maytansinoid DM4, are mostly in the 3 mg/kg and 5 mg/kg range, respectively [7]. Further evidence that linker/payload-driven off-target toxicities dictate the clinical MTD is that the dose-limiting toxicities (DLT) of most ADCs are more consistent with those of the free toxin, such as myelosuppression and peripheral neuropathy, than with those expected from the antibody alone [5]. For example, a DLT for the anti-Her2 antibody trastuzumab is cardiotoxicity that is thought to be an on-target toxicity derived from Her2 expression in the heart. In contrast, the DLT for T-DM1, the mcc-DM1-conjugated version of trastuzumab, is reversible thrombocytopenia that is thought to be an off-target toxicity from the linker/payload [8]. These data point to reducing linker/payload-driven off-target toxicity as a way to improve the clinical MTD and boost ADC efficacy. A surrogate marker that has been used for predicting off-target toxicity, albeit still unproven given the limited data, is the use pharmacokinetic (PK) properties of ADCs. Greater circulating half-life and exposure correlate with less off-target toxicity and better tolerability. Since ADC linker/payloads are largely hydrophobic, numerous strategies have been proposed to increase the solubility of ADCs and thereby improve their PK properties. These approaches include limiting the number of linker/payloads per antibody molecule with site-specific conjugation (e.g. conjugation to engineered cysteines, non-natural amino acids, or specific sequence motifs) and improving the solubility of the linker-payloads (e.g. PEGylated, quaternary ammonium, or beta-glucuronic acid linkers). These efforts are described in more detail in a recent review [9] and in other chapters of this book.

In contrast to addressing the linker/payload-driven off-target toxicities of ADCs, a complementary approach is to increase the potency of the ADC within the existing confines of the linker/payload-driven MTD (Fig. 1c). One approach is to use more potent linker/payloads (e.g. DNA-alkylating toxins and ADCs with high drug-antibody ratios, or DAR) that could conceivably target lower-expressing tumor antigens; however, given that many of these potent next-generation linker/toxins are also accompanied by a reduction in MTD, it remains to be seen whether there will be an increased therapeutic window. Another approach is to redefine the ADC target space and target tumor antigens that would yield a more potent effect. Current ADCs are severely hampered by the availability of suitable tumor antigens that have all of the desired features: high expression in tumors to drive high uptake of the drug, high differential expression between tumor and normal tissues to avoid on-target toxicity, efficient internalization to deliver maximal toxin to the tumor cells, homogeneously expression on all tumor cells to reduce the likelihood of drug resistance, and sufficient prevalence in different tumors to warrant its development. The dearth of suitable ADC targets, especially for solid tumors, is exemplified by the large number of ADCs targeting the Her2 antigen and competing to be the best T-DM1 "biobetter" drug. In contrast, a few attempts to target high prevalence and high expression tumor antigens have resulted in on-target off-tumor toxicities, including ADCs targeting the Lewis-Y

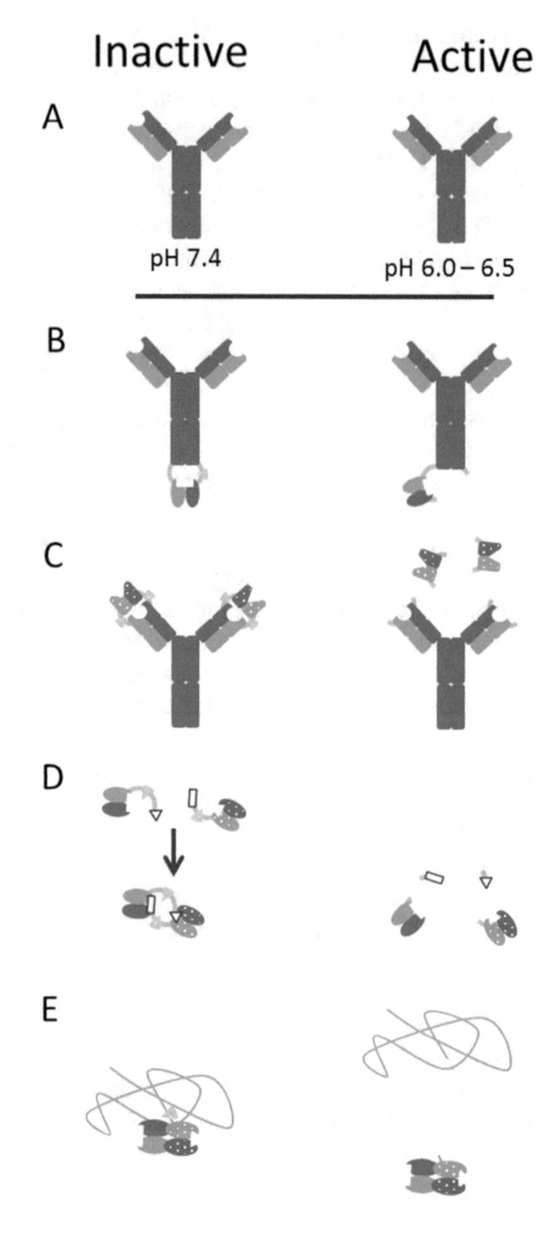

Fig. 2 Diagram of various antibody and antibody fragment formats that may localize to tumors. The left column shows the less active format and the right column shows the more active format of (**a**) pH dependent binding, (**b**) trivalent antibodies, (**c**) dual variable domain antibodies, (**d**) cross-masking antibodies, and (**e**) ProTIA formats

antigen [10], CD44v6 [11], and EphA2 [12]. One proposed solution to safely expand the addressable target space for ADCs to more desirable antigens is the use of antibody drug conjugates that are designed to be preferentially active in the tumor microenvironment, and thus spare normal tissues.

In this chapter, we will review two general strategies for making antibody prodrugs that have been or could be used to selectively deliver drug to a tumor: differential pH-sensitivity and protease activatability (Fig. 2). As discussed below, these strategies exploit two common attributes of the tumor microenvironment that differ from normal tissues: the slightly acidic pH in the tumor (Fig. 2a) and the dysregulated proteolytic tumor milieu (Fig. 2b–e).

Acidic Tumor Microenvironment

Various imaging modalities have confirmed that tumor microenvironments are slightly more acidic than normal tissues [13, 14]. Two interrelated mechanisms contribute to the acidic tumor microenvironment: hypoxia and tumor metabolism [15]. Hypoxia, from inadequate vascularization in tumors, leads to the induction of hypoxia inducible factor 1 (HIF1α) that in turn upregulates the expression of carbonic anhydrase IX, glucose transporters, and glycolytic enzymes. This permits tumor cells to adopt different metabolic processes than normal cells. Normal cells utilize glycolysis under anaerobic conditions and mitochondrial oxidative phosphorylation under aerobic conditions to maximize the generation of ATP per glucose molecule. In contrast, tumor cells preferentially depend on glycolysis even under aerobic conditions, a phenomenon known as aerobic glycolysis or the “Warburg effect” (reviewed in [16, 17], and [18]). The reliance on aerobic glycolysis ultimately results in the accumulation of lactic acid as a byproduct which contributes to the tumor environment being more acidic than that of normal tissues.

Not surprisingly, the pH differential of the tumor microenvironment has been exploited as a way to engineer antibody drug conjugates that bind preferentially under these conditions. The concept of engineering pH-dependent conditional binding proteins by the incorporation of “histidine switches” was first demonstrated for cytokines [19] and subsequently in antibodies [20, 21]. Of the 20 naturally occurring amino acids, histidine is the preferred choice for this approach because its pKa confers the ability to ionize and de-ionize its side chains around physiological pH. With an antibody library enriched with histidine residues within the complementarity determining regions and with an appropriate screening strategy, one could identify antibodies that preferentially engage target either under acidic pH or at neutral pH conditions. The first pH-dependent antibodies were engineered for lower affinity at the pH of the endosome (5.5–6.0) compared to the pH of plasma (7.4) in order to decrease target-mediated degradation and promote antibody recycling from the endosomal compartment, thereby increasing circulating antibody half-life [20, 21].

To take advantage of the acidic tumor microenvironment, the opposite pH-switch is required: antibodies that bind with higher affinity at the acidic pH 6.0 compared to neutral pH 7.4. This arrangement would have an antibody that preferentially engages its targets in the acidic tumor microenvironment, while sparing normal tissues under neutral pH conditions. For an ADC, the tighter binding at the lower pH may facilitate binding in the endosomal/lysosomal compartment and target-mediated degradation of the ADC, enhancing the release of toxin payload. Halozyme and BioAtla have exploited the pH differential between normal tissue vs. tumor microenvironment to engineer an auristatin-based ADC that binds to EGFR with an approximately tenfold stronger affinity under acidic pH 6.0–6.5 than under neutral pH 7.4 [22]. The goal is to preferentially target EGFR-expressing tumor cells in the acidic tumor environment while sparing other EGFR-expressing healthy tissues such as skin under neutral pH conditions. This ADC induced tumor regressions in cetuximab-resistant mouse xenograft models at 15 mg/kg and was well tolerated at 8 mg/kg in cynomolgus monkeys.

Potential challenges with designing pH-sensitive antibody drug conjugates are (1) the biophysical limitations on designing a highly tumor-selective targeting antibody given the relatively small pH difference (pH 6–6.5 in tumors vs. pH 7.4 in normal tissues), with possibly an even smaller pH differential in micro-metastatic tumor lesions that may be well vascularized; (2) balancing the trade-off between the need for optimal antibody sequence with the need for incorporation of histidines; and (3) the need for having the flexibility to fine-tune the desired affinity-differential between tumor vs. normal tissue.

Proteolytic Tumor Microenvironment

Proteolysis is a highly regulated process under normal physiological conditions. Many proteases work in series as part of proteolytic cascades with large amplification effects (e.g. coagulation and complement pathways); therefore, an aberrant proteolytic event could trigger devastating consequences if not for the intricate network of protease activators and inhibitors required to maintain proteolytic homeostasis. Consequently, dysregulated proteolytic activity is often the hallmark of many pathophysiological conditions, and protease inhibitors have been successfully approved to treat a number of indications including hypertension, thrombosis, viral infection, and inflammation [23].

Dysregulated extracellular proteolytic activity is also an important hallmark of most human cancers because it is required to maintain key elements of the transformed phenotype, including growth, invasion, and metastasis [24, 25]. Of the more than 500 human proteases, examples identified to be involved in cancer include serine proteases such as the type II transmembrane serine proteases [26] and urokinase plasminogen activator (uPA) systems [27]; metalloproteases such as MMPs [24] and ADAMs [28]; and cysteine proteases such as cysteine cathepsins [29]. While the importance of proteases in maintaining a proteolytic pro-tumorigenic environment is widely established, no inhibitors to extracellular proteases have been successful in treating solid tumors to date. Especially notable have been the multiple unsuccessful attempts to target extracellular MMPs with broad spectrum small molecule inhibitors (reviewed in [30]), and highly specific allosteric antibodies [31, 32]. This likely reflects the difficulty of effectively inhibiting a wide spectrum of different proteases necessary to deliver a therapeutic effect while avoiding toxicity.

Instead of neutralizing these tumor-associated proteases for direct therapeutic effect, an alternate approach is to exploit this unique proteolytic milieu in the tumor microenvironment to better target therapy to tumors. This rich proteolytic environment could be used to preferentially activate antibodies and other protein-based therapeutic agents in the tumor while sparing normal healthy tissues. Like the pH-sensitive antibodies described above, there are also general protein engineering trade-offs associated with the entire class of protease-activatable antibodies. Some common concerns include (1) the risk of immunogenicity from additional sequence extensions from the antibody scaffold, (2) the possibility that the proteolytic milieu in mouse xenograft tumors might not adequately model those in human tumors, and (3) the identification of suitable protease substrates that are efficiently cleaved in the tumor microenvironment but not within normal tissues. These issues will be monitored as this class of protease-activatable therapeutics advance into the clinical setting. We outline below some of the different protease-activatable antibody formats that have been described.

Protease Activatable Antibody Formats

Several protease-activatable antibody- or antibody fragment-based platforms have been described in the literature or are in preclinical development. The Probody platform has been extensively used to selectively target the activity of antibody drug conjugates to tumors and will therefore be described in detail. It is not the goal of this chapter to provide a comprehensive review of protease activatable antibody formats. However, several examples of formats that could potentially be applied to ADCs will be highlighted.

Activatable Trivalent Antibodies

Metz et al. [33] describe an engineered antibody in which a disulfide-stabilized Fv (dsFv) is expressed on the C-terminus of the heavy chain. In this design, the dsFv is sterically inhibited from binding its target antigen by the Fc portion of the antibody. If a protease site is introduced between one of the Fc and dsFv portions of the protein, cleavage would result in the ability of the dsFv to swivel open and become competent to bind to its target (Fig. 2b). To demonstrate the potential of this approach, a cMET dsFv was engineered onto an anti-Her3 IgG. If substrates for MMP2, MMP9, or uPA were incorporated into one arm of the construct, the resulting protein's affinity for cMET could be increased by cleavage with the respective enzyme. Using this approach, the authors were able to demonstrate an approximately 1000-fold difference in affinity between the precursor and activated molecules in vitro. While these trivalent antibodies wouldn't provide a strict on/off switch because of the binding capabilities of the IgG portion, one could imagine that this approach could result in increased tumor targeting as a result of the enhanced avidity that would be restricted to the tumor microenvironment.

Activatable Dual Variable Domain Antibodies

Similar to the activatable trivalent antibody approach, Onuoha [34] engineered an activatable dual variable domain (aDVD) antibody on two different anti-TNF-α antibodies (adalimumab and infliximab). This was achieved by linking the variable domains of an anti-ICAM to the N-terminus of the anti-TNF- α antibody via an MMP9 substrate/linker. In this format, the ICAM variable domain retains the ability to bind ICAM while effectively blocking the ability of adalimumab or infliximab to bind TNF-α. Upon removal of the ICAM variable domains by treatment with MMP9, the TNF- α binding was restored to that of the parental anti-TNF- α antibody. A diagram of this approach is shown in Fig. 2c. This method was capable of producing a greater than 1000-fold difference in K_D between the cleaved and uncleaved aDVDs, as measured by SPR in vitro. As with the trivalent approach, tumor protease-driven targeting could be achieved by the tumor-specific enhancement of affinity for the target.

Cross-masking Antibodies

The cross-masking antibody approach involves attaching the cognate antigen epitope of one antibody via a protease substrate-containing linker to a second antibody or antibody fragment and vice versa (Fig. 2d). Donaldson, et al. [35] demonstrated in vitro proof of concept for this approach using scFvs based on two anti-EGFR antibodies, cetuximab and matuzumab. The epitope used was a portion of soluble EGFR domain III with point mutations introduced to reduce the potential for intramolecular binding of the EGFR fragment. The individual constructs were purified, mixed together allowing the assembly of the cross-masked heterodimeric complex, followed by removal of monomer and misassembled complexes by chromatography. The authors showed that the binding of the heterodimeric complex to sEGFRvIII was significantly attenuated as compared to the MMP9-treated complex.

XTEN Platform

The XTEN platform was originally described by Amunix as a way to extend the in vivo half-life of biologics and small molecules (reviewed in [36]). The XTEN polypeptides consist of polymers of the amino acids alanine, glycine, glutamic acid, proline, serine, and threonine. These were selected for their solubility and lack of potential immunogenicity and propensity to aggregate. The original XTEN polypeptide was 864 amino acids long but XTEN polypeptides of different lengths and compositions have been subsequently evaluated. Importantly, various chemical functionalities can be engineered into XTEN peptides enabling the conjugation of different classes of molecules through various chemistries. Recently Amunix has engineered T-cell bispecifics conjugated to XTEN peptides (referred to as "XTENylation") via a protease linker and is referred to as Protease Triggered Immune Activators or ProTIA (Fig. 2e). These molecules are proposed to selectively target activity to tumors in several different ways, including preferred extravasation due to leaky tumor vasculature and removal of the XTEN polypeptide by tumor specific proteases (www.amunix.com).

Probody™ Therapeutics

The most advanced protease-activatable antibody drug conjugates are based on Probody therapeutics. Probody therapeutics are a novel class of recombinant antibody-based therapeutics that target antibody activity to the tumor by taking advantage of the dysregulation of proteases in diseased tissues. The key components are two peptide sequences encoded on the N-terminus of the light chain of antibodies collectively called the Prodomain (Fig. 3a). The first sequence is a "masking" peptide which physically blocks the ability of the antibody to bind antigen. This sequence is connected to the rest of the light chain by a second peptide sequence designed to be preferentially cleaved by proteases with increased activity in tumors. The addition of the Prodomain results in a molecule with significantly reduced affinity for its target antigen which, upon exposure to proteases, recovers the parental antibody binding affinity (Fig. 3b).

A Probody therapeutic based on the anti-EGFR antibody cetuximab was used to demonstrate the ability of the Probody technology to expand the therapeutic window of an antibody therapy [37]. Using in vivo imaging in mouse xenograft models, it was shown that the protease substrate-containing EGFR Probody therapeutic localized to the xenograft tumor and could achieve efficacy comparable to that of the naked EGFR antibody in tumor xenograft models. In contrast, a masked Probody therapeutic lacking a protease substrate showed reduced localization to xenograft tumors and no significant efficacy in tumor models. These data show that the substrate-containing anti-EGFR Probody therapeutic is capable of being activated and binding to its target antigen in the xenograft tumor microenvironment in a protease dependent manner. Desnoyers, et al. also showed that, in cynomolgus monkeys, the EGFR Probody therapeutic remained largely intact in circulation, had increased exposure due to avoidance of target-mediated drug disposition (TMDD), and reduced the dose limiting skin toxicity associated with cetuximab. It was estimated that the safety factor of the Probody therapeutic was increased over that of the antibody by between 3- to 15-fold. Taken together, the mouse and cynomolgus data demonstrate that the Probody approach is capable of expanding the therapeutic window of an antibody therapy.

Probody Drug Conjugates

The potential of Probody Drug Conjugates (PDC) to widen the therapeutic index for highly expressed targets has been proposed previously [38] and preclinical data for PDCs targeting the highly expressed antigens CD166 and CD71 have been reported [39, 40]. Here we will describe two examples of Probody Drug Conjugates. The first is an anti-Jagged PDC for which efficacy and on-target toxicity can be measured within the same in vivo mouse model system. The second example is a family of anti-CD166 PDCs that show how the interplay between mask strength, substrate choice, and efficacy can be used to fine-tune a PDC. Finally, we show that an anti-CD166 PDC that has similar efficacy as the corresponding ADC in mouse, is

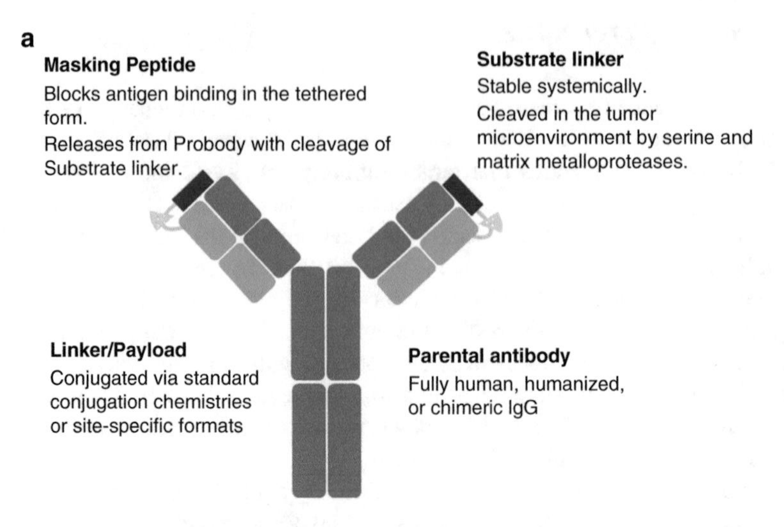

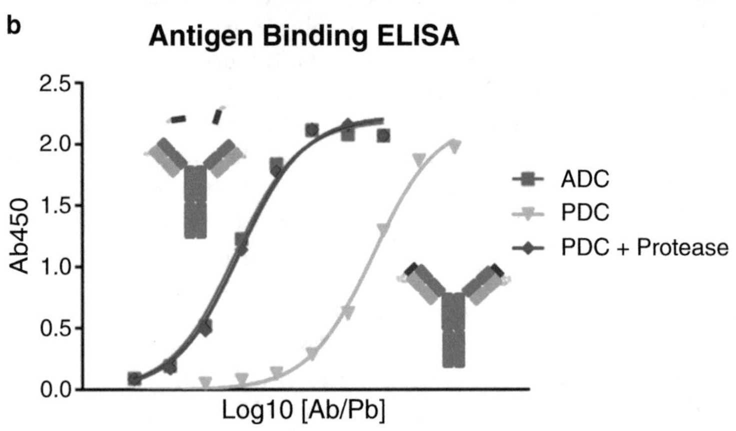

Fig. 3 The Probody Platform. (**a**) Probody drug conjugate components include a parental antibody; the Prodomain, which is comprised of a masking peptide linked to the N-terminus of the light chain of the parental antibody via a protease substrate; and finally the linker/toxin. (**b**) In their inactive form, PDCs have reduced binding for their antigen and upon activation by proteases, recover the binding equivalent to that of the parental antibody

physically stable in circulation in a nonhuman primate, and avoids the TMDD observed with the ADC, suggesting that the PDC remains functionally masked in circulation. A CD166-targeting PDC is currently being evaluated in a Phase 1 trial.

Anti-Jagged Probody Drug Conjugates

The Notch ligands Jagged 1 and Jagged 2 are attractive therapeutic targets because of the importance of the Notch pathway in cancer and tumor initiating cells [41]. We developed an antibody that binds both human and rodent Jagged 1 and 2 Notch ligands with similar affinity and inhibits their interaction with the Notch receptors. In mice, the antibody shows on-target toxicity evidenced by significant body weight loss, hair loss and elevated serum plasma thymic stromal lymphopoietin (TSLP), consistent with what has been previously reported for Notch pathway inhibition by gamma secretase inhibitors [42] and in conditional Notch knockout animals [43]. In general, the toxicities elicited by the antibody are dose dependent and most severe at dose levels greater than 10 mg/kg. It has previously been shown that a Probody therapeutic derived from this antibody is active as monotherapy and in combination with chemotherapy in a preclinical model of pancreatic cancer [44]. The anti-Jagged Probody therapeutic dosed at 20 mg/kg results in toxicities that are mild and comparable to the 5 mg/kg dose of the antibody, demonstrating an approximately fourfold safety advantage on a dose basis for the Probody therapeutic compared to the antibody.

An anti-Jagged ADC generated from this antibody using the linker-toxin combination SPDB-DM4 shows potent in vitro cytotoxicity in several cell lines and in vivo anti-tumor activity in several xenograft models, for example the HCC1806 subcutaneous tumor xenograft model in SCID mice [45]. Tumor bearing mice were dosed on day 1 and 8 with 10 mg/kg of either the SPDB-DM4 isotype control (Isotype), anti-Jagged antibody (Ab), anti-Jagged SPDB-DM4 (ADC), or the anti-Jagged Probody SPDB-DM4 (PDC) and subsequently monitored for tumor growth and body weight change. By day 30, the Isotype-DM4 control and anti-Jagged antibody groups had similar mean tumor volumes of 863 ± 136 (average ± SEM) and 852 ± 100 mm^3, respectively (Fig. 4a). All animals in the ADC and PDC treated groups showed tumor regressions by day 9 of the study and mean tumor volumes of 13.1 ± 1.2 and 20.3 ± 3.6 mm^3, respectively, at day 30. The antibody and ADC treated animals both showed weight loss, with weights of 87 ± 5 and 82 ± 5 percent, respectively, of their starting weight at day 20 (Fig. 4b). In contrast, both the isotype-DM4 and PDC treated animals showed undetectable weight loss. As expected, the observed weight loss in the ADC treated animals was similar to that observed for the non-conjugated antibody treated group, suggesting that the toxicity was due to target (Jagged) inhibition rather than to the conjugated toxin. These results demonstrate that the PDC is capable of antitumor activity comparable to the ADC but with significantly less on-target toxicity when measured in the same animals.

Anti-Jagged Probody Therapeutic Pharmacokinetics in Non-tumor Bearing Mice

To demonstrate that the anti-Jagged Probody therapeutic is stably masked in circulation and avoids binding target in normal tissues, we conducted a 14-day single dose pharmacokinetic study in non-tumor bearing mice comparing the non-conjugated antibody with the Probody therapeutic. The PK curves and the calculated pharmacokinetic values are summarized in Fig. 5. The anti-Jagged antibody and Probody therapeutic had comparable Cmax values at 35 and 45 ug/ml, respectively.

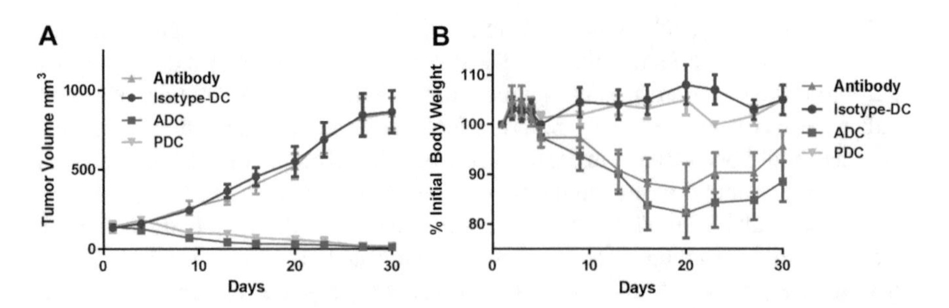

Fig. 4 Anti-Jagged ADC and PDC in the HCC1806 tumor xenograft model in SCID mice. (**a**) Tumor growth curves showing the average ± SEM tumor volumes for HCC1806 xenograft-bearing mice treated with the anti-Jagged antibody (antibody), isotype drug conjugate (isotype-DC), anti-Jagged drug conjugate (ADC), and Probody drug conjugate (PDC). (**b**) Average of percent of initial body weight ± SEM for the same animals with HCC1806 tumors in panel (**a**). All test articles were dosed at 10 mg/kg on day 1 and day 8 and each group consisted of 8 mice

The anti-Jagged antibody was more rapidly cleared to below the lower limit of detection of the assay by day 10, while the anti-Jagged Probody therapeutic showed significantly increased serum half-life (4.6 vs 1.0 days) with the Probody therapeutic concentration remaining above 4 μg/mL at day 14. The increased half-life and greater systemic exposure is consistent with the avoidance of target mediated drug disposition by the masked Probody therapeutic.

The pharmacokinetic and in vivo efficacy and safety data for the anti-jagged Probody therapeutic in preclinical studies support two main conclusions. First, the extended half-life of the PDC and lack of weight loss in PDC-treated animals compared to the ADC demonstrates that the PDC avoids target binding in healthy tissues and, therefore, on-target toxicities. Second, the PDC is capable of antitumor activity comparable to the ADC.

CD166 Probody Drug Conjugates

A second example of an attractive target for Probody drug conjugates is activated leukocyte cell adhesion molecule (ALCAM), also known as CD166. CD166 is reported to be a cell adhesion molecule expressed on many cell types including activated leukocytes, neurons, and epithelial cells. Although CD166 has been identified as a ligand for the CD6 receptor, which is expressed on T lymphocytes and implicated in T cell proliferation and activation [46], its biological functions and the consequences of its inhibition are not understood. CD166 is also highly and homogenously overexpressed in many types of cancer at high prevalence among patients. The high tumor expression and broad normal tissue expression make CD166 an example of an attractive ADC target that would be difficult to develop with traditional ADC technology, but can be addressed by Probody drug conjugates. We developed a panel of anti-CD166 Probody drug conjugates with different masks and substrates and evaluated their efficacy in a xenograft model to identify the preferred PDC design.

Antibody and Probody Tx mouse PK

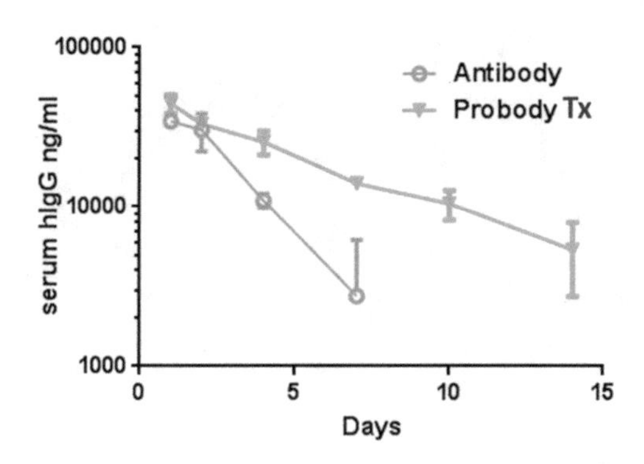

Article	Half life (Days)	Cmax (ug/mL)	AUClast (day*ug/mL)
Antibody	1.0	35	129
Probody Tx	4.6	45	278

Fig. 5 Total human IgG plasma levels and calculated PK parameters in nude mice dosed with either 5 mg/kg of anti-Jagged antibody (Antibody) or anti-Jagged Probody therapeutic (Probody Tx)

CD166 Probody and PDC Characterization

A humanized anti-CD166 antibody that has equivalent affinity for human and cynomolgus monkey CD166 was developed. When conjugated to SPDB-DM4, the ADC is potently cytotoxic in vitro across a large panel of human cancer cell lines [40]. A panel of CD166 Probody therapeutics was developed in which the strength of the masking peptide was varied as measured by binding to HCC1806 cells, referred to as "Low", "Medium", and "High" masked Probody therapeutics (Fig. 6a). When conjugated to SPDB-DM4, and in the absence of protease activity, all but the Low masked PDC protects against target-dependent cytotoxicity in vitro. Although the Low masked PDC does show reduced cytotoxicity as compared to the ADC, it is not completely masked and does show some level of on-target activity as compared to that of the isotype control. Upon protease treatment to remove the mask, all the activated PDCs demonstrated the same cytotoxicity as the ADC (Fig. 6b).

In Vivo Efficacy of CD166 PDCs

To determine the preferred mask/substrate combination for CD166 PDC efficacy, a panel of anti-CD166 Probody SPDB-DM4 drug conjugates was assessed in the H292 xenograft model. Besides varying the mask strength, the "Medium" mask was

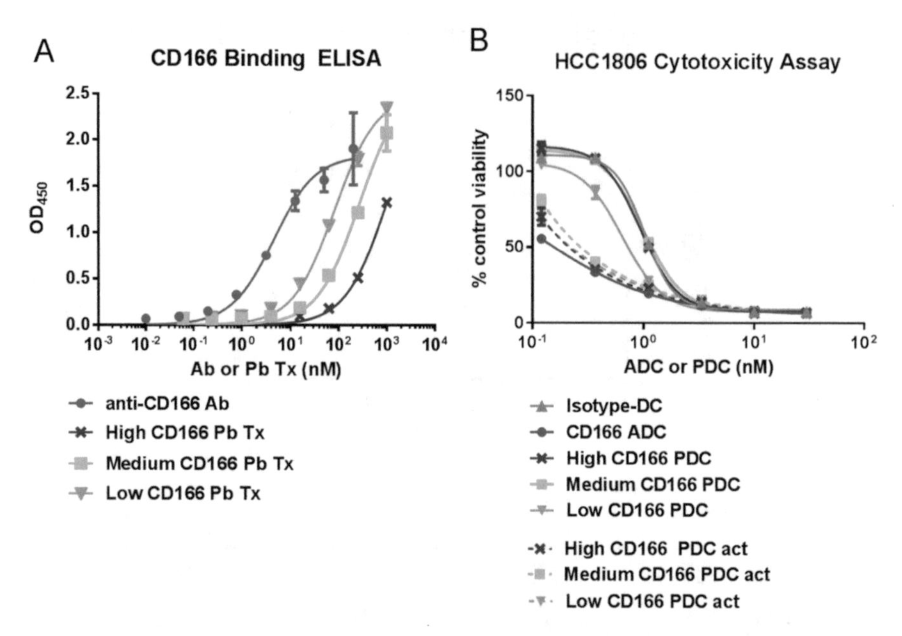

Fig. 6 ELISA binding curves (**a**) for the anti-CD166 antibody (anti-CD166 Ab) and three anti-CD166 Probody therapeutics (Pb Tx) with different masking strengths: High-CD166 Pb Tx, Medium-CD166 Pb Tx, and Low-CD166 Pb Tx. Cytotoxicity assay results (**b**) for anti-CD166 drug conjugate (CD166 ADC) and Probody drug conjugates (High-CD166 PDC, Medium-CD166 PDC, and Low-CD166 PDC) show a range of masking strengths. The High and Medium masked PDCs have similar cytotoxicity as the Isotype-DC while the Low masked PDC shows some level of on-target cytotoxicity. Each data point shows the average ± SD. When activated with a protease (act), all of the PDCs recovered the activity of the CD166 ADC. All Probody therapeutics and PDCs described here contain protease substrate 1 (see text)

evaluated with two different protease substrates, referred to as Substrate 1 (Sub1) and Substrate 2 (Sub2). Both substrates are capable of being cleaved by MMP and serine proteases, however, the substrates differ in their kinetic reactivity, with Sub2 generally being more reactive and cleavable than Sub1. The "Medium" mask was chosen to compare the two substrates as it was sufficient to avoid on-target toxicities in the vitro cytotoxicity assay.

Figure 7a shows the efficacy of the isotype control, the Low-, Medium-, and High-masked Sub1 CD166 PDCs, and the parental ADC. As might be expected, the High masked PDC showed the least efficacy and the Low masked PDC showed the most efficacy in the H292 model. Using the less cleavable Sub1, none of the PDCs achieved equivalent efficacy as the ADC. Within the same study, CD166 PDCs comprising Sub1 or Sub2 with the Medium mask were compared as described above (Fig. 7b). In this configuration, PDCs containing the more cleavable Sub2, but not the less cleavable Sub1, were capable of achieving tumor regressions similar to that of the ADC. These data together demonstrate that the activity of a PDC can be modulated by varying both the mask strength and sub-

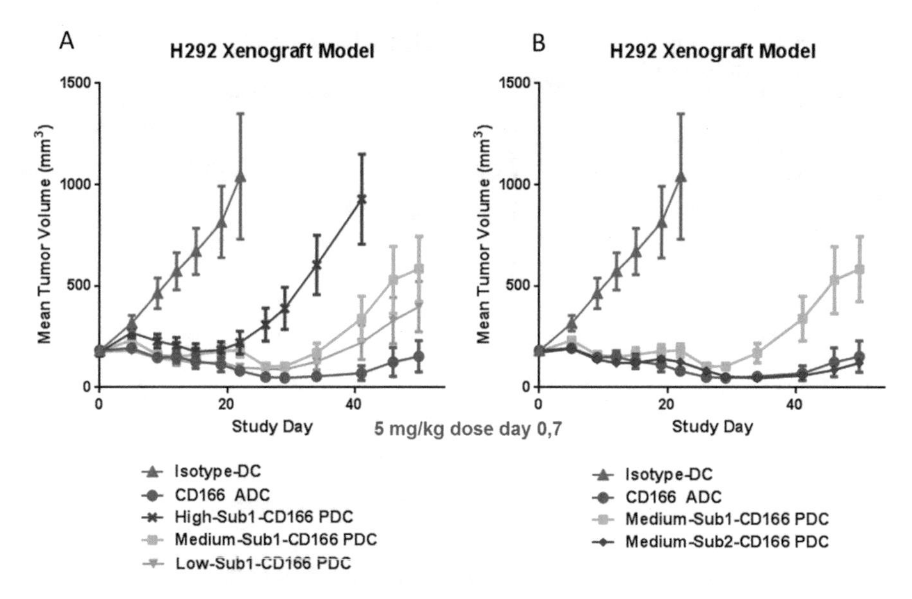

Fig. 7 H292 xenograft tumor bearing mice treated with anti-CD166 PDCs with High, Medium, and Low masks (**a**) and comparing substrates Sub1 and Sub2 in PDCs having the Medium mask (**b**). Each data point shows the average ± SEM tumor volume for each group (N = 8). Efficacy was inversely proportional with the masking strength (**a**) with the Low masked PDC showing the greatest efficacy. While the Medium masked PDC with Substrate 1 (Sub1) did not achieve efficacy similar to that of the CD166 ADC, the Medium masked PDC with Substrate 2 (Sub2) showed efficacy comparable to that of the ADC

strate composition, and that a PDC can be selected that can achieve efficacy similar to that of the unmasked ADC.

Stability of CD166 PDCs in NHP

As described above, if a PDC is sufficiently masked and the substrate is sufficiently stable in circulation to avoid binding to target in normal tissues, it would be expected that the PDC would show prolonged half-life and increased serum exposure as compared to the parental ADC. The pharmacokinetics of the two most efficacious CD166 PDCs (Low mask with the less cleavable substrate "Low-Sub1" and Medium mask with the more cleavable substrate "Medium-Sub2") and the ADC were evaluated at 5 mg/kg in non-human primate (NHP) cynomolgus monkeys. As expected, the PDCs show slower clearance than the ADC (Fig. 8). Further, as in tumor xenograft models, the PK in monkeys can be tuned by modulating the two key components of a Probody therapeutic, the mask and substrate.

Using PDCs targeting CD166, we have shown that a preferred mask/substrate pair can be identified for a PDC targeting an antigen that is expressed on both tumor and normal tissues. Using a xenograft model, we demonstrated that that

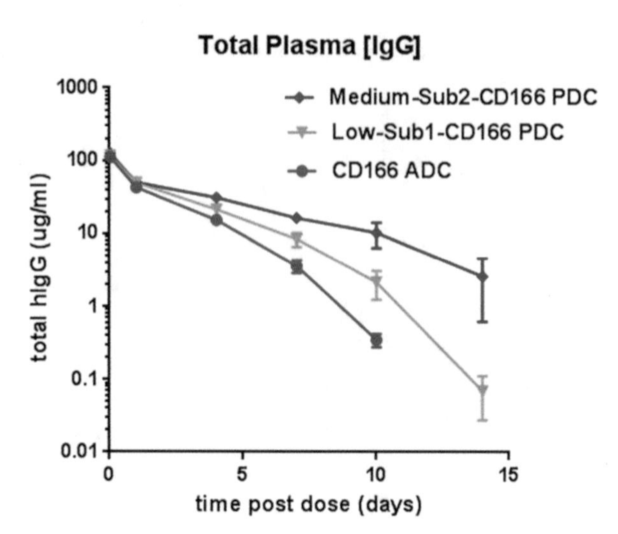

Fig. 8 Plasma human IgG concentrations measured in cynomolgus monkeys (n = 2 per test article) treated at single dose of 5 mg/kg with the Medium-Sub2 CD166 PDC, the Low-Sub1 CD166 PDC, or the anti-CD166 ADC. The average ± SD is shown for each time point. Both PDCs showed extended half-life and exposure compared to the ADC with the Medium-Sub2-PDC showing the largest increase

PDC has similar anti-tumor activity and superior PK compared to that of the parental ADC.

Summary/Future Perspectives

The development of new approaches to address the problems of on-target and off-target toxicities has generated a renewed sense of optimism in the ADC field. After a drought of ADC approvals in the past several years, there are multiple ADCs in pivotal trials for various solid and hematological cancer indications, and new ADC technologies are also being tested in early clinical trials. In the near future, it is possible that a combination of technologies may be needed to achieve the widest therapeutic window and realize the vision of ADCs replacing traditional chemotherapy as the backbone of oncology care.

References

1. Bross PF et al (2001) Approval summary: gemtuzumab ozogamicin in relapsed acute myeloid leukemia. Clin Cancer Res 7(6):1490
2. de Claro RA et al (2012) U.S. Food and Drug Administration approval summary: brentuximab vedotin for the treatment of relapsed Hodgkin lymphoma or relapsed systemic anaplastic large-cell lymphoma. Clin Cancer Res 18(21):5845
3. Amiri-Kordestani L et al (2014) FDA approval: ado-trastuzumab emtansine for the treatment of patients with HER2-positive metastatic breast cancer. Clin Cancer Res 20(17):4436
4. Rowe JM, Lowenberg B (2013) Gemtuzumab ozogamicin in acute myeloid leukemia: a remarkable saga about an active drug. Blood 121(24):4838
5. Donaghy H (2016) Effects of antibody, drug and linker on the preclinical and clinical toxicities of antibody-drug conjugates. MAbs 8(4):659

6. de Goeij BE, Lambert JM (2016) New developments for antibody-drug conjugate-based therapeutic approaches. Curr Opin Immunol 40:14
7. Saber H, Leighton JK (2015) An FDA oncology analysis of antibody-drug conjugates. Regul Toxicol Pharmacol 71(3):444
8. Krop IE et al (2010) Phase I study of trastuzumab-DM1, an HER2 antibody-drug conjugate, given every 3 weeks to patients with HER2-positive metastatic breast cancer. J Clin Oncol 28(6):2698
9. Beck A et al (2017) Strategies and challenges for the next generation of antibody–drug conjugates. Nat Rev Drug Discov 16:315
10. Saleh MN et al (2000) Phase I trial of the anti-Lewis Y drug Immunoconjugate BR96-doxorubicin in patients with Lewis Y-expressing epithelial tumors. J Clin Oncol 18:2282–2292
11. Tijink BM et al (2006) A phase I dose escalation study with anti-CD44v6 bivatuzumab mertansine in patients with incurable squamous cell carcinoma of the head and neck or esophagus. Clin Cancer Res 12(20 Pt 1):6064
12. Annunziata CM et al (2013) Phase 1, open-label study of MEDI-547 in patients with relapsed or refractory solid tumors. Investig New Drugs 31(1):77
13. Tannock IF, Rotin D (1989) Acid pH in tumors and its potential for therapeutic exploitation. Cancer Res 49(16):4373
14. Zhang X et al (2010) Tumor pH and its measurement. J nuclear. Medicine 51:1167
15. Gatenby RA, Gillies RJ (2004) Why do cancers have high aerobic glycolysis? Nat Rev Cancer 4(11):891
16. Liberti MV, Locasale JW (2016) The Warburg effect: how does it benefit Cancer cells? Trends Biochem Sci 41(3):211
17. Vander Heiden MG et al (2009) Understanding the Warburg effect: the metabolic requirements of cell proliferation. Science 324(5930):1029
18. Bhattacharya B et al (2016) The Warburg effect and drug resistance. Br J Pharmacol 173(6):970
19. Sarkar CA et al (2002) Rational cytokine design for increased lifetime and enhanced potency using pH-activated "histidine switching". Nat Biotechnol 20(9):908
20. Chaparro-Riggers J et al (2012) Increasing serum half-life and extending cholesterol lowering in vivo by engineering antibody with pH-sensitive binding to PCSK9. J Biol Chem 287:11090
21. Igawa T et al (2010) Antibody recycling by engineered pH-dependent antigen binding improves the duration of antigen neutralization. Nat Biotechnol 28(11):1203
22. Huang L et al (2016) Preclinical evaluation of a next-generation, EGFR targeting ADC that promotes regression in KRAS or BRAF mutant tumors. Presented at American Association for Cancer Research Annual Meeting, New Orleans, Louisiana, April 16 - 20, 2016 http://www.abstractsonline.com/Plan/ViewAbstract.aspx?sKey=43ef76fe-c845-4b4b-8531-601f2b1c2c32&cKey=bb5dcf16-e379-432f-a72c-191183729d7b&mKey=%7b1D10D749-4B6A-4AB3-BCD4-F80FB1922267%7d
23. Turk B (2006) Targeting proteases: successes, failures and future prospects. Nat Rev Drug Discov 5:785
24. Kessenbrock K et al (2010) Matrix metalloproteinases: regulators of the tumor microenvironment. Cell 141(1):52
25. Sevenich L, Joyce JA (2014) Pericellular proteolysis in cancer. Genes Dev 28(21):2331
26. Bugge TH et al (2009) Type II transmembrane serine proteases. J Biol Chem 284(35):23177
27. Dass K et al (2008) Evolving role of uPA/uPAR system in human cancers. Cancer Treat Rev 34(2):122
28. Murphy G (2008) The ADAMs: signalling scissors in the tumour microenvironment. Nat Rev Cancer 8(12):929
29. Olson OC, Joyce JA (2015) Cysteine cathepsin proteases: regulators of cancer progression and therapeutic response. Nat Rev Cancer 15(12):712
30. Coussens LM et al (2002) Matrix metalloproteinase inhibitors and cancer: trials and tribulations. Science 295(5564):2387
31. Appleby TC et al (2017) Biochemical characterization and structure determination of a potent, selective antibody inhibitor of human MMP9. J Biol Chem 292(16):6810–6682

32. Marshall DC et al (2015) Selective allosteric inhibition of MMP9 is efficacious in preclinical models of ulcerative colitis and colorectal Cancer. PLoS One 10(5):e0127063
33. Metz S et al (2012) Bispecific antibody derivatives with restricted binding functionalities that are activated by proteolytic processing. Protein Eng Des Sel 25:571–580
34. Onuoha SC (2015) Rational design of Antirheumatic Prodrugs specific for sites of inflammation. Arthritis Rheumatol 67:2662–2672
35. Donaldson JM et al (2009) Design and development of masked therapeutic antibodies to limit off-target effects: application to an anti-EGFR antibodies. Cancer Biol Ther 8:2147–2152
36. Podust VN (2016) Extension of in vivo half-life of biologically active molecules by XTEN protein polymers. J Control Release 240:52–66
37. Desnoyers LR et al (2013) Tumor-specific activation of an EGFR-targeting Probody enhances therapeutic index. Sci Transl Med 5:207ra144
38. Polu KR, Lowman HB (2014) Probody therapeutics for targeting antibodies to diseased tissue. Expert Opin Biol Ther 14:1049–1053
39. Singh S et al (2016) Preclinical development of a probody drug conjugate (PDC) targeting CD71 for the treatment of multiple cancers. Presented at American Association for Cancer Research Annual Meeting, New Orleans, Louisiana, April 16 - 20, 2016. http://cytomx.com/wp-content/uploads/2016/04/Preclinical-Development-of-a-ProbodyTM-Drug-Conjugate-PDC-Targeting-CD71-for-the-Treatment-of-Multiple-Cancers-AACR-2016.pdf
40. Weaver AY et al (2015) Development of a probody drug conjugate (PDC) targeting CD166 for the treatment of multiple cancers. Presented at AACR-NCI-EORTC International Conference on Molecular Targets and Cancer Therapeutics Boston, Massachusetts, November 5 - 9, 2015 http://cytomx.com/wp-content/uploads/2015/11/20151104_CD166_AACR_NCI_EORTC_poster_TO_PRINT_FINAL.pdf
41. Takebe N et al (2014) Targeting notch signaling pathway in cancer: clinical development advances and challenges. Pharmacol Ther 141:140–149
42. Wei P et al (2010) Evaluation of selective gamma-secretase inhibitor PF-03084014 for its antitumor efficacy and gastrointestinal safety to guide optimal clinical trial design. Mol Cancer Ther 9(6):1618–1628
43. Dumortier A et al (2010) Atopic dermatitis-like disease and associated lethal myeloproliferative disorder arise from loss of notch signaling in the murine skin. PLoS One 5(2):e9258
44. Sagert J et al (2013) Tumor-specific inhibition of Jagged-dependent notch signaling using a Probody™ Therapeutic. Presented at AACR-NCI-EORTC International Conference on Molecular Targets and Cancer Therapeutics, Boston, MA, October 19-23, 2013. Mol Cancer Ther 2013;12(11 Suppl):C158
45. Sagert J et al (2014) Transforming Notch ligands into tumor-antigen targets: a probody-drug conjugate (PDC) targeting Jagged 1 and Jagged 2. Presented at AACR Annual Meeting, San Diego, CA April 5-9, 2014. Cancer Res 2014;74(19 Suppl):Abstract 2665
46. Weidle UH et al (2010) ALCAM/CD166: cancer-related issues. Cancer Genomics Proteomics 7(5):231–243

Antibody-Drug Conjugates: Targeting the Tumor Microenvironment

Alberto Dal Corso, Samuele Cazzamalli, and Dario Neri

Abstract Antibody-drug conjugates (ADCs) have been used for more than two decades as tools for the selective delivery of cytotoxic agents to the tumor site, with the aim to increase anti-cancer activity and spare normal tissues from undesired toxicity. Until recently, most ADC development activities have focused on the use of monoclonal antibodies, capable of selective binding and internalization into the target tumor cells. However, in principle, it would be conceivable to develop non-internalizing ADC products, which liberate their toxic payload in the extracellular environment. In this Chapter, we review previous work performed on non-internalizing ADC products, with a special emphasis on drug conjugates which selectively localize to the modified extracellular matrix in the neoplastic mass.

Keywords Non-internalizing ADCs · Extracellular tumor antigens · Tumor microenvironment · Vascular targeting

Introduction

Conventional pharmacological approaches for the chemotherapy of cancer are mostly based on the administration of cytotoxic agents, which promote cell death by blocking biological pathways that are essential for cell proliferation. The efficacy of this class of antitumor agents is often limited by their inability to preferentially accumulate at the tumor site, as demonstrated both in preclinical biodistribution studies and in positron-emission tomography (PET) imaging of cancer patients [1]. Drug accumulation in healthy tissues may give rise to side effects, which prevent dose escalation to therapeutically active regimens. For this reason, the covalent

A. Dal Corso · S. Cazzamalli · D. Neri (✉)
Swiss Federal Institute of Technology (ETH Zürich), Department of Chemistry and Applied Biosciences, Zürich, Switzerland
e-mail: neri@pharma.ethz.ch

M. Damelin (ed.), *Innovations for Next-Generation Antibody-Drug Conjugates*, Cancer Drug Discovery and Development,
https://doi.org/10.1007/978-3-319-78154-9_13

conjugation of potent cytotoxic payloads to suitable vehicles (e.g., antibodies), capable of binding to tumor-associated antigens (e.g., receptors or other proteins that are overexpressed at the site of disease), has been proposed as a general strategy to improve the therapeutic index of cancer chemotherapy [2].

ADC products result from the conjugation of a cytotoxic agent and a monoclonal antibody (mAb), using a suitable linker. Most of the antibodies that have been used for ADC development display insufficient anti-tumor activity, when administered as "naked" immunoglobulins [3]. On the other hand, the role of the mAb moiety in ADC products mainly consists in the selective delivery of a cytotoxic compound at the tumor site, where the latter is released and acts on cellular targets causing direct damage. According to this mechanism of action, ADCs can be considered as prodrugs, for which the release of the cargo is of fundamental importance for therapeutic activity.

While ADC products specific to internalizing receptors have shown encouraging clinical responses in patients bearing non-solid tumors, the therapeutic activity against the most frequent solid malignancies (e.g., tumors of breast, lung and colon) is still far from optimal [4]. The emerging clinical results are often less favorable than the preclinical data obtained in tumor-bearing mice, where several internalizing ADC products have led to cancer cures. The higher permeability of interstitial tissues in mice xenografts, compared to solid malignancies in human patients, may partially account for this observed discrepancy [5]. A suboptimal penetration of ADC products within the tumor mass may result in an insufficient delivery of suitable payload concentrations. The limited diffusion properties of monoclonal antibodies emerged from immunofluorescence detection studies, which revealed the striking accumulation of mAbs in IgG formats on perivascular tumor cells, with a substantial inability to penetrate the tumor mass and to reach the majority of neoplastic cells [6].

Since the birth of the ADC technology, it has commonly been assumed that the mAb should preferably be directed against tumor-associated antigens expressed on the surface of cancer cells. Ideally, the ADC would internalize upon binding to its cognate target, thus facilitating the delivery and release of the cytotoxic cargo inside the malignant cell. This receptor-mediated endocytosis represents the most exploited mechanism for ADC activation, as discussed extensively in different reviews [7].

In principle, it is conceivable that also ADC products, based on internalizing antibodies, may display at least part of their activity through drug release in the extracellular space. The internalization efficiency is typically variable and rarely reaches 100%. Furthermore, while antibody internalization can be easily studied *in vitro*, an *in vivo* characterization of the process is hindered by many technical limitations, associated with the processing of the tumor mass and with the specific detection of individual antibody, linker and payload components. As a result, the need to use internalizing mAbs for ADC development has recently been questioned and the availability of novel antibodies, with exquisite tumor-targeting properties, has prompted the investigation of ADC products based on non-internalizing ligands.

In the following sections, the development and *in vivo* testing of non-internalizing ADC products is described, with a special focus on molecules targeting the modified extracellular matrix within tumor lesions.

Non-internalizing ADC Products: Mechanism of Action

As an alternative to the traditional receptor-mediated endocytic process, the drug release from tumor-targeting devices could ideally take place in the tumor microenvironment, allowing the subsequent diffusion of the active payload and its internalization into neighboring neoplastic cells. Since passive diffusion is a non-specific process, the cytotoxic agent has the potential to reach antigen-negative cancerous cells within the tumor mass (a mechanism often referred to as "bystander effect"). In principle, non-internalizing ADCs may display potent therapeutic activity against tumors with high mutation rates or characterized by antigen loss, where certain cell populations can develop resistance to conventional internalizing ADCs. Potentially, the bystander killing effect could also impair structures which support tumor growth, such as stromal cells, leukocytes and tumor blood vessels, thus enhancing the anti-tumor effect of the product [8].

Ideally, this alternative strategy could be potentially pursued using monoclonal antibodies specific to both tumor-specific extracellular structures and poorly/non-internalizing transmembrane antigens. However, due to the identical localization of the target protein, mAbs targeting non-internalizing transmembrane receptors would show similar features in terms of tumor accumulation, as compared to antibodies specific to internalizing antigens. Together with the mAb development and the choice of a suitable payload, the design of a proper linker is crucially important for the generation of efficacious and well-tolerated ADCs. While both cleavable and non-cleavable linkers have found application in internalizing ADC products, only cleavable bonds have been so far used as linkers of choice, for the development of non-internalizing drug delivery systems. This can be easily explained by the intrinsic nature of the endocytic process, which leads to the proteolytic degradation of the antibody structure in the intracellular compartments, followed by the release of an active drug metabolite. Various cleavable linkers have been proposed for the preferential drug release in the tumor interstitium. A main requirement to prevent premature drug release and the related side effects is a high linker stability in plasma, after ADC administration. Provided that a sufficient amount of the ADC reaches intact the tumor microenvironment, a second key attribute of the linker is the ability to efficiently release the payload at the tumor site. Glutathione (GSH) represents the most abundant thiol and reducing agent in the intracellular space, both in normal cells and in tumors, which often contain higher concentrations of this species [9, 10]. While disulfide-based linkers have been designed for the intracellular release of anti-cancer drugs, the same chemical structures can be considered for the extracellular drug release, as a consequence of tumor cell death and increased GSH concentration. Disulfides are typically stable in the absence of free thiols at physiological pH, with a serum half-life that can be longer than 1 week. *In vivo*, certain disulfide-based ADCs have exhibited stability in blood for 2–4 days. Moreover, this stability can be dramatically improved by increasing the steric hindrance of substituents at the cleavage site [11]. Several ADCs and small molecule-targeted cytotoxics that incorporate reducible linker systems such as disulfide bridges have been considered for clinical development [2, 12]. Most of these new products have been designed to release the payload through receptor-mediated endocytosis. However, it is conceivable to assume that the tumor environment *in vivo* is a more complex scenario, in which dying cells are constantly releasing reducing agents to the surrounding areas. Therefore, non-internalizing ADC products based on disulfide bonds can potentially be cleaved in the tumor extracellular milieu, releasing the payload and promote apoptosis in cancer cells. The release of GSH to the extracellular environment may generate a self-amplifying cycle of cell death and subsequent drug release (Fig. 1).

In addition to disulfides, certain peptide sequences have been used as linkers for the generation of ADC products. These functional groups combine a high systemic stability with a rapid release of the drug at the site of disease. Indeed, proteolytic enzymes such as cathepsin B, urokinase-type plasminogen activator and matrix metalloproteinases (MMPs), which are involved in cancer progression features like angiogenesis, invasion and metastasis [13], may be over-expressed at the tumor site, both in intra- and extra-cellular compartments [14]. In particular, the Valine-Citrulline (Val-Cit) dipeptide had shown promising features for the development of internalizing ADCs. This line of research led to the use of a Val-Cit-containing linker in the marketed Adcetris™ product and in other clinical-stage candidates [15, 16]. Similarly to the cleavage of disulfide bonds, proteolytically-cleavable linkers could be exploited also for the release of drugs in the extracellular tumor microenvironment. Indeed, the protease-mediated release of payloads from non-internalizing ADCs can be amplified by tumor cell death, which sheds a large number of proteolytic activities into the cancer microenvironment (Fig. 1).

Non-internalizing ADC Products: Early Evidence of Biological Activity

Studies on non-internalizing (or poorly internalizing) ADC products have been performed both against targets expressed on the cell membrane (such as CD20, CD21, CAIX and FAP) and against components of the modified extracellular matrix in the neoplastic mass (e.g., splice variants of fibronectin and tenascin-C, fibrin and collagen IV). CD20 and CD21 are well-known cell-surface markers of B-cell derived non-Hodgkin's Lymphomas (NHLs) and have been intensively investigated as antigens for ADC products [17, 18]. NHLs have been extensively studied as targets for ADC development, providing insights into the mechanism of action, the anti-tumor potential and limiting toxicities. NHLs are often successfully treated with a combination of chemotherapeutic agents and antibody-based products [19]. However, there is a need for improved medications, especially for patients who relapse from previous pharmacological interventions. CD19 and CD22 have been described as internalizing NHL antigens, while anti-CD20 and anti-CD21 antibodies typically remain on the membrane of B cells and lymphoma cells [20]. Polson and coworkers generated ADCs against different NHL antigens (i.e. CD19, CD20, CD21, CD22, CD72, CD79b, and

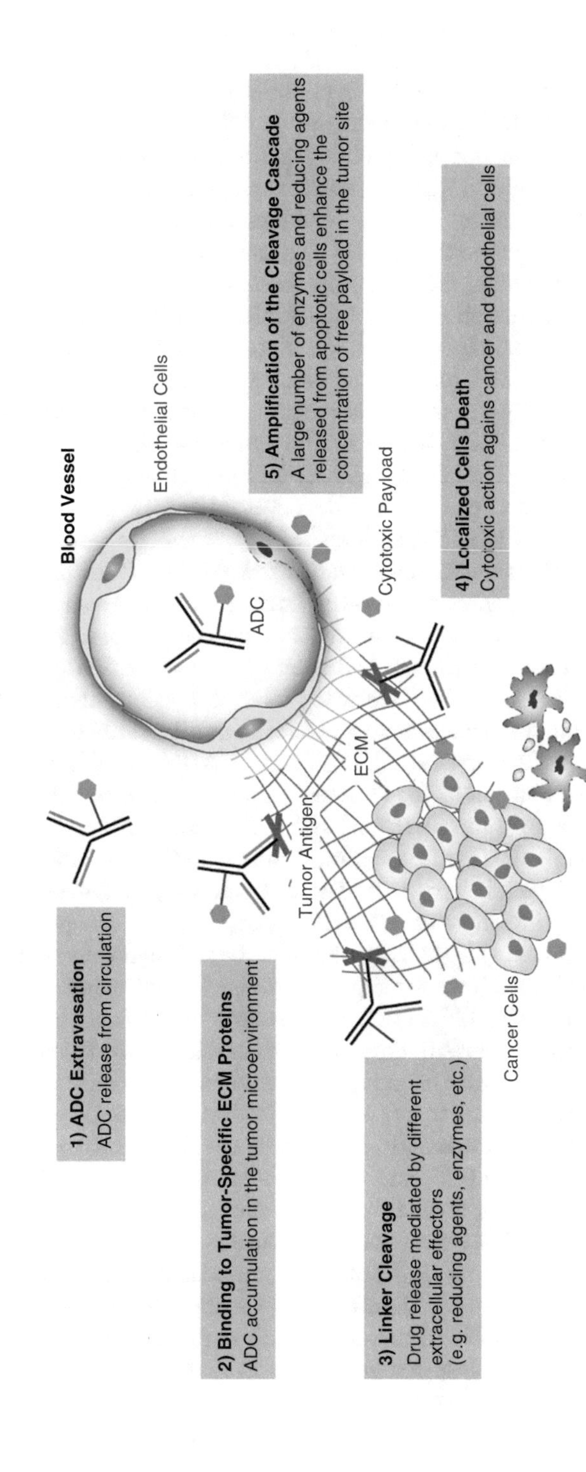

Fig. 1 Schematic representation of possible mechanisms for the drug release and cytotoxic activity of non-internalizing ADCs

CD180), in which potent anti-tubulin agents (DM1 or MMAE) were conjugated to the parental antibodies through either cleavable (disulfide or peptide bonds) or non-cleavable linkers [17]. Therapy experiments performed in tumor-bearing mice showed that all ADCs featuring cleavable linkers (i.e., both products based on internalizing and on non-internalizing antibodies) exhibited a therapeutic effect *in vivo*. By contrast, when non-cleavable linkers were used, only the products directed against internalizing antigens showed a therapeutic activity. Similar results were reported for an anti-CD20 antibody coupled to calicheamicin through both cleavable and non-cleavable linkers [21]. These observations are compatible with the assumption that the cleavable linker is processed in the tumor extracellular space after ADC localization. Subsequently, the drug may diffuse through the cell membrane, reaching its biochemical target. This mechanism of action was reinforced by the observation that the substitution of MMAE with its charged analogue MMAF (i.e., membrane-impermeable) led to a lower antitumor activity, for ADC products directed against non-internalizing antigens [22].

Investigated as tumor marker for the development of targeted cytotoxics, Carbonic Anhydrase IX (CAIX) has long been considered to be an internalizing antigen. However, recent studies have clearly shown that CAIX displays extremely poor internalization properties and resides virtually exclusively on the cell membrane. Carbonic Anhydrases are metalloenzymes that can be found in most of living organisms, where they catalyze the hydration of carbon dioxide to bicarbonate. Among all the CA isoforms, CAIX (formerly referred to as MN antigen) is a transmembrane homodimeric enzyme overexpressed in more than 90% of clear cell renal cell carcinoma (ccRCC) subtypes [23]. In addition, CAIX is one of the best markers of hypoxia and, as such, can be found in many tumor types, especially those characterized by a low oxygen concentration [24]. The pattern of expression of CAIX in healthy organs is limited on the first portion of the gastro-intestinal tract (e.g., stomach, duodenum and gallbladder) [25], These encouraging immunohistochemical results stimulated the investigation of CAIX as a target for ADC products. Although in the early development anti-CAIX therapeutics were designed to be internalized by tumor cells, our group recently reported the inefficient internalization of the protein upon ligand binding [26, 27]. Petrul and coworkers explored the conjugation of an anti-CAIX mAb to MMAE, through the cleavable Val-Cit linker, to generate the ADC BAY 79–4620 [28]. The group demonstrated the selective affinity of this product to the CAIX isoform and its ability selectively kill CAIX-positive cancer cells *in vitro*, by tubulin disruption. BAY 79–4620 was also shown to be effective *in vivo* in mice grafted with HT-29 and Colo205 colorectal tumors or with cervix carcinoma HeLa-MaTu tumors, at doses between 5 and 10 mg/kg. A modest anticancer activity was reported against other cancer models, albeit at higher doses (30–60 mg/kg). However, while free MMAE (0.2 mg/kg, equivalent to 10 mg/kg of ADC) was less effective than BAY 79–4620, the efficacy of paclitaxel administered at the dose of 15 mg/kg was comparable to the one described for the ADC. In 2014, BAY 79–4620 entered a phase I dose-escalation clinical study with 12 patients, bearing histologically or cytologically confirmed solid tumors [29]. The product was administered at doses ranging from 0.3 to 4.6 mg/kg. While no complete or partial response were reported, treatment-related side effect occurred in the majority of patients and the highest dose led to patient death due to cardiac arrest and pancreatitis. This tragic event underlined the importance of an accurate preliminary evaluation of the antigen expression in patients, since data of CAIX expression in the studied tumors were available for only 50% of patients, among whom only 2 showed more than 10% antigen-positive cells in the tumor mass.

Antigens that localize in the tumor microenvironment, or on the surface of stromal cells have also been studied as targets for non-internalizing ADCs. The extravascular deposition of fibrin has been described in different human solid tumors as a consequence of the disruption of vascular barriers, which allows the extravasation of fibrinogen and other substrates of the coagulation cascade [30]. Indeed, after tumor transplantation in animal models of cancer, fibrin deposition is one of the first morphological changes that can be observed [31]. While in wound healing processes fibrin is progressively replaced by collagen fibers in few weeks, fibrin clot formation persists in cancer until living tumor cells are present [32]. Yasunaga and coworkers exploited this tumor-specific pathophysiological feature to develop the first fibrin-specific ADC [33]. This immunotoxin comprised a chimeric IgG1 mAb coupled to the active metabolite of Irinotecan (SN-38) as payload. Cysteine residues of the immunoglobulin were coupled to dendrimeric structures bearing 3 SN-38 molecules, individually bound to a PEG spacer via ester linkers. Such a complex design allowed a heavy functionalization of the mAb scaffold, achieving a drug/antibody ratio (DAR) of approximately 24. The resulting anti-fibrin immunoconjugate was stable at acidic pH values, but released gradually and effectively SN-38 at physiological pH in saline buffer and in mouse serum. As expected, this so-called AFCA-branched-PEG-(SN-38)$_3$ ADC acted as a pro-drug *in vitro*, displaying no substantial direct activity against tumor cells. By contrast, four injections per week of the product into tumor-bearing mice at a dose of 13.3 mg/kg were able to suppress tumor growth for more than 1 month. This potent anti-tumor activity was remarkable, especially when compared to the administration of Irinotecan (injected daily at the MTD) which was largely inefficacious. A long-term observation of side-effects revealed that the ADC product was well tolerated in mice, with no signs of bone marrow, liver or kidney dysfunction at the recommended dose. Immunohistochemistry and *in vivo* fluorescence endomicroscopy indicated that the antitumoral activity was mainly due to tumor vessel disruption.

The same group working on anti-fibrin ADCs also reported activity for products directed against murine collagen IV [34]. The naked antibody was coupled to eight molar equivalents of SN-38 cytotoxic agent via a PEG spacer and a cleavable ester linker. The group compared the anti-collagen-4 conjugate and another ADC product, targeting the EpCAM, an antigen expressed on the cancer cell membrane. The comparative evaluation of the two products highlighted the potential of ADCs targeting the tumor stroma to localize and efficiently release their toxic cargo within the tumor microenvironment. Indeed, some cell-targeting products are hindered by stromal barriers, preventing access to the antigen on the cell membrane. When comparing the two products, the anti-collagen IV ADC was found to be superior in two different EpCAM-positive murine models of carcinoma. Since the treatment with the collagen-targeted ADC resulted in a higher SN-38 concentration in the tumor and with the death of vascular endothelial cells, the authors concluded that the uneven distribution of the anti-EpCAM product within the tumor mass may have led to an inferior performance and lower efficacy.

The work by Yasunaga and colleagues highlighted the potential of stromal-targeting ADCs. Metastasis and tumor invasion are usually linked to adaptation of mesenchyme-derived stromal cells (fibroblasts, myofibroblasts, endothelial cells, pericytes, smooth muscle, and hematopoietic cells) of the neighboring healthy organs [35, 36]. Fibroblasts respond to cancer progression producing Fibroblast Activation Protein α (FAPα), a serine protease involved in tissue remodeling and wound healing [37]. This antigen has been initially proposed as a possible target for cancer therapy with unconjugated antibodies in colorectal cancer patients. Sibrotuzumab, a humanized anti-FAPα antibody, was found to be well tolerated and to exhibit a selective tumor uptake 24–48 h after i.v. administration. No anticancer activity, however, was detected in patients [38]. Ostermann and colleagues conjugated an anti-FAPα mAb to different maytansinoid payloads using both cleavable and non-cleavable linkers [39]. The internalizing behavior of the FAPα antigen was demonstrated by cell antiproliferative assays *in vitro*, where all the ADC products, including the ones featuring non-cleavable linkers, were found to be active against FAPα-transfected cells. However, the *in vivo* administration of the ADCs in mice bearing a panel of FAPα-positive tumors (i.e., pancreatic, a non-small cell lung, a head and neck squamous cell and a colorectal carcinoma) revealed that cleavable linkers are required to induce a potent anticancer effect. These data suggested that the efficacy of the anti-FAP ADC products was due to a bystander effect, associated with the diffusion of the active payload within the tumor microenvironment. In line with this proposed mechanism of action, histological analysis and biomarker studies identified the death of malignant cells surrounding stromal cells as an early therapeutic event.

Another example of a tumor-associated antigen expressed on fibroblasts in the tumor stromal environment is LRRC15 (i.e., leucine rich repeat containing 15). Also known as Lib, this protein is a transmembrane member of the leucine-rich repeat superfamily, which are involved in cell-cell and cell-ECM interactions. Showing weak expression in healthy tissues, LLRC15 was initially detected in astrocytes in response to pro-inflammatory cytokines [40]. It was then found to be frequently overexpressed in many solid tumors, such as aggressive breast cancer [41] and prostate tumors [42]. The anti-LRRC15 ADC product ABBV-085, based on the linker-toxin combination ValCit-MMAE, has recently entered Phase I clinical trial, after showing promising activity against different murine tumor models, administered both as single agent and in combination with chemotherapy, radiation or checkpoint inhibitors [43].

In general, it is technically challenging to quantify internalization rates *in vivo*, even for products directed against cell surface targets. While the examples reviewed below relate to non-internalizing ADC targets (e.g., extracellular matrix antigens), it is reasonable to assume that a substantial portion of putative internalizing ADCs may not reach the corresponding intracellular compartments *in vivo* as intact conjugates.

Targeting the Modified Extracellular Matrix in Tumors

Among the clinically-validated tumor markers, specific isoforms of ECM proteins represent ideal targets for biopharmaceutical intervention. The generation of these tumor-specific proteins can be considered as an end-product of the abnormal proliferative rates of cancer cells, which is not only sustained by several defections in fundamental inhibitory functions of neoplastic cells (e.g. contact inhibition, apoptosis, autophagy, cellular homeostasis) but it is also favored by substantial alterations of the extracellular environment [44]. In particular, the high proliferation rate and the irregular vascularization of a fast-growing tumor mass lead to inadequate oxygen supply to the tumor tissue. It is now well established that cancer cells modify their metabolism to adapt to hypoxia: cellular respiration runs under anaerobic conditions, causing high glucose consumption and production of large quantities of respiratory end-products (i.e. CO_2 and H^+-lactate) [45]. The latter are released in the extracellular environment, resulting in a substantial acidification of the tumor interstitium (the pH can shift from the usual values of 6.5–7.0 to values as low as 6.0). While this phenomenon may lead to apoptosis in normal cells, it acts as a Darwinian selection process for cancer cells, which eventually develop resistance to the altered environmental conditions. For instance, the enzymes carbonic anhydrase IX and XII are over-expressed in many tumors to catalyze the CO_2 hydration in the extracellular environment. This process minimizes the passive diffusion of CO_2 through the membrane, thus allowing the cell to maintain a slightly alkaline intracellular pH (pH 7.2–7.4), which results from increased metabolism and supports cell proliferation [46].

Anomalies in pH values at both side of the cell membrane have been associated with the expression of proteins in mutated isoforms, generated by alternative splicing of their primary RNA transcript. Although the latter is a fundamental process in many physiological functions (e.g. in tissue and organ development) [47], the understanding of alternative splicing in cancer is a field of growing interest in oncology, to such an extent that aberrant alternative splicing is now commonly included in the list of the hallmarks of cancer [48, 49]. Alternative splicing events can generate protein isoforms that help tumors to acquire therapeutic resistance. Moreover, protein splice variants have been associated with particular diagnostic and prognostic features for certain types of cancers, even though their functional/mechanistic role is often not understood [50]. For instance, acidification of the tumor microenvironment have been shown to influence the alternative splicing of vascular endothelial growth factor (VEGF-A) in by endometrial cancer cells [51]. The produced isoforms are known to activate signaling pathways that stimulate tumor progression (e.g. angiogenesis and metastasis) and thus represent a mechanism of tumor cells adaptation to the acidic stress.

A basic intracellular pH may lead to the modulation of splice variants for certain extracellular matrix (ECM) components, such as fibronectin and tenascin C [52, 53]. Fibronectins (FNs) are glycoproteins, which are present either in soluble form in plasma and other body fluids or in cellular form in the ECM and basement membranes of tissues. Acting as a bridge between the cell surface and the extracellular

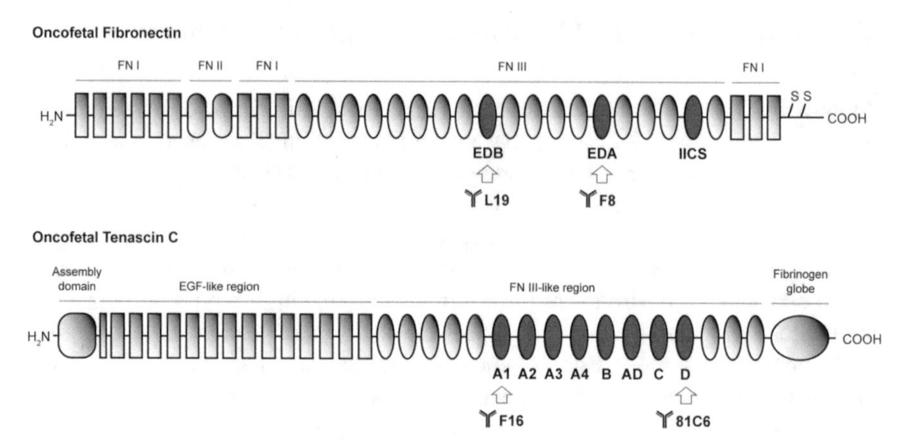

Fig. 2 Modular structure of oncofetal variants of ECM proteins fibronectin and tenascin C. Different shapes are given to different types of protein repeats. Alternatively-spiced domains are shown in red. Arrows show clinically-evaluated domains and their relative antibodies

material, FN is involved in various cell-ECM interactions, such as adhesion, cell migration, hemostasis, thrombosis and wound healing [54]. FN is secreted from cells as a dimer consisting of two 250 kDa subunits covalently linked by two disulfide bonds near their C-termini. Although FN is encoded by a single gene, it exists in multiple isoforms which result from the combination of three alternatively-spliced domains: EDA, EDB and IIICS (see Fig. 2) [55]. While EDA and EDB show constant structures, composed respectively by 90 and 91 amino acids, the extra domain IIICS can be expressed in multiple variants in humans, ranging from 64 to 120 amino acids [56]. The group of Luciano Zardi firstly reported the over-expression of FN extra-domains in tumor-derived or SM40-transformed human cells, compared to normal human fibroblasts [57].

This discovery stimulated an intense research activity around FN splice variants, aimed at understanding their expression pattern and pathological role. In particular, the EDB of FN was found to be virtually absent in all normal adult tissues, but abundantly expressed in the proximity of angiogenic blood vessels and in the stroma of various types of aggressive tumors, including brain, lung, skin, kidney and bladder [58, 59]. Similarly to EDB, the EDA domain was found to be expressed in subendothelial ECM of proliferating tumors, while being undetectable in human plasma and healthy tissues [60]. The singular expression profile of EDA and EDB led to the identification of these markers of angiogenesis as "oncofetal" domains of fibronectin [61, 62].

Tenascin C (TnC) is another cell-binding, large oligomeric glycoprotein of the ECM, composed by 240 kDa subunits that assembly in oligomers (mainly hexamers) through disulfide bonds [63]. A functional antagonism between TnC and FN have emerged from different observations: (i) TnC shows poor binding affinity of to ECM components (FN, collagen, laminin), thus supporting only a weak cell attachment to ECM; (ii) TnC promotes cell rounding and detachment, whereas FN promotes cell-substrate adhesion; (iii) FN is ubiquitously distributed while TnC expression is restricted to morphogenesis and remodeling events [64]. Two main human TnC isoforms are generated by alternative splicing of the single TnC primary mRNA, resulting in the inclusion (or omission) of eight extra domains (Fig. 2) in the final transcript. The expression of these two isoforms was proposed to be dependent to intracellular pH, as a result of adaptation to environmental conditions. In particular, while TnC alternative splicing in normal cultured fibroblasts showed a sensitivity towards small variation of extracellular pH [65], malignantly-transformed cells mainly expressed the large TnC variant (i.e., bearing the 8 extra domains). This observation was explained by the ability of malignant cells to maintain a basic intracellular pH even in an acidic environment, which promotes the alternative splicing event [53].

The abundant and tumor-specific expression of oncofetal FN and TnC stimulated the investigation of these proteins as ideal targets for biomolecular intervention. For instance, ^{131}I-labeled murine and chimeric antibodies specific to A1 and D domains of TnC have been evaluated in the clinic for the treatment of glioma and lymphoma [66, 67]. Moreover, the human recombinant antibodies L19 and F16 were generated upon selections of a phage display library against the EDB and A1 antigens [68, 69]. The two antibodies have been produced in different formats (scFv, diabody, SIP, IgG) and their tumor-targeting properties were studied by quantitative biodistribution analysis, revealing promising *in vivo* tumor targeting performances [69, 70]. Importantly, quantitative biodistribution data are available for L19 and F16 both in mice and in man. The ^{131}I-L19 and ^{131}I-F16 antibodies in SIP format have been evaluated for radio-immunotherapy applications in patients bearing Hodgkin's lymphoma [71, 72] and head and neck cancer [73]. In addition to radiopharmaceutical applications, a variety of immunocytokines composed by the L19 and F16 antibodies fused with either interleukin 2 or TNF are currently evaluated in the clinic for the treatment of different solid tumors (i.e. melanoma, soft tissue sarcoma, diffuse large B-cell lymphoma, oligometastatic solid tumor, Merkel cell carcinoma, acute myeloid leukemia and non-small cell lung cancer) in combination with chemotherapy. Similarly to L19 and F16, also the F8 antibody (specific to the EDA domain of FN) may be considered as a delivery vehicle for pharmaceutical applications. F8 displayed encouraging tumor-targeting properties in mouse models and a characteristic ability to stain neo-vascular structures not only in aggressive solid tumors, but also of solid masses of hematological malignancies [74]. EDA is expressed not only in cancer, but also in other pathological conditions, characterized by extensive tissue remodeling. The observation of an intense and diffuse staining pattern of F8 in synovial tissue biopsies obtained from rheumatoid arthritis patients led to the development of the immunocytokine F8-IL10, which is currently evaluated in the clinic [75].

The L19, F8 and F16 antibodies, specific to non-internalizing ECM antigens, have been instrumental for the selective delivery of cytotoxic compounds to the tumor environment. Initial studies involved the functionalization of the anti-EDA F8 antibody with cemadotin, a tubulin inhibitor [76]. A thiol derivative of this dolastatin analogue, with low-nanomolar cytotoxic activity, was coupled in a site-specific manner to two C-terminal Cys residues of the F8 antibody in SIP format. The resulting ADC showed a drug-antibody ratio (DAR) of 2 and the disulfide linker displayed acceptable stability in mouse plasma (half-life of approximately 48 h). On the other hand, the ADC incubation with glutathione resulted in a fast and "traceless" release of the drug in its active thiol form. Therapy experiments performed in immunocompetent mice, subcutaneously grafted with F9 teratocarcinoma cells, showed a substantial tumor growth inhibition. Most probably, the disulfide linker can be cleaved by glutathione [77], which is released from apoptotic cells, promoting an exponential increase of the free payload concentration in the tumor environment. However, despite the high dose (43 mg/kg) and the frequent administration schedule, no complete responses were observed, suggesting that more potent cytotoxic payloads should be used. Indeed, the maytansinoid DM1 payload led to the generation of more potent ADC products based on the F8 antibody [78]. As for cemadotin, DM1 was connected to the SIP(F8) antibody through a cleavable disulfide linker and administered to immunocompetent mice bearing different cancer models (e.g., F9 teratocarcinomas and CT26 colon carcinoma). When administered in three doses of 7 mg/kg, the SIP(F8)-SS-DM1 ADC cured 60% of the treated mice bearing F9 tumors, but not mice bearing the CT26 carcinoma model. These data reflected the 100-fold higher *in vitro* cytotoxicity of free DM1 against F9 cells, as compared to the CT26 cell line. This correlation between the *in vitro* and *in vivo* observations suggested that the tumor cells, rather than the endothelial cells, may be the primary target for the activity of the ADC, despite the selective expression of the EDA antigen around tumor blood vessels.

Coupling of the DM1 payload to F8 did not alter biodistribution profiles when the antibody was used in IgG or SIP format. However, the stability of disulfide linkers was substantially longer for ADC products based on the IgG format [79]. The longer residence time of IgG(F8)-SS-DM1 in the tumor did not result in better anticancer properties. A comparative evaluation of IgG(F8)-SS-DM1 and SIP(F8)-SS-DM1, administered to tumor-bearing mice in equimolar doses, revealed a more potent anti-cancer activity for the ADC product in SIP format, even though the IgG product exhibited a slower clearance and a higher tumor accumulation. These data suggest that a suitable (i.e., not too slow) rate of drug release in the tumor environment may be beneficial, in order to expose malignant cells to sufficiently high concentrations of the cytotoxic agent.

The F16 antibody, specific to the A1 extra-domain of tenascin C, has been also investigated as vehicle for cytotoxic agents in both IgG and SIP format. In particular, the antibodies were equipped with the microtubule-disrupting agent monomethyl auristatin E (MMAE) and the protease-sensitive linker Val-Cit [80]. Also in this case, the IgG antibody showed higher absolute accumulation in three different tumor models (A431, U87 and MDA MB 231) as compared to its SIP counterpart. The latter product, however, displayed better tumor/organ ratios, as a result of an efficient tumor uptake combined with a rapid clearance from blood and normal tissues. The administration of IgG(F16)-Val-Cit-MMAE led to complete tumor eradication in mice, bearing either A431 or U87 human tumors. Mice treated with SIP(F16)-Val-Cit-MMAE experienced a significant and prolonged tumor regression, but tumors eventually started growing again. The different anticancer properties of the ADC products based on the two formats may be explained by considering that: (i) the highly stabile peptide linker is compatible with the long half-life in circulation of the IgG-formatted ADC; (ii) the IgG shows a higher absolute accumulation in the tumor than the SIP analogue (i.e., %ID/g of ca. 30 and 10 at 24 h, respectively) indicating that large quantities of payload are necessary to achieve complete response. More recently, other peptide linkers have been investigated for the delivery of MMAE from the IgG(F16) antibody, with the Val-Ala sequence showing similar anticancer activity and *in vivo* metabolic profile to the Val-Cit counterpart [81]. The Val-Cit-MMAE module represents the linker-payload combination used in the approved pharmaceutical product brentuximab vedotin (Adcetris™) and in many others ADCs which are currently in clinical development [16]. Historically, the Val-Cit peptide had been designed as a protease-sensitive linker for products based on internalizing antibodies [82]. The linker should be sufficiently stable in circulation, while being efficiently cleaved by certain intracellular proteases (in particular, cathepsin B) after receptor-mediated endocytosis. This mechanism is supported by *in vitro* cytotoxicity data, whereby only antigen-positive cell lines were efficiently killed by the cognate ADC product [83]. However, the evaluation of the F16-Val-Cit-MMAE product revealed that a more complex series of events may occur *in vivo*, involving an extracellular cleavage and release of the linker-payload combinations.

Improving the Potency and Selectivity of Non-internalizing ADC Products

All three moieties in ADC products (antibody, linker and payload) contribute to activity and selectivity. When non-internalizing antibodies are used, lipophilic payloads capable of rapid diffusion through the cell membrane may be preferred. While proteolytic degradation of the antibody moiety may be a release mechanism for internalizing products with non-cleavable linkers, this option does not apply for agents with long residence in the extracellular space [84]. Non-cleavable linkers have gained increasing research interest in the recent past, also in light of the approval of T-DM1 (Kadcyla™), a product that relies on this technology. The use of non-cleavable linkers is, in principle, attractive for very hydrophilic payloads, as one would expect to confine the cytotoxic agent either to the extracellular space (in which it would not be toxic) or to those cells capable of target-based antibody internalization. Unfortunately, *in vitro* experiments provide insufficient information regarding antigen accessibility and accumulation at the tumor site *in vivo*. Quantitative biodistribution experiments may be combined with other investigations (e.g., plasma stability and immunohistochemistry), in order to gain a detailed information regarding the mechanism of action of ADC products. Other structural innovations in the ADC field, such as the use of polymeric linkers, may result compatible with the use of non-internalizing mAbs. These highly functionalized linkers allow the macromolecule labelling with a large number of cytotoxic payloads (DAR > 10). While high DARs have often been associated to poor pharmacokinetic properties [85], the hydrophilic nature of these biodegradable polymers has shown favorable plasma PK profiles [86]. However, the potential immunogenicity of these highly functionalized structures may represent an important aspect during clinical investigations.

The use of ADC products may benefit from combination with immunostimulatory drugs. In the recent past, immune-mediated cancer treatment has become an important area of pharmaceutical oncology, thanks to the clinical advance of immunological checkpoint inhibitors, immunocytokines, bispecific antibodies, CAR T cells, vaccines and other products. There are different pathways that may lead to cancer cell death, upon exposure to different types of cytotoxic agents. Some drugs are particularly active for dendritic cell activation and in promoting immunogenic cell death. It is still not clear how tubulin drugs promote direct activation of dendritic cells. Anthracyclines and other DNA-targeting cytotoxics have been found to promote the expression of the so-called damage-associated molecular patterns (DAMPs) [87, 88]. When certain markers (e.g., calreticulin, HMGB1, ATP and type I interferon) are released into the extracellular environment by dying cells, they may stimulate dendritic cell maturation and activation, leading to an increased infiltration of $CD8^+$ T cells into the tumor mass, followed by cytotoxic activity. In many instances, immunological check-point inhibitors (e.g., anti-PD-1 antibodies) are used in patients that had progressed after treatment with conventional anti-cancer drugs, but use of pembrolizumab or nivolumab in first line is becoming more and more frequent [89, 90]. The use of ADC products in combination with certain immunotherapeutic agents can lead to synergistic activity, as damage to cancer cells may result in improved antigen presentation (with subsequent recognition by $CD8^+$ T cells) or surface expression of proteins such as MIC-A, which trigger NK cell activation through NKG2D receptors [91, 92]. Specifically, it would be interesting to understand whether non-internalizing ADC products could give significant advantages over internalizing analogues in enhancing the activity of the immunotherapeutic partner. Indeed, considering the more widespread cytotoxic action that non-internalizing ADCs could promote in the tumor microenvironment, a more heterogeneous area of the solid mass could efficiently lead to inflammation and to an increase of the population of infiltrating lymphocytes in the tumor mass. It is now becoming increasingly evident that this process, often described as the conversion of "immunologically cold" tumors into "hot", is a key parameter to extend the efficacy of immunotherapy to a larger number of patients and indications [93].

Conclusions and Outlook

The possibility to develop non-internalizing ADCs is, by now, firmly established, at least at the preclinical level. Splice isoforms of tenascin-C and of fibronectin represent ideal targets for pharmacodelivery applications, but it is possible that other tumor-associated antigens may be considered [94]. ECM components offer unique opportunities for pharmacodelivery applications, as these targets are often abundant and stable, thus allowing a long residence time of ADC products at the tumor site. The field of ADC research, both for internalizing and non-internalizing products, will continue to face an important scientific challenge, namely the translation of preclinical data into a prediction of efficacy in patients.

In this context, the therapeutic widows of marketed ADC products were found to be much smaller in human patients than in rodents. For instance, while early clinical studies of MMAE-based ADCs reported MTD values between 1.2 and 2.4 mg/kg [95], administrations of Tenfold higher doses are commonly well tolerated in mice. This important aspect is due to several factors (e.g., the different tumor size in mice and humans, the number of antigen copies in the tumor and their accessibility by ADCs, etc.) and it limits the progression of promising ADC candidates through the clinical stages. The pharmaceutical relevance of this "bottleneck" is reflected in the fact that only two ADC products are currently available on the market, whereas more than 40 ADC candidates are currently being investigated in clinical trials [96]. The use of tumor-associated ECM proteins as targets for ADC development takes the internalization process out of the mechanism of action, thus potentially promoting an easier and more rational design of future ADC products.

One of the most challenging issues for future developments in the ADC field relates to the quantification of product uptake in mouse and man, as well as to the comparative evaluation of drug release kinetics in different species. In particular, a quantitative evaluation of the targeting properties of ADCs in human patients is often missing, which negatively impacts on the clinical development of drug candidates. In principle, initial information about antibody biodistribution, pharmacokinetics, tumor targeting properties and interpatient variability could be obtained from microdosing (phase 0) PET clinical studies [73]. However, these trials are normally performed with drug dosages that are substantially lower than the ones used for therapy purposes. A more systematic and accurate use of imaging techniques for the analysis of antibody performances in patients, as well as the real-time monitoring of ADC fragments at preclinical level (e.g. through the labeling of drug and antibody with different radioisotopes) [97], may provide important insights for the optimal pharmaceutical development of targeted cytotoxics.

In summary, while most academic and industrial efforts have so far been devoted to the development of internalizing ADC products, there is a strong rationale for the design and optimization of antibody-drug conjugates, which do not directly internalize into the target cells. ADC products directed against splice isoforms of fibronectin and tenascin-C are particularly attractive, as those targets are abundantly expressed in the majority of solid tumors and lymphomas, while being virtually undetectable in the majority of normal adult tissues.

References

1. (a) van der Veldt AA, Hendrikse NH, Smit EF, Mooijer MP, Rijnders AY, Gerritsen WR, et al (2010) Biodistribution and radiation dosimetry of 11C-labelled docetaxel in cancer patients. Eur J Nucl Med Mol Imaging 37:1950–1958; (b) van der Veldt AA, Lubberink M, Mathijssen RH, Loos WJ, Herder GJ, Greuter HN, et al (2013) Toward prediction of efficacy of chemotherapy: a proof of concept study in lung cancer patients using 11C-docetaxel and positron emission tomography. Clin Canc Res 19:4163–4173; (c) Kesner AL, Hsueh WA, Htet NL, Pio BS, Czernin J, Pegram MD, et al (2007) Biodistribution and predictive value of 18F-fluorocyclophosphamide in mice bearing human breast cancer xenografts. J Nucl Med 48:2021–2027; (d) Abe Y, Fukuda H, Ishiwata K, Yoshioka S, Yamada K, Endo S, et al (1983) Studies on 18F-labeled pyrimidines. Tumor uptakes of 18F-5-fluorouracil, 18F-5-fluorouridine, and 18F-5-fluorodeoxyuridine in animals. Eur J Nucl Med 8:258–261; (e) Kuchar M, Oliveira MC, Gano L, Santos I, Kniess T (2012) Radioiodinated sunitinib as a potential radiotracer for imaging angiogenesis-radiosynthesis and first radiopharmacological evaluation of 5-[125I] Iodo-sunitinib. Bioorg Med Chem Lett 22:2850–2855
2. (a) Senter PD (2009) Potent antibody drug conjugates for cancer therapy. Curr Opin Chem Biol 13:235–244; (b) Srinivasarao M, Galliford CV, Low PS (2015) Principles in the design of ligand-targeted cancer therapeutics and imaging agents. Nat Rev Drug Disc 14:203–219; (c) Krall N, Scheuermann J, Neri D (2013) Small targeted cytotoxics: current state and promises from DNA-encoded chemical libraries. Angew Chem Int Ed 52:1384–1402
3. (a) Gurcan HM, Keskin DB, Stern JN, Nitzberg MA, Shekhani H, Ahmed AR (2009) A review of the current use of rituximab in autoimmune diseases. Int Immunopharmacol 9:10–25; (b) Wu AM, Senter PD (2005) Arming antibodies: prospects and challenges for immunoconjugates. Nat Biotechnol 23:1137–1146; (c) Carter P (2001) Improving the efficacy of antibody-based cancer therapies. Nat Rev Cancer 1:118–129
4. Kim EG, Kim KM (2015) Strategies and advancement in antibody-drug conjugate optimization for targeted Cancer therapeutics. Biomol Ther 23:493–509
5. Ricart AD, Tolcher AW (2007) Technology insight: cytotoxic drug immunoconjugates for cancer therapy. Nat Clin Pract Oncol 4:245–255
6. Dennis MS, Jin H, Dugger D, Yang R, McFarland L, Ogasawara A et al (2007) Imaging tumors with an albumin-binding fab, a novel tumor-targeting agent. Cancer Res 67:254–261
7. (a) Gerber HP, Senter PD, Grewal IS (2009) Antibody drug-conjugates targeting the tumor vasculature: Current and future developments. mAbs 1:247–253;(b) Teicher BA, Chari RV (2011) Antibody conjugate therapeutics: challenges and potential. Clin. Canc. Res. 7:6389-6397; (c) Sievers EL, Senter PD (2013) Antibody-drug conjugates in cancer therapy. Annu. Rev. Med. 64:15-29; d) Chari RV, Miller ML, Widdison WC (2014) Antibody-drug conjugates: an emerging concept in cancer therapy. Angew Chem Int Ed 53:3796–3827
8. Lambert JM (2013) Drug-conjugated antibodies for the treatment of cancer. Br J Clin Pharmacol 76:248–262
9. Gamcsik MP, Kasibhatla MS, Teeter SD, Colvin OM (2012) Glutathione levels in human tumors. Biomarkers 17:671–691
10. Mills BJ, Lang CA (1992) Differential distribution of free and bound glutathione and cysteine in human blood. Biochem Pharmacol 52:401–406
11. (a) Thorpe PE, Wallace PM, Knowles PP, Relf MG, Brown AN, Watson GJ, Knyba RE, Wawrzynczak EJ, Blakey DC (1987) New coupling agents for the synthesis of immunotoxins containing a hindered disulfide bond with improved stability in vivo. Cancer Res 47:5924–5931;(b) Kellogg BA, Garrett L, Kovtun Y, Lai KC, Leece B, Miller M, et al (2011) Disulfide-linked antibody-maytansinoid conjugates: optimization of in vivo activity by varying the steric hindrance at carbon atoms adjacent to the disulfide linkage. Bioconjugate Chem 22:717–727
12. Kovtun YV, Audette CA, Mayo MF, Jones GE, Doherty H, Maloney EK et al (2010) Antibody-maytansinoid conjugates designed to bypass multidrug resistance. Cancer Res 70:2528–2537

13. Zucker S (1988) A critical appraisal of the role of proteolytic enzymes in Cancer invasion: emphasis on tumor surface proteinases. Cancer Investig 6:219–231
14. Choi KY, Swierczewska M, Lee S, Chen X (2012) Protease-activated drug development. Theranostics 2:156–178
15. Senter PD, Sievers EL (2012) The discovery and development of brentuximab vedotin for use in relapsed Hodgkin lymphoma and systemic anaplastic large cell lymphoma. Nat Biotechnol 30:631–637
16. Jain N, Smith SW, Ghone S, Tomczuk B (2015) Current ADC linker chemistry. Pharm Res 32:3526–3540
17. Polson AG, Calemine-Fenaux J, Chan P, Chang W, Christensen E, Clark S et al (2009) Antibody-drug conjugates for the treatment of non-Hodgkin's lymphoma: target and linker-drug selection. Cancer Res 69:2358–2364
18. Hong EE, Erickson H, Lutz RJ, Whiteman KR, Jones G, Kovtun Y et al (2015) Design of Coltuximab Ravtansine, a CD19-targeting antibody-drug conjugate (ADC) for the treatment of B-cell malignancies: structure-activity relationships and preclinical evaluation. Mol Pharm 12:1703–1716
19. Armitage JO, Gascoyne RD, Lunning MA, Cavalli F (2017) Non-Hodgkin lymphoma. Lancet 390:298
20. Press OW, Farr AG, Borroz KI, Anderson SK, Martin PJ (1989) Endocytosis and degradation of monoclonal antibodies targeting human B-cell malignancies. Cancer Res 49:4906–4912
21. Dijoseph JF, Dougher MM, Armellino DC, Kalyandrug L, Kunz A, Boghaert ER et al (2007) CD20-specific antibody-targeted chemotherapy of non-Hodgkin's B-cell lymphoma using calicheamicin-conjugated rituximab. Cancer Immunol Immunother 56:1107–1117
22. Li F, Emmerton KK, Jonas M, Zhang X, Miyamoto JB et al (2016) Intracellular released payload influences potency and bystander-killing effects of antibody-drug conjugates in preclinical models. Cancer Res 76:2710–2719
23. Bui MH, Seligson D, Han KR, Pantuck AJ, Dorey FJ, Huang Y et al (2003) Carbonic anhydrase IX is an independent predictor of survival in advanced renal clear cell carcinoma: implications for prognosis and therapy. Clin Cancer Res 9:802–811
24. Wykoff CC, Beasley NJ, Watson PH, Turner KJ, Pastorek J, Sibtain A et al (2000) Hypoxia-inducible expression of tumor-associated carbonic anhydrases. Cancer Res 60:7075–7083
25. Thiry A, Dogne JM, Masereel B, Supuran CT (2006) Targeting tumor-associated carbonic anhydrase IX in cancer therapy. Trends Pharmacol Sci 27:566–573
26. Krall N, Pretto F, Decurtins W, Bernardes GJ, Supuran CT, Neri D (2014) A small-molecule drug conjugate for the treatment of carbonic anhydrase IX expressing tumors. Angew Chem Int Ed 53:4231–4235
27. (a) Cazzamalli S, Dal Corso A, Neri D (2016) Acetazolamide serves as selective delivery vehicle for dipeptide-linked drugs to renal cell carcinoma. Mol Cancer Ther 15:2926-2935; (b) Cazzamalli S, Dal Corso A, Neri D (2017) Linker stability influences the anti-tumor activity of acetazolamide-drug conjugates for the therapy of renal cell carcinoma. J Control Release 246:39–45
28. Petrul HM, Schatz CA, Kopitz CC, Adnane L, TJ MC, Trail P et al (2012) Therapeutic mechanism and efficacy of the antibody-drug conjugate BAY 79-4620 targeting human carbonic anhydrase 9. Mol Cancer Ther 11:340–349
29. Clinical Study Report No. PH-37705, BAY 79-4620 / 12671: Bayer HealthCare (2014)
30. Nagy JA, Brown LF, Senger DR, Lanir N, Van de Water L, Dvorak AM et al (1989) Pathogenesis of tumor stroma generation: a critical role for leaky blood vessels and fibrin deposition. Biochim Biophys Acta 948:305–326
31. Dvorak HF, Dvorak AM, Manseau EJ, Wiberg L, Churchill WH (1979) Fibrin gel investment associated with line 1 and line 10 solid tumor growth, angiogenesis, and fibroplasia in Guinea pigs. Role of cellular immunity, myofibroblasts, microvascular damage, and infarction in line 1 tumor regression. J Natl Cancer Inst 62:1459–1472

32. Dvorak HF (1986) Tumors: wounds that do not heal. Similarities between tumor stroma generation and wound healing. N Engl J Med 315:1650–1659
33. Yasunaga M, Manabe S, Matsumura Y (2011) New concept of cytotoxic immunoconjugate therapy targeting cancer-induced fibrin clots. Cancer Sci 102:1396–1402
34. Yasunaga M, Manabe S, Tarin D, Matsumura Y (2011) Cancer-stroma targeting therapy by cytotoxic immunoconjugate bound to the collagen 4 network in the tumor tissue. Bioconjug Chem 22:1776–1783
35. Huber MA, Kraut N, Beug H (2005) Molecular requirements for epithelial-mesenchymal transition during tumor progression. Curr Opin Cell Biol 17:548–558
36. Joyce JA (2005) Therapeutic targeting of the tumor microenvironment. Cancer Cell 7:513–520
37. (a) Scanlan MJ, Raj BK, Calvo B, Garin-Chesa P, Sanz-Moncasi MP, Healey JH, et al (1994) Molecular cloning of fibroblast activation protein alpha, a member of the serine protease family selectively expressed in stromal fibroblasts of epithelial cancers. Proc Natl Acad Sci USA. 91:5657–5661;(b) Rettig WJ, Garin-Chesa P, Beresford HR, Oettgen HF, Melamed MR, Old LJ. (1988) Cell-surface glycoproteins of human sarcomas: differential expression in normal and malignant tissues and cultured cells. Proc Natl Acad Sci USA 85:3110–3114; (c) Rettig WJ, Garin-Chesa P, Healey JH, Su SL, Ozer HL, Schwab M, et al (1993) Regulation and heteromeric structure of the fibroblast activation protein in normal and transformed cells of mesenchymal and neuroectodermal origin. Cancer Res 53:3327–3335
38. (a) Welt S, Divgi CR, Scott AM, Garin-Chesa P, Finn RD, Graham M, et al (1994) Antibody targeting in metastatic colon cancer: a phase I study of monoclonal antibody F19 against a cell-surface protein of reactive tumor stromal fibroblasts. J Clin Oncol 12:1193–1203; (b) Hofheinz RD, al-Batran SE, Hartmann F, Hartung G, Jager D, Renner C, et al (2003) Stromal antigen targeting by a humanised monoclonal antibody: an early phase II trial of sibrotuzumab in patients with metastatic colorectal cancer. Onkologie 26:44–48; (c) Scott AM, Wiseman G, Welt S, Adjei A, Lee FT, Hopkins W, et al (2003) A Phase I dose-escalation study of sibrotuzumab in patients with advanced or metastatic fibroblast activation protein-positive cancer. Clin Cancer Res. 9:1639–1647
39. Ostermann E, Garin-Chesa P, Heider KH, Kalat M, Lamche H, Puri C et al (2008) Effective immunoconjugate therapy in cancer models targeting a serine protease of tumor fibroblasts. Clin Cancer Res 14:4584–4592
40. Satoh K, Hata M, Yokota H (2002) A novel member of the leucine-rich repeat superfamily induced in rat astrocytes by beta-amyloid. Biochem Biophys Res Commun 290:756–762
41. Satoh K, Hata M, Yokota H (2004) High lib mRNA expression in breast carcinomas. DNA Res 11:199–203
42. Stanbrough M, Bubley GJ, Ross K, Golub TR, Rubin MA, Penning TM, Febbo PG, Balk SP (2006) Increased expression of genes converting adrenal androgens to testosterone in androgen-independent prostate cancer. Cancer Res 66:2815–2825
43. Gish KC, Hickson JA, Purcell JW, Morgan-Lappe SE (2015) Anti-huLRRC15 Antibody Drug Conjugates and methods for their use. WO2017095805A1
44. Hanahan D, Weinberg RA (2011) Hallmarks of cancer: the next generation. Cell 144:646–674
45. Gatenby RA, Gillies RJ (2004) Why do cancers have high aerobic glycolysis? Nat Rev Cancer 4:891–899
46. Swietach P, Vaughan-Jones RD, Harris AL, Hulikova A (2014) The chemistry, physiology and pathology of pH in cancer. Philos Trans R Soc B 369:–20130099
47. (a) Yamada K, Nomura N, Yamano A, Yamada Y, Wakamatsu N (2012) Identification and characterization of splicing variants of PLEKHA5 (Plekha5) during brain development. Gene 492:270–275;(b) Yousaf N, Deng Y, Kang Y, Riede H (2001) Four PSM/SH2-B alternative splice variants and their differential roles in mitogenesis. J Biol Chem 276:40940–40948
48. Ladomery M (2013) Aberrant alternative splicing is another hallmark of cancer. Int J Cell Biol 2013:463786
49. Venables JP (2004) Aberrant and alternative splicing in cancer. Cancer Res 64:7647–7654
50. Oltean S, Bates DO (2014) Hallmarks of alternative splicing in cancer. Oncogene 33:5311–5318

51. Elias AP, Dias S (2008) Microenvironment changes (in pH) affect VEGF alternative splicing. Cancer Microenviron 1:131–139
52. Gaus G, Demir-Weusten AY, Schmitz U, Bose P, Kaufmann P, Huppertz B, Frank HG (2002) Extracellular pH modulates the secretion of fibronectin isoforms by human trophoblast. Acta Histochem 104:51–63
53. Borsi L, Allemanni G, Gaggero B, Zardi L (1996) Extracellular pH controls pre-mRNA alternative splicing of tenascin-C in normal, but not in malignantly transformed, cells. Int J Cancer 66:632–635
54. Hynes RO, Yamada KM (1982) Fibronectins: multifunctional modular glycoproteins. J Cell Biol 95:369–377
55. Colombi M, Barlati S, Kornblihtt A, Baralle FE, Vaheri A (1986) A family of fibronectin mRNAs in human normal and transformed cells. Biochim Biophys Acta 868:207–214
56. Paul JI, Schwarzbauer JE, Tamkun JW, Hynes RO (1986) Cell-type-specific fibronectin subunits generated by alternative splicing. J Biol Chem 261:12258–12265
57. (a) Borsi L, Carnemolla B, Castellani P, Rosellini C, et al (1987) Monoclonal antibodies in the analysis of fibronectin isoforms generated by alternative splicing of mRNA precursors in normal and transformed human cells. J Cell Biol 104:595–600;(b) Zardi L1, Carnemolla B, Siri A, Petersen TE, et al (1987) Transformed human cells produce a new fibronectin isoform by preferential alternative splicing of a previously unobserved exon. EMBO J 6:2337–2342
58. Castellani P, Viale G, Dorcaratto A, Nicolo G, Kaczmarek J, Querze G, Zardi L (1994) The fibronectin isoform containing the ED-B oncofetal domain: a marker of angiogenesis. Int J Cancer 5:612–618
59. Carnemolla B, Balza E, Siri A, Zardi L, Nicotra MR, Bigotti A, Natali PG (1989) A tumor-associated fibronectin isoform generated by alternative splicing of messenger RNA precursors. J Cell Biol 108:1139–1148
60. Borsi L, Castellani P, Allemanni G, Neri D, Zardi L (1998) Preparation of phage antibodies to the ED-A domain of human fibronectin. Exp Cell Res 240:244–251
61. Matsuura H, Hakomori S (1985) The oncofetal domain of fibronectin defined by monoclonal antibody FDC-6: its presence in fibronectins from fetal and tumor tissues and its absence in those from normal adult tissues and plasma. Proc Natl Acad Sci U S A 82:6517–6521
62. Kumra H, Reinhardt DP (2016) Fibronectin-targeted drug delivery in cancer. Adv Drug Deliv Rev 97:101–110
63. Erickson HP (1989) Tenascin: an extracellular matrix protein prominent in specialized embryonic tissues and tumors. Annu Rev Cell Biol 5:71–92
64. Sage EH, Bornstein P (1991) Extracellular proteins that modulate cell-matrix interactions. SPARC, tenascin, and thrombospondin. J Biol Chem 23:14831–14834
65. Borsi L, Balza E, Gaggero B, Allemagni I, Zardi L (1995) The alternative splicing pattern of the tenascin-C pre-mRNA is controlled by the extracellular pH. J Biol Chem 270:6243–6245
66. Reardon DA, Akabani G, Coleman RE, Friedman AH et al (2002) Phase II trial of murine (131) I-labeled antitenascin monoclonal antibody 81C6 administered into surgically created resection cavities of patients with newly diagnosed malignant gliomas. J Clin Oncol 20:1389–1397
67. Rizzieri DA, Akabani G, Zalutsky MR, Coleman RE et al (2004) Phase 1 trial study of 131I-labeled chimeric 81C6 monoclonal antibody for the treatment of patients with non-Hodgkin lymphoma. Blood 104:642–648
68. Pini A, Viti F, Santucci A, Carnemolla B, Zardi L, Neri P, Neri D (1998) Design and use of a phage display library. Human antibodies with subnanomolar affinity against a marker of angiogenesis eluted from a two-dimensional gel. J Biol Chem 21:21769–21776
69. Brack SS, Silacci M, Birchler M, Neri D (2006) Tumor-targeting properties of novel antibodies specific to the large isoform of tenascin-C. Clin Cancer Res 12:3200–3208
70. Borsi L, Balza E, Bestagno M, Castellani P, Carnemolla B et al (2002) Selective targeting of tumoral vasculature: comparison of different formats of an antibody (L19) to the ED-B domain of fibronectin. Int J Cancer 102:75–85

71. Sauer S, Erba PA, Petrini M, Menrad A et al (eds) (2009) Expression of the oncofetal ED-B-containing fibronectin isoform in hematologic tumors enables ED-B-targeted 131I-L19SIP radioimmunotherapy in Hodgkin lymphoma patients. Blood 113:2265–2274
72. Aloj L, D'Ambrosio L, Aurilio M, Morisco A et al (2014) Radioimmunotherapy with Tenarad, a 131I-labelled antibody fragment targeting the extra-domain A1 of tenascin-C, in patients with refractory Hodgkin's lymphoma. Eur J Nucl Med Mol Imaging 41:867–877
73. Heuveling DA, de Bree R, Vugts DJ, Huisman MC, Giovannoni L, Hoekstra OS, Leemans CR, Neri D, van Dongen GA (2013) Phase 0 microdosing PET study using the human mini antibody F16SIP in head and neck cancer patients. J Nucl Med 54:397–401
74. Villa A, Trachsel E, Kaspar M, Schliemann C, Sommavilla R, Rybak JN, Rösli C, Borsi L, Neri D (2008) A high-affinity human monoclonal antibody specific to the alternatively spliced EDA domain of fibronectin efficiently targets tumor neo-vasculature *in vivo*. Int J Cancer 122:2405–2413
75. Schwager K, Kaspar M, Bootz F, Marcolongo R, Paresce E, Neri D, Trachsel E (2009) Preclinical characterization of DEKAVIL (F8-IL10), a novel clinical-stage immunocytokine which inhibits the progression of collagen-induced arthritis. Arthritis Res Ther 11:R142
76. Bernardes GJ, Casi G, Trüssel S, Hartmann I, Schwager K, Scheuermann J, Neri D (2012) A traceless vascular-targeting antibody-drug conjugate for cancer therapy. Angew Chem Int Ed 51:941–944
77. Austin CD, Wen X, Gazzard L, Nelson C, Scheller RH, Scales SJ (2005) Oxidizing potential of endosomes and lysosomes limits intracellular cleavage of disulfide-based antibody-drug conjugates. Proc Natl Acad Sci U S A 102:17987–17992
78. Perrino E, Steiner M, Krall N, Bernardes GJ, Pretto F, Casi G, Neri D (2014) Curative properties of noninternalizing antibody-drug conjugates based on maytansinoids. Cancer Res 74:2569–2578
79. Gébleux R, Wulhfard S, Casi G, Neri D (2015) Antibody format and drug release rate determine the therapeutic activity of noninternalizing antibody-drug conjugates. Mol Cancer Ther 14:2606–2612
80. Gébleux R, Stringhini M, Casanova R, Soltermann A, Neri D (2016) Non-internalizing antibody-drug conjugates display potent anti-cancer activity upon proteolytic release of monomethyl auristatin E in the subendothelial extracellular matrix. Int J Cancer 140:1670–1679
81. Dal Corso A, Cazzamalli S, Gébleux R, Mattarella M, Neri D (2017) Protease-cleavable linkers modulate the anticancer activity of noninternalizing antibody-drug conjugates. Bioconjug Chem 28:1826–1833
82. Doronina SO, Toki BE, Torgov MY, Mendelsohn BA, Cerveny CG et al (2003) Development of potent monoclonal antibody auristatin conjugates for cancer therapy. Nat Biotechnol 21:778–784
83. Dal Corso A, Pignataro L, Belvisi L, Gennari C (2016) αvβ3 integrin-targeted peptide/Peptidomimetic-drug conjugates: in-depth analysis of the linker technology. Curr Top Med Chem 16:314–329
84. Verma VA, Pillow TH, DePalatis L, Li G, Phillips GL, Polson AG, Raab HE, Spencer S, Zheng B (2015) The cryptophycins as potent payloads for antibody drug conjugates. Bioorg Med Chem Lett 25:864–868
85. Sun X, Ponte JF, Yoder NC, Laleau R, Coccia J et al (2017) Effects of drug-antibody ratio on pharmacokinetics, biodistribution, efficacy, and tolerability of antibody-Maytansinoid conjugates. Bioconjug Chem 28:1371–1381
86. Yurkovetskiy AV, Yin M, Bodyak N, Stevenson CA, Thomas JD et al (2015) A polymer-based antibody-Vinca drug conjugate platform: characterization and preclinical efficacy. Cancer Res 75:3365–3372
87. Bianchi ME (2014) Killing cancer cells, twice with one shot. Cell Death Differ 21:1–2
88. Gerber HP, Sapra P, Loganzo F, May C (2016) Combining antibody-drug conjugates and immune-mediated cancer therapy: what to expect? Biochem Pharmacol 12:1–6

89. Litterman AJ, Zellmer DM, Grinnen KL, Hunt MA, Dudek AZ, Salazar AM, Ohlfest JR (2013) Profound impairment of adaptive immune responses by alkylating chemotherapy. J Immunol 190:6259–6268
90. Mahoney KM, Rennert PD, Freeman GJ (2015) Combination cancer immunotherapy and new immunomodulatory targets. Nat Rev Drug Discov 14:561–584
91. List T, Casi G, Neri D (2014) A chemically defined Trifunctional antibody-cytokine-drug conjugate with potent antitumor activity. Mol Cancer Ther 13:2641–2652
92. Gutbrodt KL, Schliemann C, Giovannoni L, Frey K, Pabst T, Klapper W, Berdel WE, Neri D (2013) Antibody-based delivery of Interleukin-2 to Neovasculature has potent activity against acute myeloid leukemia. Sci Transl Med 5:201ra118
93. Sharma P, Hu-Lieskovan S, Wargo JA, Ribas A (2017) Primary, adaptive, and acquired resistance to Cancer immunotherapy. Cell 168:707–723
94. Hynes RO (2014) Stretching the boundaries of extracellular matrix research. Nat Rev Mol Cell Biol 15:761–763
95. Donaghy H (2016) Effects of antibody, drug and linker on the preclinical and clinical toxicities of antibody-drug conjugates. MAbs 8:659–671
96. Bakhtiar R (2016) Antibody drug conjugates. Biotechnol Lett 38:1655–1664
97. Cohen R, Vugts DJ, Visser GW, Stigter-van Walsum M et al (2014) Development of novel ADCs: conjugation of tubulysin analogues to trastuzumab monitored by dual radiolabeling. Cancer Res 74:5700–5710

Next Horizons: ADCs Beyond Oncology

Shan Yu, Andrew Lim, and Matthew S. Tremblay

Abstract Most ADCs developed thus far have been explored for oncology indications. Emerging ADC technologies present many opportunities to apply the modality beyond oncology. The key variables for oncology ADCs in terms of the targeted cell type, targeting strategy, and payload are often clearer while the corresponding elements for non-oncology indications are more complex. Challenges in designing such non-oncology ADCs include selecting the targeting cell type(s) from among potentially several contributing to the disease, a distinct surface marker expressed on the targeting cells, which often overlaps healthy cells, and a potent, non-cytotoxic payload drug. So far, only a few ADCs were designed for non-oncology indications, with none yet successfully progressing through clinical trials. Here, we summarize those that have been reported. In addition, we discuss some considerations to be taken into account for designing ADCs for non-oncology indications, including payload and antibody selection. With the evolution of ADC platform and technology, more ADCs for non-oncology indications are yet to be developed.

Keywords Non-oncology ADC · Inflammation · Anti-inflammatory · Steroid · Anti-infective · Antibiotic · Antibiotic-antibody conjugate · Payload selection · Antigen selection · Antibody-drug conjugate

As extensively reviewed elsewhere in this edition, antibody-drug conjugates (ADCs) have been an intense focus of research into targeted oncology therapies with improved selectivity and efficacy, wherein monoclonal antibodies are used to selectively deliver potent cytotoxic agents to antigen-expressing tumor cells, with several such agents translating successfully into human clinical efficacy. However, very few studies have extended the ADC paradigm outside the field of oncology with non-cytotoxic small molecules. Given the seeming generality and breadth of the

S. Yu · A. Lim · M. S. Tremblay (✉)
California Institute for Biomedical Research (Calibr), La Jolla, CA, USA
e-mail: mtremblay@calibr.org

M. Damelin (ed.), *Innovations for Next-Generation Antibody-Drug Conjugates*, Cancer Drug Discovery and Development,
https://doi.org/10.1007/978-3-319-78154-9_14

technology paradigm, broader disease indications outside of oncology could clearly benefit by delivering intracellular-acting small molecules to target tissues of interest, while enhancing their therapeutic index relative to on-target effects in other tissues. Theoretically, this platform could be developed for any disease wherein pharmacological manipulation is desirable in particular tissue(s) and cell type(s) that express cell surface markers with some degree of selectivity. We will begin this chapter by describing several examples of ADCs developed for non-oncology indications, followed by generalization of certain considerations in payload and antibody selection that are distinct from designing ADCs for oncology indications.

Existing Examples of ADCs for Non-oncology Applications (Table 1)

αCD163-Dexamethasone Conjugate

Synthetic glucocorticoids are potent anti-inflammatory drugs, although their widespread use in chronic disease treatment is limited by serious side effects such as bone mobilization, muscle mass loss, strong immunosuppression, and metabolic dysregulation. The anti-inflammatory effect of glucocorticoids relies on suppressing release of TNF and other cytokines at the inflammatory sites and reducing cell division and survival of immune cells [43].

In order to capture the potent anti-inflammatory effects of glucocorticoids on immune cells (primarily macrophages) and avoid side effects driven by action in other tissue compartments, a biodegradable anti-CD163 antibody conjugated with dexamethasone was generated and characterized [18]. CD163 is a glucocorticoid-regulated surface protein expressed by monocytes and macrophages that imparts various biological functions, including clearance of debris and balancing immune responses [17]. As a scavenger receptor, CD163 mediates the clearance of the hemoglobin-haptoglobin (Hb-Hp) complex from circulation by macrophages to prevent the toxic effect of the heme molecule during hemolysis. As an innate immune response mediator, CD163 internalizes the tumor necrosis factor (TNF)-superfamily cytokine TWEAK to block pro-inflammatory signaling mediated by TWEAK [7, 45]. CD163 also binds to certain viruses and bacteria (e.g. *S. mutans*, *S. aureus*, and *E. coli*), resulting in the initiation of host defense mechanisms and pro-inflammatory signaling, as evidenced by an increase in TNF release [13]. As the expression of CD163 on macrophages is detected at the inflammatory sites of a variety of pro-inflammatory diseases, such as rheumatoid arthritis, inflammatory bowel disease, non-alcoholic steatohepatitis, atherosclerosis, etc. [17, 33, 60], it has been explored as a target of tissue-specific delivery of anti-inflammatory small molecules using ADCs.

To generate the **αCD163-Dexamethasone**, the reaction of an N-hydroxysuccinimide (NHS) ester of a hemisuccinate-modified dexamethasone analog with free amines on an anti-CD163 antibody yielded a conjugate with an average drug-antibody ration (DAR) of four (Fig. 1). The resultant ADC **αCD163-**

Table 1 Summary of emerging ADCs and exemplary constructs for non-oncology indications

Example ADC	Antibody	Drug-linker	Conjugation site	References
αCD163-Dexamethasone (macrophage-targeted)	αCD163 monoclonal antibody Ed-2	Hemisuccinate-NHS ester-Dexamethasone derivative	Surface lysines, DAR ~4	[18]
αCD70-Budesonide (Immune cell-targeted)	Humanized αCD70 2 h5, IgG1	Phosphate containing Budesonide Cathepsin B	Inserted *p*-azido-phenylalanine non-natural amino acid, DAR = 1.9	[25]
αCXCR4-Dasatinib (T cell-targeted)	Humanized IgG1 αCXCR4 antibody	Pentapeptide-SS-dasatinib derivative	Surface lysines, DAR ~3	[70]
αCD11a-LXR agonist (macrophage-targeted)	Humanized αCD11a modified with pAcF	PEG4-Phe-Lys-LXR agonist derivative	Inserted *p*-acetyl-phenylalanine non-natural amino acid, DAR = 2	[35]
αCD11a-PDE4 inhibitor (macrophage-targeted)	Humanized αCD11a modified with pAcF or mouse αCD11a	PEG4-Phe-Lys-LXR agonist or NHS ester-PDE4 inhibitor	Inserted *p*-acetyl-phenylalanine non-natural amino acid, DAR = 2 (for human antibody) and surface lysines, DAR ~3 (for mouse antibody)	[74]
αS. Aureus-Antibiotic (pathogen-targeted)	β-N-acetylglucosamine cell-wall teichoic acid (β-GlcNAc-WTA) antibody	MC-ValCit-PABQ-dmDNA31	Engineered to contain unpaired cysteine residues ("THIOMAB" technology)	[31]

DAR drug-antibody ratio

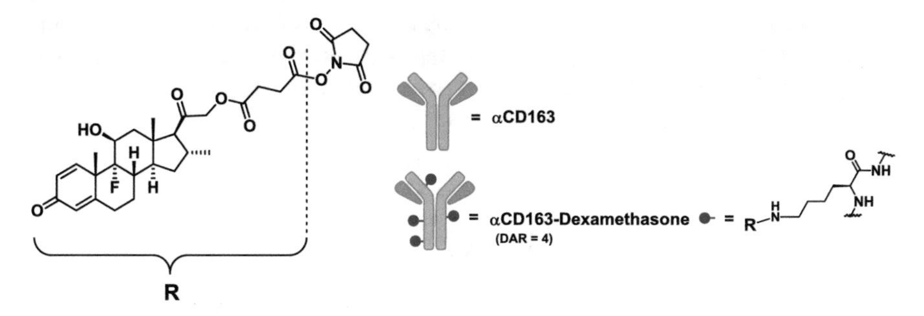

Fig. 1 αCD163-Dexamethasone conjugate

Dexamethasone exhibited a strong anti-inflammatory effect in an *in vivo* rat model using LPS-induced TNF secretion as a readout. In contrast to a strong systemic effect of dexamethasone, the ADC had no such effect as measured by thymocyte apoptosis, body weight loss, and suppression of endogenous cortisol levels, suggesting the side effects were greatly attenuated by this targeted delivery method. In fact, Cytoguide ApS and Affinicon are developing this ADC for non-alcoholic steatohepatitis indication. The authors also proposed that the use of CD163-mediated targeting of macrophages may not be restricted to inflammation, but could be extended to treatment of infectious diseases, where the pathogen uses the macrophage as host cell, CD163-expressing cancers, and lysosomal storage diseases.

αCD70-Budesonide Conjugate

Budesonide is a potent corticosteroid that is available as an inhaler, pill, nasal spray and rectal forms for various inflammatory diseases, including respiratory tract inflammation and inflammatory bowel diseases. The common side effects of long-term systemic exposure to this drug include vomiting, joint pain, loss of bone strength, cataracts and adrenal insufficiency. To expand the potential indications of this drug, budesonide was conjugated to αCD70 antibody, which specifically target a subset of immune cells [25]. CD70 is a type II transmembrane receptor, normally expresses on a subset of B, T and NK cells, where it plays a co-stimulatory role in immune cell activation, while it is also found to be aberrantly elevated in multiple human carcinoma types and tumor-derived cells line [25].

To conjugate Budesonide to αCD70 antibody, a novel, site specific, phosphate based cathepsin B sensitive linker (CatPhos Linker) approach was developed to attach via the aliphatic alcohol of the payload (Fig. 2). These CatPhos linkers were demonstrated to have high stability with human blood, rapid cleavage when incubated with rat lysosomal lysates and good aqueous solubility. A cell-based assay with CD70-expressing 786-O cells measuring glucocorticoid-induced leucine zipper (GILZ) mRNA expression was developed to determine glucocorticoid receptor target engagement by the ADCs carrying budesonide payload. Both **αCD70-Budesonide** ADCs potently induced GILZ mRNA expression, while the negative control ADCs, which had the same drug-linkers but conjugated to αRSV (a Synagis-based antibody), were inactive. This phosphate linker approach provide an alternative approach for internalizing ADC construction as well as other targeted delivery platforms [25].

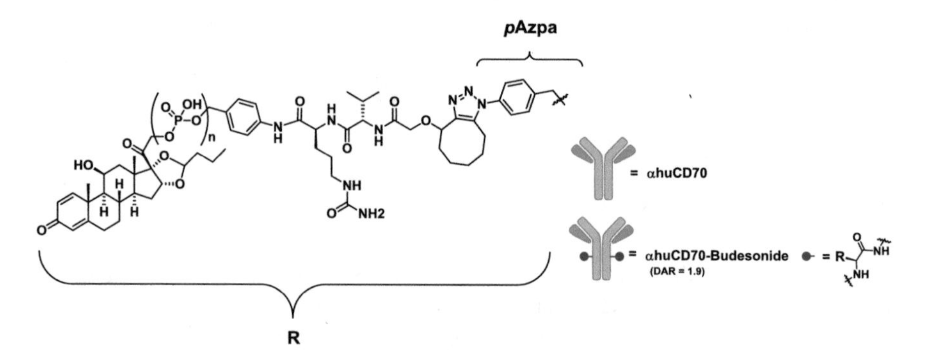

Fig. 2 αCD70-Budesonide conjugate

αCXCR4-Dasatinib Conjugate

Dasatinib (Sprycel®, Bristol-Myers Squibb), a potent inhibitor of the Bcr-Abl and Src families of tyrosine kinases, is an oral drug used to treat chronic myelogenous leukemia and certain forms of acute lymphoblastic leukemia. Dasatinib also potently inhibits the T cell receptor (TCR) signaling kinase Lck and thereby inhibits T cell activation and proliferation [30, 62], suggesting potential utility in T cell-driven autoimmune diseases. However, dasatinib's lack of selectivity for related kinase family members leads to side effects, such as pulmonary arterial hypertension, neutropenia, myelosuppression, diarrhea, peripheral edema, and headache [10], which would be incompatible with its use as an immune therapy.

To expand the potential utility and improve the safety and efficacy of dasatinib, we conjugated dasatinib to a novel anti-CXCR4 antibody. CXCR4 is highly expressed on the surface of human T cells and less abundantly expressed on other hematopoietic cells, while it has minimal to no expression on non-hematopoietic cells and resting neutrophils. The anti-CXCR4 antibody used for conjugation was generated by fusion of a CXCR4 inhibitory peptide into the CDR3H loop of Herceptin using the antibody CDR fusion approach developed at Calibr [70].

In order to create a conjugate of dasatinib with an anti-CXCR4 antibody, the hydroxyl group of dasatinib was modified to display an aminooxy-terminated appendage containing either a non-cleavable, tetra-poly-ethylene glycol linker, or a reductively cleaved, highly water soluble peptide-based linker (Fig. 3, R1 versus R2, respectively). Using Solulink chemistry, these moieties were non-specifically conjugated to produce **αhuCXCR4-Dasatinib** with drug-to-antibody ratios (DAR) of around 3 (Fig. 3). Disulfide bonds are relatively stable in serum and undergo reduction by intracellular glutathione to release the small molecule, while non-cleavable linkers rely on intracellular degradation of the antibody (choice of linkers is discussed further herein). The resultant ADC **αhuCXCR4-Dasatinib** was able to selectively deliver dasatinib into human T cells with excellent *in vitro* immunosuppressive activity as demonstrated in αCD3/αCD28-induced T cell activation assays, where production of IL-2 and TNFα was effectively suppressed. A limitation of studying CXCR4 in preclinical models is the significant differences in CXCR4 expression levels and distribution in rodent and human T cells. Thus, in order to evaluate the preclinical *in vivo* efficacy, non-human primate studies would likely be necessary to determine the therapeutic potential and safety of **αhuCXCR4-Dasatinib** [70].

αCD11a-LXR Agonist Conjugate

Liver X Receptor (LXR), a nuclear hormone receptor, is an essential regulator of both lipid metabolism and immune responses. Activation of LXR-mediated transcription by synthetic agonists, such as T0901317 and GW3965, promotes lipid

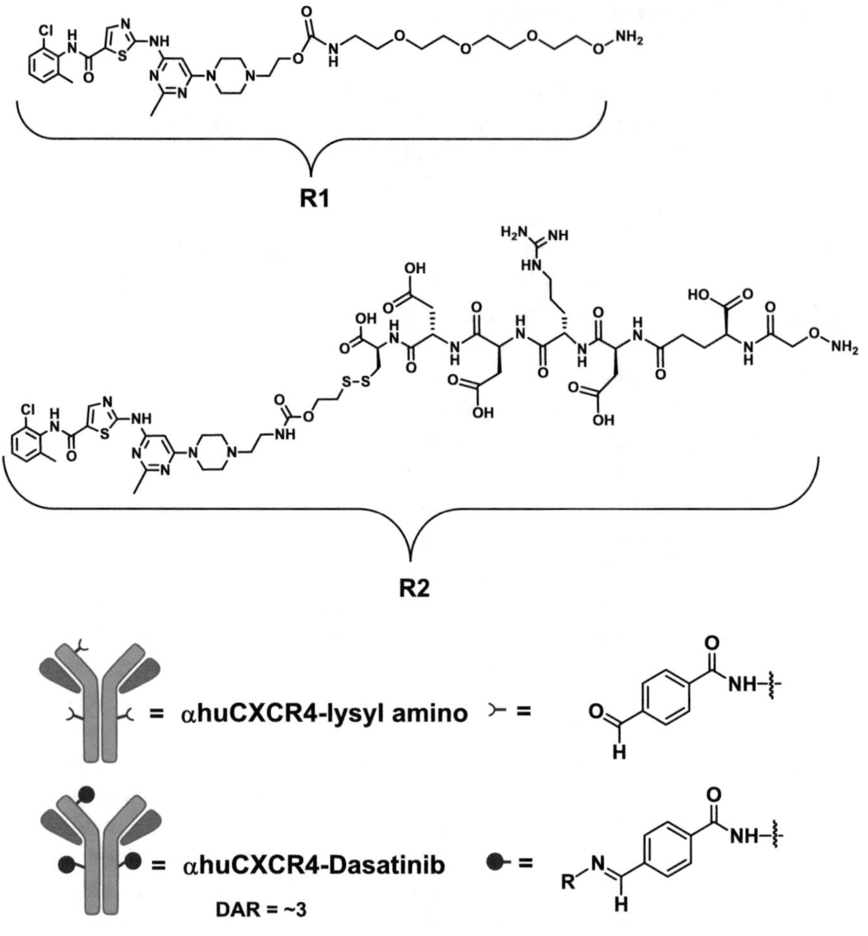

Fig. 3 αCXCR4-Dasatinib conjugate

efflux from lipid-laden macrophages and attenuates progression of inflammatory disease in animal models. These agonists have demonstrated preclinical efficacy in treating many diverse types of chronic inflammatory diseases, including atherosclerosis [32], contact dermatitis [28], rheumatoid arthritis [58], and ulcerative colitis [18]. However, traditional LXR agonists unfavorably elevate liver triglycerides via increasing transcriptional levels of genes regulating lipogenesis, such as Srebf1 and Fas [34, 57]. As a result, the side effects of LXR agonism-induced liver lipid synthesis have impeded exploitation of this intriguing mechanism for chronic therapy. To specifically deliver the LXR agonists into disease-related effector cells while sparing the liver, we sought to employ ADC technology wherein a potent LXR agonist (from Wyeth) was conjugated with antibodies against CD11a, a pan-immune cell surface marker [35].

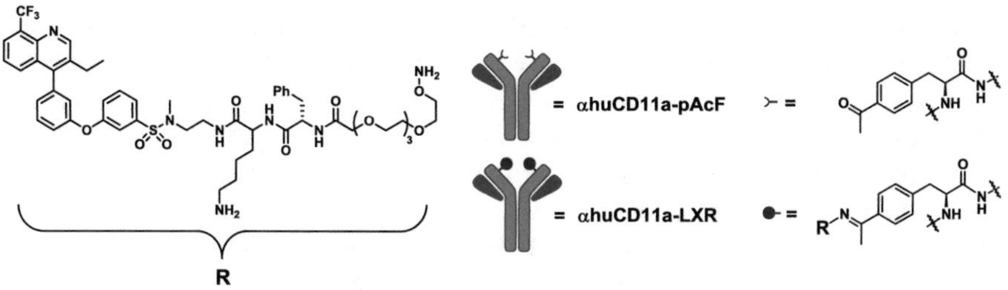

Fig. 4 αCD11a-LXR agonist conjugate

CD11a, an integrin playing a central role in leukocyte trafficking, is abundantly expressed by most leukocytes. Efalizumab, a commercial humanized CD11a antibody, was used for treating multiple sclerosis but was subsequently withdrawn from the market due to increased incidence of progressive multifocal leukoencephalopathy. To demonstrate the concept of broadly targeting the immune system, a synthetic LXR agonist analog was designed that could accommodate modification with a protease cleavable phenylalanine-lysine (Phe-Lys) dipeptide linker, which is readily hydrolyzed by the endosomal enzyme Cathepsin B, and a terminal aminooxy (Fig. 4). Efalizumab was engineered to introduce two para-acetylphenylalanine (pAcPhe) for site-specific conjugation, a method which has been extensively reviewed elsewhere [26], leading to the resultant ADC **αhuCD11a-LXR**. To assess the cell type-specificity of **αhuCD11a-LXR**, activity was compared in THP-1 (human monocyte/macrophage-derived cell line) and HepG2 (human hepatocyte cell line) cells. **αhuCD11a-LXR** showed dramatic selectivity and enhanced activity in these two cell lines compared with conventional LXR agonists, such as T0901317. These results represent an important proof-of-concept for the use of ADCs to deliver LXR agonists specifically to immune cells to safely treat diseases driven by lipid-laden and inflamed macrophages.

αCD11a-PDE4 Inhibitor Conjugate

Payload potency has been a constraining factor for the exploration of ADCs outside of oncology, as few small molecules possess the potency of cytotoxins used for cytotoxic ADCs. With this constraint in mind, we were drawn to the highly potent small molecule inhibitor GSK256066, which inhibits phosphodiesterase 4 (PDE4) enzymatic activity at sub-picomolar concentrations [68]. PDE4 is a key enzyme regulating the amplitude and duration of the signal of cyclic adenosine monophosphate (cAMP), a key second messenger involved in dampening inflammatory responses. Increased or dysregulated PDE4 activity promotes the inappropriate hydrolysis of cAMP, thus amplifying pro-inflammatory signals. Various PDE4 inhibitors had demonstrated preclinical efficacy in models of chronic inflammatory diseases, such as inflammatory bowel disease [61], rheumatoid arthritis [42], and psoriasis [49] and several have progressed to clinical studies and marketed products. However, dose-limiting side effects, including nausea, emesis, diarrhea, and headache, resulting from inhibiting PDE4 in the central nervous system (CNS) and gastrointestinal tract (GI), have impeded the clinical development of more potent members of this class of drugs for a broad range of inflammatory disease indications. Many potent PDE4 inhibitors were developed through an alternative path as inhaled or topical drugs to eliminate systemic exposure. To overcome these dose-limiting side effects in a way that was compatible with a systemic drug, which we felt could have greater efficacy and more widespread utility, we sought to create pan-immune cell-targeted PDE4 inhibitors [74].

We first designed and characterized an analog of GSK256066 that supported chemo-selective conjugation to anti-CD11a antibody using available structural information. A non-cleavable linker was attached to the small molecule to provide the conjugate with better stability and specificity; based on the structure of GSK256066 bound to PDE4, we believed a polar, peptide fragment could be accommodated outside of the binding pocket with a suitable linker. The humanized αCD11a antibody efalizumab was mutated to incorporate two pAcPhe residues for site-specific conjugation (Fig. 5). Following conjugation, the resultant ADC **αhuCD11a-PDE4** was assessed in human peripheral blood mononuclear cells (PBMCs) isolated from fresh blood, which were treated with LPS to induce pro-inflammatory cytokine secretion. This ADC significantly attenuated LPS-induced TNFα secretion in a concentration-dependent manner, while treatment with αCD11a

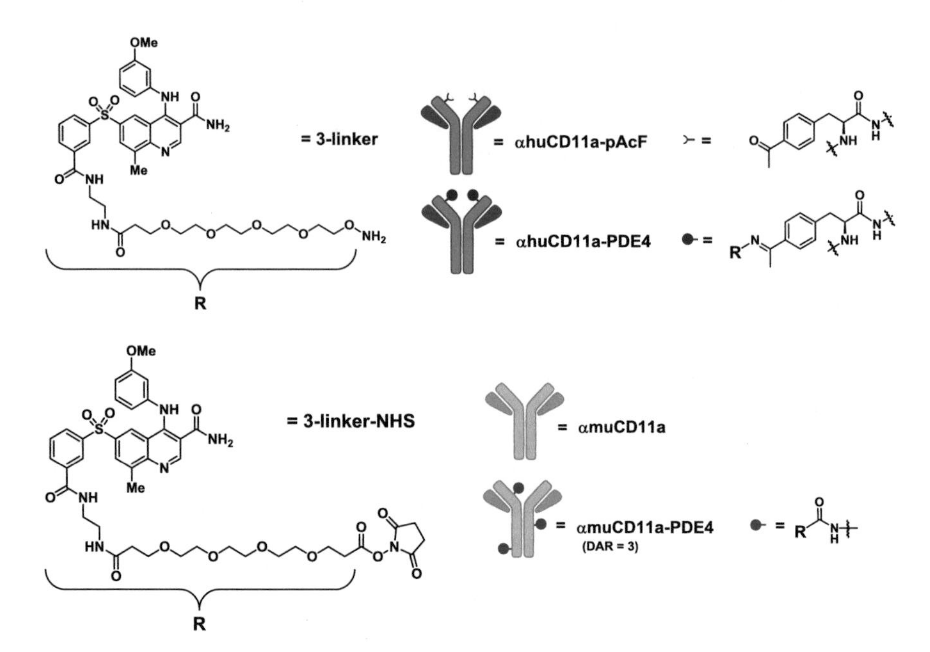

Fig. 5 αCD11a-PDE4 inhibitor conjugate

antibody alone did not. Because efalizumab does not cross react with rodent cells, in order to evaluate this concept *in vivo* we generated a preclinical tool using a mouse surrogate αCD11a antibody, using in this case non-site-specific conjugation technology to generate **αmuCD11a-PDE4** with an average DAR of three. The anti-inflammatory effect of **αmuCD11a-PDE4** was first demonstrated in mouse peritoneal macrophages treated with LPS, where treatment with the ADC significantly reduced TNFα secretion. This anti-inflammatory effect was clearly shown to be mediated through the CD11a receptor, based on a competition assay with excess amount of αCD11a antibody and the lack of activity in a CD11a-negative cell type. We next investigated the translation of these effects into an *in vivo* setting using a mouse carrageenan air pouch model. Treatment with **αmuCD11a-PDE4**, but not αCD11a antibody itself, significantly attenuated pro-inflammatory cytokine production induced by carrageenan in the air pouch. This anti-inflammatory effect was well-correlated with the exposure of the ADC in the air pouch exudate and serum, and was also accompanied by clear evidence of the binding of **αmuCD11a-PDE4** to CD11a positive immune cells. This novel tissue-targeted PDE4 inhibitor conjugate provides evidence that ADCs are feasible and attractive approaches to next-generation therapies for inflammatory diseases with a best-in-class balance of safety and efficacy.

αS. Aureus-Antibiotic Conjugate

Non-oncology applications of ADCs have also been explored in treating infectious disease. It is widely known that certain pathogens bypass immune surveillance and find refuge in the intracellular compartments of various cells [59, 67]. During the lifecycle of these cells, the pathogen is disseminated via the bloodstream, facilitating the establishment of persistent infections. Most conventional antibiotics are not effective in killing intracellular pathogens due to poor intracellular penetration and lack of action under intracellular conditions, pointing to significant unmet medical needs [31, 40, 67].

Scientists from Genentech reported an antibody-antibiotic conjugate (AAC) with improved therapeutic effect against intracellular *Staphylococcus aureus* in animal models [31]. This AAC consists of an antibiotic tethered to an antibody against β-N-acetylglucosamine cell-wall teichoic acid (β-GlcNAc-WTA) to target delivery of the payload to the surface of bacteria. The AAC was proposed to work for both phagocytic and non-phagocytic host cells. Despite having no direct affinity for the host cell, the AAC gains entry into the host cell by opsonizing circulating or escaped bacteria, and then infiltrating the host cell via the Fc receptor (on phagocytic cells) or via binding to fibronectin (on non-phagocytic cells, e.g., epithelial and endothelial cells). Once internalized, the AAC is processed in phagolysosomes leading to subsequent release of antibiotic, which eliminates tagged or by-standing untagged resident bacteria (Fig. 6b).

Two members of the ansamycin class of antibiotics, rifampicin and dimethyl DNA31 (dmDNA31) were explored for the construction of AACs. These antibiotics were modified chemically to attach the MC-Val-Cit-PABQ linker, which consists of maleimide and caproic acid (MC) for attachment to the antibody, valine citrulline (Val-Cit) as a protease-cleavable dipeptide, and a novel p-aminobenzyl quaternary ammonium salt (PABQ) for attachment to dmDNA31 (Fig. 6a). The antibiotic is released upon cathepsin-mediated cleavage of Val-Cit. The activities of these constructs were analyzed by the standard minimal inhibitory concentration (MIC) assay at neutral and acidic pH to determine their antibacterial potency. It was found that only dmDNA31 was active as an AAC [31].

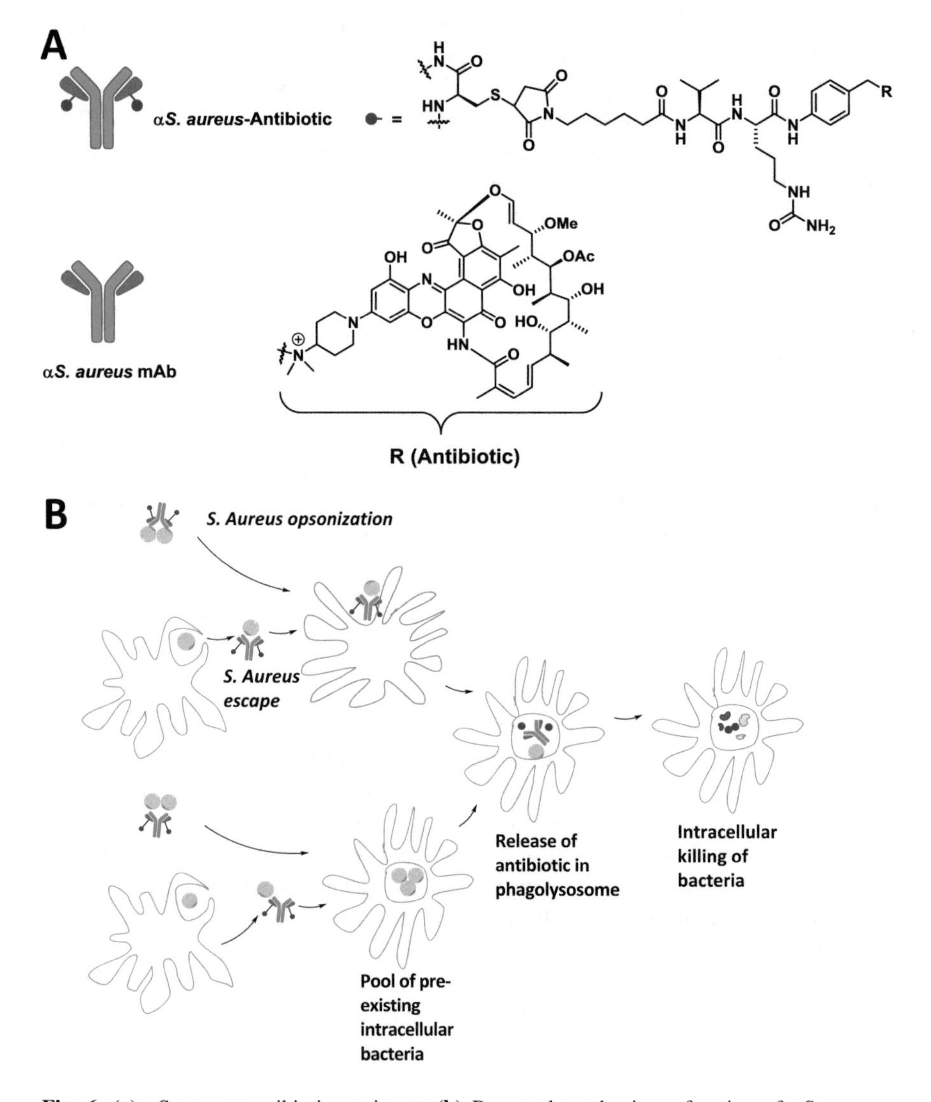

Fig. 6 **(a)** αS. aureus-antibiotic conjugate **(b)** Proposed mechanism of action of αS. aureus-antibiotic conjugate killing intracellular bacteria

From an *in vivo* pharmacokinetics perspective, AAC molecules showed similar profiles to the unconjugated mAb, including a short distribution phase, a long elimination phase, and a long half-life. Very low level of unconjugated dmDNA31 was detected in plasma, suggesting *in vivo* stability of the linker. Furthermore, AAC clearance in infected mice was only marginally increased compared to non-infected mice, and this might have resulted from the expected increase in deconjugation associated with uptake of the AAC-bacteria complexes [75]. The efficacy of this AAC was studied in a *S. aureus* infected mouse model. In this model, vancomycin was not effective in eliminating intracellular bacteria, while the AAC was able to kill intracellular bacteria as well as tagged bacteria that escaped from lysed cells by internalization and intracellular killing. This suggested the capability of intracellular delivery of the effective antibiotic into the infected cells by this AAC. A single dose administration of this AAC at 24-h post-infection could reduce the presence of *S. aureus*, and was found to be superior to the clinically equivalent, twice-daily dosing of vancomycin. [31].

This study opened a new field to expand to other hard-to-treat bacterial infections by re-constructing some previous potent anti-bacterials which had failed in development due to poor cell penetrance, pharmacokinetic properties and/or undesired host toxicity. This technology platform promises to enhance the anti-bacterial efficacy against infectious diseases.

αCD45-Saporin (SAP) Conjugate

Different cytotoxins have been utilized for immune-conjugation for targeting cancer cells. SAP is one of the cytotoxins that has been widely explored in cancer therapy by conjugating into protein-based immunotoxins [5, 50, 53]. SAP is a catalytic N-glycosidase ribosome-inactivating protein that inhibits protein synthesis. As a small molecule and unlike other ricin family members, it lacks a general cell entry domain and is non-toxic unless conjugated to a targeting antibody or ligand capable of receptor-mediated internalization. The more detailed information regarding the pharmacological characteristics of saporin has been reviewed in the previous chapters.

Recently, SAP was conjugated with αCD45 antibody to generate a hematopoietic-cell-specific immunotoxin. This immunotoxin was proposed to be used as a conditioning regimen in patients that need to receive hematopoietic stem cell transplantation (HSCT). Comparing to the conventional approaches, including total body irradiation and/or non-specific cytotoxic drugs, which may be genotoxic and have multiple short- and long-term adverse effects, this **αCD45-SAP conjugate** approach has been demonstrated in the animal models of improved the safety profiling of conditioning by specifically targeting hematopoietic stem cells (HSCs) and other hematopoietic cells and spare non-hematopoietic cells and minimizing off-target toxicity and immunosuppression while enabling efficient engraftment and rapid immunological recovery [48].

αCD30-Vedotin Conjugate (Adcetris)

Embracing a similar concept as the αCD45-saporin conjugate to deliver cytotoxic agent to the immune cells to inhibit immune responses, **Adcetris**, a FDA approved **αCD30-vedotin conjugate** for treating relapsed Hodgkin lymphoma and systemic anaplastic large cell lymphoma, has been tested in clinical trials for a few non-oncology indications. The previous chapter has extensively reviewed the composition and characteristics of **Adcetris** from the oncology perspective. CD30, other than being a marker of a subset of lymphoma cells, it is also expressed on the membrane of CD8+ T cells or secreted as a soluble form. As CD30+ cells and soluble CD30s have been detected in the circulation of some patients with inflammatory conditions, **Adcetris** has been clinically tested in a few immune disease contexts.

Adcetris was tested as an agent for treating steroid refractory acute GVHD. Brentuximab (αCD30 antibody) directs vedotin to target activated CD8+ T cells, which have elevated CD30 expression at diagnosis of acute GVHD. In the phase I trial, the maximum tolerated dose and the preliminary outcome of Adcetris treatment in 24 patients was established. In an abstract published in Blood in 2015, it was mentioned that this ADC was tolerable and had promising activity in steroid refractory acute GVHD. However, the phase II clinical trial was withdrawn prior to enrollment (ClinicalTrials.gov identifier NCT01616680). Other than GVHD, a phase II clinical trial for adult lupus was initiated in 2015 but was terminated due to unknown reason.

Recently, a phase II clinical trial evaluating the efficacy of **Adcetris** in early diffuse cutaneous systemic sclerosis and systemic sclerosis was initiated (ClinicalTrials.gov identifier NCT03198689 and NCT03222492). Systemic sclerosis is a multisystem autoimmune disease characterized by widespread vascular injury and progressive fibrosis of the skin and internal organs. Although no effective treatment is available for the majority of patients with this disease, the systemic inflammation in the early stage of their disease may be reversed and reduce the probability of irreversible fibrosis via significant immune modulation. The efficacy of **Adcetris** in treating systemic sclerosis will be interesting to be revealed.

αTNF-Steroid Conjugate

Steroids, exemplifying a series of four-ring arranged organic compounds, include dietary lipid cholesterols, the sex hormones and some anti-inflammatory drugs. The anti-inflammatory steroids working by reducing immune cell activity are used for treating various inflammatory diseases for a short term, while long term treatment is usually not recommended due to its systemic side effect of long exposure. The most common side effects of steroids include insomnia, weight gain, impaired vision, osteoporosis, mood swings and body water retention. To minimize the size effect of this class of drugs for long term use, the ADC approach was taken by AbbVie Inc. to specifically conjugate the steroid to an αTNF antibody, which specifically delivers the steroid to TNF receptor expressing cells. Due to being at the discovery phase, not much information regarding this **αTNF-steroid conjugate** has been disclosed, including the name of the steroid, linker chemistry, and efficacy of the ADC.

TNF exists as soluble and membrane forms and both forms interact with two types of TNF receptors, TNF-R1 and TNF-R2, each with distinct signaling pathways and biologic outcomes [1]. The membrane form of TNF also exists in 2 forms, either as membrane-anchored transmembrane TNF (TmTNF; ~25 kDa) or as TACE-cleaved soluble TNF bound to its cognate cell surface receptors (mTNF;15 kDa) [39]. The αTNF antibody may interact with either TmTNF or mTNF, and forms complexes with TNF-R1 or TNF-R2 and subsequently being taken up by cells [11]. Thus, the targeting profile of this **αTNF-steroid conjugate** will depend on which αTNF antibody was used by AbbVie in this conjugate. The bottom line of this approach is to deliver anti-inflammatory steroid into TNF receptor expressing cells for inflammatory disease indication. However, due to lack of detailed information of **αTNF-steroid conjugate**, we cannot further comment on the specific mechanism of this approach.

αCXCR4-Tacrolimus Conjugate

Tacrolimus (FK506) is a very potent immunosuppressant used to prevent organ rejection post-transplantation and it reduces inflammation in various autoimmune diseases. Despite its approval, severe off-target effects and generalized immune suppression are observed after prolonged treatment, which limit its therapeutic application. To address this problem, Ambrx developed a novel ADC consisting of a chimeric αhuCXCR4 antibody and two FK506 drug molecules using Ambrx's proprietary site-specific conjugation technology. CXCR4 was chosen as the targeting antibody as it is upregulated on activated human lymphocytes and metastatic tumor cells but is only expressed at low levels on normal cells. The naked CXCR4 antibody was able to internalized and processed in the lysosomes of activated human T cells for optimal intracellular drug delivery. The potency of the **αCXCR4-tacrolimus conjugate** was assessed by measuring inhibition of NFAT activation in Jurkat-NFAT-luciferase reporter cells. It was shown that the ADC was able to deliver active FK506 into the target cells. The ADC significantly reduced pro-inflammatory cytokines released by anti-CD3/anti-CD28 activated primary human T cells. This ADC was described in an abstract of 2015 Federation of Clinical Immunology Societies conference and no detailed experimental information was published.

Antibody-siRNA Conjugate

Small interfering RNA (siRNA) is one of the most commonly used RNA interference (RNAi) tools for inducing short-term silencing of protein-coding genes. To utilize RNAi to inhibit gene expression, siRNAs may be directly introduced into cells. Alternatively, plasmids or viral vectors can be used to express short hairpin RNAs (shRNAs) that are processed by endogenous cellular machinery into siRNAs. However, because of the limitations associated with both direct uptake of siRNA, as well as viral transduction, the methods mentioned above have not been met with widespread generality. The ability to use ADCs as vehicles for efficient targeting and cellular uptake has sparked interest in accelerating the siRNA paradigm into the creation therapeutics [36].

The first antibody-mediated targeted delivery of siRNA *in vivo* was demonstrated using HIV-suppressing siRNAs fused with anti-HIV envelope protein. This antibody was an antigen-binding fragment (Fab) conjugated to protamine to facilitate entry into CD4 T cells. This antibody-siRNA conjugate was effective in inhibiting HIV replication in these cells [64]. In addition to being explored for the suppression of viral infection and cancer growth [4, 73], antibody-mediated siRNA delivery has also been explored in treating kidney disease by targeting podocytes [20], skeletal and cardiac muscle diseases by targeting muscle cells [66], and inflammatory diseases by targeting activated leukocytes [52].

Folate Conjugates in Non-Oncology Applications

Targeting moieties other than antibodies have been explored for the delivery of pharmacologically active payloads for non-oncology indications. As early as the beginning of 1990s, the concept of using a targeting molecule for specific delivery has led to the development of a series of folate conjugates, which is based on the natural high affinity of folate for the folate receptor (FR) [29]. Folate, or folic acid, is a vital nutrient and cofactor for intracellular enzymes, exhibiting a high affinity for the FR and a robust endocytosis and recycling mechanism [23]. Since FR is selectively upregulated on certain malignant cells and activated macrophages and conjugation of folate to low molecular weight drugs, genes, liposomes, nanoparticles, and imaging agents does not impair folate's ability to bind FR, folate could be exploited to specifically target both therapeutic and imaging agents to activated macrophages without promoting their uptake by other healthy cells [69].

From this mechanistic perspective, folate-targeted therapies were explored for various clinical uses. Folate-targeted chemotherapies have been developed and six folate-drug conjugates have entered clinical trials for the treatment of cancer. Taking advantage of FR overexpression on about 40% of human cancers, folate-targeted imaging therapy helps visualize FR overexpressed areas and is used as a diagnostic tool for the presence of tumors associated with ovarian, lung, breast, kidney, brain, endometrial, and colon cancer. Specifically, with this approach, folate was conjugate with radionuclide ^{99m}Tc or ^{111}In-DTPA, and it has been successfully used to imaging malignant locations of ovarian cancer patients [37, 63]. Moreover, because FRs are also overexpressed and accessible on activated macrophages, opportunities for folate targeting in the imaging and therapy of inflammatory diseases are envisioned. Folate-conjugated radionuclides were also used for imaging inflammatory sites of rheumatoid arthritis patients in the clinic ([15, 37]). Substantial pre-clinical evidence suggests the possible use of molecular imaging of FR as a prognostic tool for tissue inflammation and folate-conjugate as therapeutics for inflammatory diseases, such as ulcerative colitis, atherosclerosis, pulmonary fibrosis and acute lung injury [19, 22, 24, 56].

As folate receptor-β (FR-β) is mainly upregulated in activated macrophages, various folate-drug conjugates were developed for immune disease indications. The pharmacokinetics of binding, internalization and recycling of FR-β on activated macrophages was characterized to help to guide optimization of drug dosing regimens. In an adjuvant-induced arthritis model, the saturation of macrophage FR was achieved at injection doses of about 150–300 nmol/kg, with more rapidly perfused tissues (e.g. liver and spleen) saturating at lower doses than inflamed tissues, probably due to higher perfusion volumes in liver and spleen, whereas macrophages in RA joints are buried in collagen-rich synovium, where perfusion access was limited. Upon binding, FR-β was internalized and recycled back to the cell surface every 10–20 min, suggesting this receptor internalization might not impair FR-β-mediated physiological function. However, the short half-life of such low molecular weight folate conjugates in the vasculature (< 1 h) made these conjugate suboptimal therapeutics. Thus, further engineering and optimization is needed to provide the next generation folate conjugates with longer half-life and stability for treating chronic inflammatory diseases [69].

Nevertheless, several critical proof-of-concept studies have been carried out to demonstrate the targeted delivery of anti-inflammatory and anti-infectious drugs using folate. A study showed that EC0746, a folate-based ligand conjugated with a γ-hydrazide analog of aminopterin, was effective against experimental retinal S-antigen (PDSAg)-induced experimental autoimmune uveitis (EAU) and myelin basic protein (MBP)-induced experimental autoimmune encephalomyelitis (EAE). The activity of EC0746 was completely blocked by a folate competitor, suggesting that the therapeutic outcomes were specifically mediated by FR-β [38]. Other than simple conjugation methods, folate has been used for nanoparticle and polymer conjugation for targeted delivery to activated macrophages. For example, folate was coupled with three-layered micelles to encapsulate DNA [44], as well as coupled to methotrexate-conjugated poly(amido-amide) dendrimer [56]. In both studies, the conjugates were used as delivery systems to specifically target activated macrophages for RA. Furthermore, folate was linked to poloxamer 407-coated ritonavir-boosted atazanavir (FA-nanoATV/r) nanoparticles to specifically target HIV-infected cell reservoirs. This conjugate improved the half-life, pharmacokinetic profile and bio-distribution to infected reservoirs, and reduced local and systemic toxicities of this nanoformulation. This nanotherapy was able to reduce HIV-infected cell count in a humanized mouse model ([14, 55]). Overall, these studies suggest the potential applications of folate-FR specific interactions for chronic infectious and inflammatory diseases.

Key Considerations in Payload and Antibody Selection for Non-oncology ADCs

Payload Selection

As is the case in oncology, the nature of the small molecule payload is a critical selection criteria for ADCs in non-oncology indications. While small molecule drugs are typically designed and optimized with passive diffusion envisaged as the major cellular uptake mechanism, ADCs typically decouple the uptake process from the physicochemical properties of the molecule and instead rely upon factors such as copy number of the target surface antigen, internalization and refresh rate of the surface antigen, endosomal escape of the payload, and the potential for the payload to be re-released into the extracellular space. Thus, new design considerations become the focus of payload selection and context-specific optimization. Other than the discussion below, additional information on payload outside of oncology maybe found in the previous chapter of the next-generation payload.

Payload Pharmacology and Toxicity

In contrast to payloads used in oncology ADCs, typically cytotoxic molecules such as tubulin polymerization inhibitors and DNA damaging agents [6], the potential payloads for non-oncology indications represent a far more diverse and heterogeneous array of compounds, including receptor agonists, receptor antagonists, and enzyme inhibitors. The relative paucity of appropriate surface antigens to target with ADCs must be recognized and compensated for through the selection of a highly potent payload. While the evolution of highly potent small molecule payloads and high affinity antibodies is the purview of ADC developers, the existence of surface antigens with appropriate expression levels, tissue distribution, and internationalization kinetics is controlled by nature and must be treated as a fixed parameter. Thus, in considering what payload molecules form the basis of the greatest opportunities to impact unmet medical needs through the use of ADC technology, one is challenged to examine a number of factors. Importantly, if one limits the search for ideal payloads to drugs that have been studied as systemic treatments, one may miss related compounds that are more amenable to ADC design but for one reason or another were deprioritized for use as conventional therapeutics.

For example, the pharmacokinetics of the payload small molecule becomes irrelevant in the context of an ADC. Because the antibody component of an ADC accounts for a majority of the therapeutic agent (approximately 98% of total ADC by molecular weight), the pharmacokinetics of an ADC is dominated by the antibody backbone, eliminating conventional small molecule clearance pathways. Similarly, the proximity of the small molecule payload to the large antibody scaffold may limit conventional extracellular metabolic instability of the small molecule; intracellular metabolism must still be accounted for, but if tissue-targeting avoids highly metabolically active tissues such as the liver, these considerations may also be diminished. In addition, intrinsic membrane permeability is not a key feature of ADC payloads, since their uptake into cells will be driven by an active process mediated by the antibody carrier. When exploring a compound class for potential application in an ADC, one may largely disregard the medicinal chemistry trajectory that led to highly metabolically stable, low-clearance molecules with high cellular permeability, and instead focus on highly potent molecules with structural features that lend themselves to linker attachment. Such molecules are often reported within patents or publications describing lead optimization campaigns, but are typically not highlighted as desirable compounds in the presented context. Indeed, this thought process led us to choose the starting points for both the LXR and PDE4 ADCs from amongst their respective structure-activity relationship studies.

Along similar lines, the selectivity of the payload against related protein targets may be irrelevant if the related protein targets are not dominantly expressed in the tissue of interest. Often medicinal chemistry campaigns will be driven by achieving such selectivity, compromising along the way other properties, such as potency. By disregarding such trends in structure-activity relationships, the options for identifying an appropriate ADC payload are broadened. We employed this concept in choosing an LXR agonist that lacked selectivity for LXRβ (which drives efficacy in cardiovascular disease and inflammatory disease) over LXRα (which drives deleterious lipogenesis in the liver), relying instead on the lack of exposure of the ADC in the liver; this allowed us to focus our payload design exclusively on highly potent compounds with chemical structures that were amenable to linker attachment.

Payload Mode of Action

The potency requirements for non-oncology ADCs differ according to the mechanism of action of the payload, i.e. antagonist, agonist, inhibitor, etc. Examples such as αCXCR4-dasatinib (Bcr-Abl inhibitor) and αCD11a-PDE4 inhibitor utilized highly potent payload inhibitors with low picomolar potency, which are likely required to maintain suppression of the relevant pathologic pathways. On the other hand, the LXR agonist-based ADC incorporated a considerably less potent pharmacophore with single digit nanomolar potency. It is quite likely that agonist-based ADCs have less stringent requirements for potency and consistent intracellular exposure than antagonists or inhibitors. In the case of the CD163-targeted dexamethasone, the *in vivo* efficacy of the ADC was 50-fold greater than the non-conjugated dexamethasone, despite similar intrinsic potency, which speaks to the varied factors that contribute to pharmacodynamics of ADCs [18]. While these relative trends are likely consistent across different ADCs, the surface expression level, rate of internalization, release, and re-surfacing of the antigen target will play a dominant role in the absolute requirement of the payload potency.

Antibody Conjugation Chemistry

As with oncology payloads, non-oncology payloads can be attached through a variety of chemistries to the antibody: lysine conjugation, cysteine conjugation, unnatural amino acid conjugation, and various other emerging technologies. These various approaches are extensively reviewed elsewhere in this edition. Of note, each of these approaches has been illustrated in non-oncology ADC settings. For example, αCD163-dexamethasone, αCXCR4-dasatinib, and αCD11a-PDE4 each utilized lysine conjugation in their ADC formats whereas α*S. Aureus*-antibiotic utilizes cysteine conjugation. αCD11a-LXR, as well as an alternative αCD11a-PDE4 construct, utilized the unnatural amino acid pAcPhe to effect site-specific conjugation. With a lack of published data suggesting one mode of linker attachment over another in directly comparable settings, it seems that an empirical approach is utilized to determine the best method for linker attachment. Other considerations, such as freedom-to-operate, may also factor into this decision.

Linker Design and Chemistry

The factors leading up to the choice of a cleavable versus non-cleavable linker are similar for oncology and non-oncology ADCs, and are extensively reviewed elsewhere in this edition. The desire to capture potency and efficacy by releasing a payload intracellularly that can engage its target without the encumbrance of a linker remnant must be balanced against the risk of premature, extracellular cleavage or re-release of the free payload generated within the cell into the extracellular compartment. However, the consequences of extracellular release of a non-oncology ADC payload may often be less grave than that of a cytotoxic payload used in oncology. Such as in the cases of dexamethasone, LXR agonist, and PDE4 inhibitor, these molecules are all tolerated systemically to some degree and ADCs were built to dramatically expand their therapeutic index; in contrast, even small amounts of potent cytotoxic payloads could induce severe, irreversible damage if released inappropriately. This enables greater flexibility in ADC development for non-oncology ADCs and an avenue for optimizing for greater activity as cleavable linkers are generally known to have the potential for greater activity due to the bystander effect of release in target tissue, whereby some degree of re-release is leveraged (rather than avoided) to enhance a localized effect.

At least three cleavable linkers have been employed in ADCs: hydrazine cleavable linkers, disulfide cleavable linkers, and protease cleavable linkers. In the αCXCR4-dasatinib example, a disulfide cleavable and non-cleavable linker were both tested [70]. The disulfide cleavable ADC was ~2-fold more potent than the non-cleavable ADC in suppressing IL-2, TNFα, and IFNγ *in vitro*, likely owing to greater target engagement inside the cell.

Peptide-based protease cleavable linkers that were successful in oncology examples (e.g. Adcetris) can also be employed in non-oncology applications. α*S. Aureus*-antibiotic and αCD11-LXRa both incorporate peptide-based protease (Cathepsin B) cleavable linkers. In the α*S. Aureus*-antibiotic example, the non-cleavable linker was also tested and found that when opsonized, did not result in release inside macrophages after uptake of MRSA [31]. Additionally, the same bacteria that was susceptible to killing by the cleavable AAC, was not susceptible to killing by non-cleavable AAC. In this particular example, the AAC is proposed to undergo Fc-mediated uptake of bacteria and the release of antibiotic in the phagolysosome is central to killing of the bacteria highlighting how mechanism can play a key role in dictating non-oncology ADC construct requirements. These observations further show that while certain principles can be generalized for non-oncology ADCs, there may be limited utility for broad design rules. Rather, depending on the mechanism of action of the payload, one can customize certain properties to achieve optimal activity and a profile that balances efficacy and safety.

Antigen Selection

Perhaps the core feature upon which all other design elements are based is the choice of surface antigen to which the ADC will home and gain entry into its target compartment. Once a desired target tissue is identified, a variety of factors shall be taken into consideration for the selection of an appropriate surface antigen.

Antigen Specificity on Tissue and Cell Types

A foundational criteria for antigen selection is the presence of the antigen on cell type(s) of interest and the absence on other cell type(s), particularly if the latter is known to mediate specific unwanted pharmacology. In non-oncology applications especially, a clear understanding of the disease pathogenesis is critical to selecting an appropriate antigen, since host cells such as immune cells are highly adaptable and often change their phenotype dramatically in the disease state. While a more selectively expressed antigen has the theoretical ability to deliver a safer ADC, a critical threat to *efficacy* is that a surface antigen reported as highly selective for a given disease state is either transient, heterogeneous, or expressed at too low of a level to facilitate the robust delivery of a payload drug.

In our studies with LXR agonists and PDE4 inhibitors, we chose to focus on CD11a as the targeting antigen because of its widely recognized expression on a variety of immune cells in various functional states. We were able to measure robust CD11a expression across multiple experimental systems and employ various tools and methods for studying it. Similarly, CD163 is a marker expressed persistently by macrophages in various functional states, including the anti-inflammatory state designated as M2, but was nevertheless used to deliver dexamethasone for treating inflammatory conditions. Folate receptor (FR) is ubiquitously expressed, but offers an opportunity to accumulate high concentrations of payload molecule inside macrophages.

We believe the consistent theme that has led to success for non-oncology ADCs is to focus on antigens with high expression levels and internalization dynamics (discussed below) that best enable efficacy, rather than emphasizing absolute specificity, which is a greater guiding principle in oncology ADCs. Where there are specific concerns based on an understanding of the toxicity and side effect potential of the small molecule payload, this can provide a practical guideline for relative specificity against the tissue that drives these untoward effects. For example, LXR agonists are known to induce liver lipogenesis and a subsequent fatty liver phenotype – thus, the antigen chosen for delivering an LXR agonist to macrophages should not be present on hepatocytes, and special consideration in the design of *in vitro* and *in vivo* experiments can be paid to ensuring this is borne out experimentally. Similarly, PDE4 inhibitors induce CNS and GI-related side effects due to the inhibition of PDE4 enzyme in neuronal cells – so the principal guiding the antigen selection for a PDE4 inhibitor-based ADC was lack of expression on the surface of neuronal cells, rather than exquisite widespread specificity.

Antigen Surface Expression and Internalization

One of the key criteria for selecting an antigen for ADC delivery is that it should be consistently abundant on the target cells and capable of maintaining a good balance of antigen internalization and recycling. The abundancy of the antigen on the cell surface is an important factor in predicting the efficiency of antibody-mediated internalization, and thus correlates to the overall effectiveness of the ADC. For example, the β-*N*-acetylglucosamine cell-wall teichoic cacid (β-GlcNAc-WTA) monoclonal antibody was selected for the AAC against *S. aureus* because the antigen that this antibody binds is highly abundant and highly expressed on *S. aureus in vitro* and during infection, and is absent from mammalian cells [31].

CD11a was selected for delivering anti-inflammatory payloads such as PDE4 inhibitors and LXR agonists, because it is constitutively highly expressed on myeloid cells and T lymphocytes, with certain activated immune populations expressing even more CD11a [51], while it is not expressed by non-hematopoietic lineages. While CD11a is widely known to internalize rapidly, the rate at which reappearance at the surface occurs is variable (and measurable) in different cell types. Cell surface CD11a on myeloid cells, including macrophages, monocytes and neutrophils, did not significantly change when mice were treated with αCD11a antibody or αCD11a-PDE4 inhibitor ADC after 48 h, while CD11a was drastically reduced on T cells in different organs of the same mice. This suggests that the internalization and recycling kinetics of CD11a receptor may vary in various immune cell types, and CD11a on T cells was significantly internalized upon αCD11a antibody binding, resulting in impairment of T cell-mediated immune responses during infection [74]. Unlike oncology ADCs designed to target and kill cancer cells, where often a short burst of drug exposure may be sufficient to induce cell death, the kinetics of the targeted antigen bears unique importance for non-oncology ADC because of the necessity of certain antigens on the cell surface for normal physiological function.

In some cases where the expression level of the surface antigen is low, the internalization efficiency is low, or intracellular processing is insufficient, high-loaded ADCs, which consists of higher number of payload drugs per antibody, have been developed to improve the therapeutic index and delivery efficacy. The application of the high-loaded ADCs has been reviewed in the previous chapter.

Antigen Physiological Function

As many cell surface antigens possess inherent physiological functions, it is essential to understand the importance of these functions when considering an antigen's appropriateness for targeting with an ADC. Unlike in oncology, where attractive antigens are often expressed at superphysiologic levels and either have no function or drive survival of the cancer cell, in non-oncology applications it is often critical that the antigen being targeted is minimally perturbed.

The integrin class of antigens has been considered, and in some cases deployed, for generating ADCs. For example, CD11a is a leukocyte integrin, which involves in cellular adhesion and costimulatory signaling. Antibody-mediated CD11a internalization results in a deficiency of CD11a present on the cell surface, thus prevents leukocytes from adhering to adhesion molecules. This results in reduced recruitment of leukocytes to inflammatory sites and subsequent dampened immune responses [16]. Similar to CD11a, other integrins including CD11b, CD11b and CD18 could also be considered as targeting antigens. However, the cell surface reduction of these receptors may results in immune suppression and increased susceptibility to serious infection [71]. Natalizumab, an α4β1 integrin blocker, acts as an inhibitor of leukocyte extravasation and was approved for the treatment of multiple sclerosis, but was reported to be associated with cases of opportunistic infections in the brain [21]. However, Vedolizumab, an antibody against gut-selective α4β7 (LPAM-1) integrin for treating inflammatory bowel diseases, has not been reported to cause serious infections in humans [9]. This suggests that more tissue specific markers should be identified and the safety of potential antibody vehicles should be evaluated in order to generate the best-in-class ADCs.

Immunoglobulin superfamily (IgSF) is the most populous family of proteins in the human genome. Other than some soluble molecules (such as immunoglobulins), this family of molecules contains a series of cell surface antigens that were considered for ADC target. These antigens include T cell receptor chains (e.g. TCRs), antigen presenting molecules (e.g. MHCs), co-receptors (e.g. CD4, CD8, CD19), antigen receptor accessory molecules (e.g. CD3s, CD79), co-stimulatory or inhibitory molecules (e.g. CD28, CD80, CD86), cell adhesion molecules (e.g. NCAMs, ICAM-1, CD2 subset), cytokine receptors (e.g. IL-1 receptor, CSF1 receptor), growth factor receptors (e.g. platelet-derived growth factor receptor, mast/stem cell growth factor receptor precursor), receptor tyrosine kinases/phosphatases (e.g. Tie-1 precursor). These IgSF cell surface antigens are involved in the recognition, binding or adhesion processes of cells, which play important role in cell-cell interaction and adaptive immune responses. The presence of these molecules on the cell surface is endogenously finely controlled, and antibody-mediated cell surface antigen internalization is likely to result in an immunosuppressing phenotype by impairing the normal function of the immune system [3, 8, 27]. Therefore, a thorough understanding of physiological functions and identification of new members of this class of molecules will help to discover potential novel antigens to target.

Scavenger receptors are expressed on phagocytic cells engaging in taking up foreign substances and waste materials. Extensive researches have been performed to characterize the expression and function of mannose receptor, CD163, CD36 and CD68, which are expressed by different subtypes of macrophages and/or other cell types with diversified physiological roles. CD163 has been explored for conjugation with dexamethasone for treatment of inflammatory diseases in preclinical models. However, the expression of both CD163 and mannose receptor are elevated in anti-inflammatory macrophages, thus targeting either antigen to deliver anti-inflammatory payload might impair the resolution of inflammation [12, 41]. Because antibody-mediated internalization of receptor will result in a temporary or prolonged deficiency of this receptor on the cell surface, understanding of the consequences of the deficiency could be important. CD36 is expressed not only by myeloid cells but also by platelets, spleen cells, adipocytes, erythrocytes and endothelial cells. Human deficiency is CD36 is mostly asymptomatic, except exhibiting refractoriness to platelet transfusion [72]. CD68 is expressed by monocytes and macrophages. Deletion of CD68 in mice does not affect innate immune response against microbes [65], but dysfunctional osteoclasts were observed [2]. Thus, both CD36 and CD68 could be potential candidates for designing an ADC specifically for targeting macrophage-mediated diseases.

Fc receptors are expressed by a range of immune cells including B cells, follicular dendritic cells, natural killer cells, monocytes, macrophages and granulocytes. Fc receptors bind to the Fc portion of antibodies that are attached to infected cells or invading pathogens. This binding stimulates the activity of antibody-mediated phagocytosis or antibody-dependent cell-mediated cytotoxicity. Fc receptors have been considered as a target for payload delivery as they are expressed mainly on antigen presenting cells and myeloid cells. Taking account there are multiple subtypes of Fc receptors and their functions being largely redundant [47, 54], it is likely that the normal immune functions will not be impaired upon antibody-mediated Fc receptor internalization [46].

Concluding Remarks

The majority of ADCs developed to date target cancer therapies, with comparably fewer examples of ADCs for non-oncology indications, most of which are still in the early discovery phase. Perhaps because of our advanced understanding of their cell surface proteome, most non-oncology ADCs were developed for targeting immune cells. However, with increased knowledge of disease pathogenesis and identification of tissue- and cell-surface specific markers, novel therapeutics emerging from ADC platforms should be developed for a broader range of diseases. With the discovery of potent small molecules for various molecular targets relevant for disease, ADCs are poised to have a major impact on new therapies.

References

1. Akassoglou K, Douni E, Bauer J, Lassmann H, Kollias G, Probert L (2003) Exclusive tumor necrosis factor (TNF) signaling by the p75TNF receptor triggers inflammatory ischemia in the CNS of transgenic mice. Proc Natl Acad Sci 100:709–714
2. Ashley JW, Shi Z, Zhao H, Li X, Kesterson RA, Feng X (2011) Genetic ablation of CD68 results in mice with increased bone and dysfunctional osteoclasts. PLoS One 6:e25838
3. Balagué C, Kunkel SL, Godessart N (2009) Understanding autoimmune disease: new targets for drug discovery. Drug Discov Today 14:926–934
4. Baumer S, Baumer N, Appel N, Terheyden L, Fremerey J, Schelhaas S, Wardelmann E, Buchholz F, Berdel WE, Muller-Tidow C (2015) Antibody-mediated delivery of anti-KRAS-siRNA in vivo overcomes therapy resistance in Colon Cancer. Clin Cancer Res 21:1383–1394
5. Bergamaschi G, Perfetti V, Tonon L, Novella A, Lucotti C, Danova M, Glennie MJ, Merlini G, Cazzola M (1996) Saporin, a ribosome-inactivating protein used to prepare immunotoxins, induces cell death via apoptosis. Br J Haematol 93:789–794
6. Bornstein GG (2015) Antibody drug conjugates: preclinical considerations. AAPS J 17:525–534
7. Bover LC, Cardó-Vila M, Kuniyasu A, Sun J, Rangel R, Takeya M, Aggarwal BB, Arap W, Pasqualini R (2007) A Previously Unrecognized Protein-Protein Interaction between TWEAK and CD163: Potential Biological Implications. J Immunol 178(12):8183–8194. https://doi.org/10.4049/jimmunol.178.12.8183
8. Chittasupho C, Siahaan TJ, Vines CM, Berkland C (2011) Autoimmune therapies targeting costimulation and emerging trends in multivalent therapeutics. Ther Deliv 2:873–889
9. Colombel JF, Sands BE, Rutgeerts P, Sandborn W, Danese S, D'Haens G, Panaccione R, Loftus EV, Sankoh S, Fox I, et al (2016) The safety of vedolizumab for ulcerative colitis and Crohn's disease. Gut gutjnl-2015-311079
10. Conchon M, Freitas CMB d M, Rego MA d C, Braga Junior JWR (2010) Dasatinib. Rev Bras Hematol E Hemoter 33:131–139
11. Deora A, Hegde S, Lee J, Choi C-H, Chang Q, Lee C, Eaton L, Tang H, Wang D, Lee D et al (2017) Transmembrane TNF-dependent uptake of anti-TNF antibodies. MAbs 9:680–695
12. Evans BJ, Haskard DO, Sempowksi G, Landis RC (2013) Evolution of the macrophage CD163 phenotype and cytokine profiles in a human model of resolving inflammation. Int J Inflamm 2013:1–9
13. Fabriek BO, Van Bruggen R, Deng DM, Ligtenberg AJ, Nazmi K, Schornagel K, Vloet RP, Dijkstra CD, van den Berg TK. The macrophage scavenger receptor CD163 functions as an innate immune sensor for bacteria. Blood 2009 113(4):887-892. doi: https://doi.org/10.1182/blood-2008-07-167064.
14. Gautam N, Puligujja P, Balkundi S, Thakare R, Liu X-M, Fox HS, McMillan J, Gendelman HE, Alnouti Y (2014) Pharmacokinetics, biodistribution, and toxicity of folic acid-coated antiretroviral Nanoformulations. Antimicrob Agents Chemother 58:7510–7519
15. Gent YY, Weijers K, Molthoff CF, Windhorst AD, Huisman MC, Smith DE, Kularatne SA, Jansen G, Low PS, Lammertsma AA et al (2013) Evaluation of the novel folate receptor ligand

[18F]fluoro-PEG-folate for macrophage targeting in a rat model of arthritis. Arthritis Res Ther 15:R37

16. Gottlieb AB, Krueger JG, Wittkowski K, Dedrick R, Walicke PA, Garovoy M (2002) Psoriasis as a model for T-cell–mediated disease: Immunobiologic and clinical effects of treatment with multiple doses of Efalizumab, an anti–CD11a antibody. Arch Dermatol 138:591
17. Graversen JH, Moestrup SK (2015) Drug Trafficking into Macrophages via the Endocytotic Receptor CD163. Membranes (Basel) 5(2):228–252. https://doi.org/10.3390/membranes5020228
18. Graversen JH, Svendsen P, Dagnæs-Hansen F, Dal J, Anton G, Etzerodt A, Petersen MD, Christensen PA, Møller HJ, Moestrup SK (2012) Targeting the hemoglobin scavenger receptor CD163 in macrophages highly increases the anti-inflammatory potency of dexamethasone. Mol Ther 20:1550–1558
19. Han W, Zaynagetdinov R, Yull FE, Polosukhin VV, Gleaves LA, Tanjore H, Young LR, Peterson TE, Manning HC, Prince LS et al (2015) Molecular imaging of folate receptor β–positive macrophages during acute lung inflammation. Am J Respir Cell Mol Biol 53:50–59
20. Hauser PV, Pippin JW, Kaiser C, Krofft RD, Brinkkoetter PT, Hudkins KL, Kerjaschki D, Reiser J, Alpers CE, Shankland SJ (2010) Novel siRNA delivery system to target Podocytes in vivo. PLoS One 5:e9463
21. Hoepner R, Faissner S, Salmen A, Gold R, Chan A (2014) Efficacy and side effects of Natalizumab therapy in patients with multiple sclerosis. J Cent Nerv Syst Dis 6:41
22. Jager, N.A., Westra, J., Golestani, R., van Dam, G.M., Low, P.S., Tio, R.A., Slart, R.H.J.A., Boersma, H.H., Bijl, M., and Zeebregts, C.J. (2014). Folate receptor- imaging using 99mTc-folate to explore distribution of polarized macrophage populations in human atherosclerotic plaque. J Nucl Med 55, 1945–1951
23. Kamen BA, Capdevila A (1986) Receptor-mediated folate accumulation is regulated by the cellular folate content. Proc Natl Acad Sci 83:5983–5987
24. Kelderhouse LE, Mahalingam S, Low PS (2016) Predicting response to therapy for autoimmune and inflammatory diseases using a folate receptor-targeted near-infrared fluorescent imaging agent. Mol Imaging Biol 18:201–208
25. Kern JC, Dooney D, Zhang R, Liang L, Brandish PE, Cheng M, Feng G, Beck A, Bresson D, Firdos J et al (2016) Novel phosphate modified Cathepsin B linkers: improving aqueous solubility and enhancing payload scope of ADCs. Bioconjug Chem 27:2081–2088
26. Kim CH, Axup JY, Schultz PG (2013) Protein conjugation with genetically encoded unnatural amino acids. Curr Opin Chem Biol 17:412–419
27. Kuhn C, Weiner HL (2016) Therapeutic anti-CD3 monoclonal antibodies: from bench to bedside. Immunotherapy 8:889–906
28. Larrede S, Quinn CM, Jessup W, Frisdal E, Olivier M, Hsieh V, Kim M-J, Van Eck M, Couvert P, Carrie A et al (2009) Stimulation of cholesterol efflux by LXR agonists in cholesterol-loaded human macrophages is ABCA1-dependent but ABCG1-independent. Arterioscler. Thromb Vasc Biol 29:1930–1936
29. Leamon CP, Low PS (1991) Delivery of macromolecules into living cells: a method that exploits folate receptor endocytosis. Proc Natl Acad Sci 88:5572–5576
30. Lee KC, Ouwehand I, Giannini AL, Thomas NS, Dibb NJ, Bijlmakers MJ (2010) Lck is a key target of imatinib and dasatinib in T-cell activation. Leukemia 24:896–900
31. Lehar SM, Pillow T, Xu M, Staben L, Kajihara KK, Vandlen R, DePalatis L, Raab H, Hazenbos WL, Hiroshi Morisaki J et al (2015) Novel antibody–antibiotic conjugate eliminates intracellular S. Aureus. Nature 527:323–328
32. Lehmann JM, Kliewer SA, Moore LB, Smith-Oliver TA, Oliver BB, Su J-L, Sundseth SS, Winegar DA, Blanchard DE, Spencer TA et al (1997) Activation of the nuclear receptor LXR by Oxysterols defines a new hormone response pathway. J Biol Chem 272:3137–3140
33. Li W, Xu LH, Yuan XM (2004) Macrophage hemoglobin scavenger receptor and ferritin accumulation in human atherosclerotic lesions. Ann N Y Acad Sci 1030:196–201. https://doi.org/10.1196/annals.1329.025

34. Liang G, Yang J, Horton JD, Hammer RE, Goldstein JL, Brown MS (2002) Diminished hepatic response to fasting/Refeeding and liver X receptor agonists in mice with selective deficiency of sterol regulatory element-binding protein-1c. J Biol Chem 277:9520–9528
35. Lim RKV, Yu S, Cheng B, Li S, Kim N-J, Cao Y, Chi V, Kim JY, Chatterjee AK, Schultz PG et al (2015) Targeted delivery of LXR agonist using a site-specific antibody–drug conjugate. Bioconjug Chem 26:2216–2222
36. Liu B (2007) Exploring cell type-specific internalizing antibodies for targeted delivery of siRNA. Brief Funct Genomic Proteomic 6:112–119
37. Low PS, Kularatne SA (2009) Folate-targeted therapeutic and imaging agents for cancer. Curr Opin Chem Biol 13:256–262
38. Lu Y, Wollak KN, Cross VA, Westrick E, Wheeler LW, Stinnette TW, Vaughn JF, Hahn SJ, Xu LC, Vlahov IR, Leamon CP (2014) Folate receptor-targeted aminopterin therapy is highly effective and specific in experimental models of autoimmune uveitis and autoimmune encephalomyelitis. Immunol 150(1):64–77. https://doi.org/10.1016/j.clim.2013.10.010
39. Luettig B, Decker T, Lohmann-Matthes ML (1989) Evidence for the existence of two forms of membrane tumor necrosis factor: an integral protein and a molecule attached to its receptor. J Immunol Baltim Md. 1950 143:4034–4038
40. Mariathasan S, Tan M-W (2017) Antibody–antibiotic conjugates: a novel therapeutic platform against bacterial infections. Trends Mol Med 23:135–149
41. Martinez FO, Gordon S (2014) The M1 and M2 paradigm of macrophage activation: time for reassessment. F1000Prime Rep 6:13
42. McCann FE, Palfreeman AC, Andrews M, Perocheau DP, Inglis JJ, Schafer P, Feldmann M, Williams RO, Brennan FM (2010) Apremilast, a novel PDE4 inhibitor, inhibits spontaneous production of tumour necrosis factor-alpha from human rheumatoid synovial cells and ameliorates experimental arthritis. Arthritis Res Ther 12:R107
43. McColl A, Michlewska S, Dransfield I, Rossi AG (2007) Effects of glucocorticoids on apoptosis and clearance of apoptotic cells. Sci World J 7:1165–1181
44. Mohammadi M, Li Y, Abebe DG, Xie Y, Kandil R, Kraus T, Gomez-Lopez N, Fujiwara T, Merkel OM (2016) Folate receptor targeted three-layered micelles and hydrogels for gene delivery to activated macrophages. J Control Release 244:269–279
45. Moreno JA, Muñoz-García B, Martín-Ventura JL, Madrigal-Matute J, Orbe J, Páramo JA, Ortega L, Egido J, Blanco-Colio LM (2009) The CD163-expressing macrophages recognize and internalize TWEAK: potential consequences in atherosclerosis. Atherosclerosis 207(1):103–110. https://doi.org/10.1016/j.atherosclerosis.2009.04.033
46. Nimmerjahn F, Ravetch JV (2008) Fcγ receptors as regulators of immune responses. Nat Rev Immunol 8:34–47
47. Otten MA, van der Bij GJ, Verbeek SJ, Nimmerjahn F, Ravetch JV, Beelen RHJ, van de Winkel JGJ, van Egmond M (2008) Experimental antibody therapy of liver metastases reveals functional redundancy between fc RI and fc RIV. J Immunol 181:6829–6836
48. Palchaudhuri R, Saez B, Hoggatt J, Schajnovitz A, Sykes DB, Tate TA, Czechowicz A, Kfoury Y, Ruchika F, Rossi DJ et al (2016) Non-genotoxic conditioning for hematopoietic stem cell transplantation using a hematopoietic-cell-specific internalizing immunotoxin. Nat Biotechnol 34:738–745
49. Papp K, Reich K, Leonardi CL, Kircik L, Chimenti S, Langley RGB, Hu C, Stevens RM, Day RM, Gordon KB et al (2015) Apremilast, an oral phosphodiesterase 4 (PDE4) inhibitor, in patients with moderate to severe plaque psoriasis: results of a phase III, randomized, controlled trial (efficacy and safety trial evaluating the effects of Apremilast in psoriasis [ESTEEM] 1). J Am Acad Dermatol 73:37–49
50. Pastan I, Hassan R, FitzGerald DJ, Kreitman RJ (2006) Immunotoxin therapy of cancer. Nat Rev Cancer 6:559–565
51. Patarroyo M (1994) Adhesion molecules mediating recruitment of monocytes to inflamed tissue. Immunobiology 191:474–477

52. Peer D, Zhu P, Carman CV, Lieberman J, Shimaoka M (2007) Selective gene silencing in activated leukocytes by targeting siRNAs to the integrin lymphocyte function-associated antigen-1. Proc Natl Acad Sci 104:4095–4100
53. Pietersz G (2005) Book Reviews. Immunol Cell Biol 83:450–450
54. van der Poel CE, Spaapen RM, van de Winkel JGJ, Leusen JHW (2011) Functional characteristics of the high affinity IgG receptor, Fc RI. J Immunol 186:2699–2704
55. Puligujja P, Araínga M, Dash P, Palandri D, Mosley RL, Gorantla S, Poluektova L, McMillan J, Gendelman HE (2015) Pharmacodynamics of folic acid receptor targeted antiretroviral nanotherapy in HIV-1-infected humanized mice. Antivir Res 120:85–88
56. Qi R, Majoros I, Misra AC, Koch AE, Campbell P, Marotte H, Bergin IL, Cao Z, Goonewardena S, Morry J et al (2015) Folate receptor-targeted Dendrimer-methotrexate conjugate for inflammatory arthritis. J Biomed Nanotechnol 11:1431–1441
57. Repa JJ (2000) Regulation of mouse sterol regulatory element-binding protein-1c gene (SREBP-1c) by oxysterol receptors, LXRalpha and LXRbeta. Genes Dev 14:2819–2830
58. Repa JJ, Mangelsdorf DJ (2002) The liver X receptor gene team: potential new players in atherosclerosis. Nat Med 8:1243–1248
59. Rogers DE (1952) The survival of staphylococci within human leukocytes. J Exp Med 95:209–230
60. de Rycke L, Verhelst X, Kruithof E, Van den Bosch F, Hoffman IE, Veys EM, De Keyser F. Rheumatoid factor, but not anti-cyclic citrullinated peptide antibodies, is modulated by infliximab treatment in rheumatoid arthritis. Ann Rheum Dis 2005 64(2):299-302. doi: https://doi.org/10.1016/j.imbio.2005.05.010
61. Salari-Sharif P, Abdollahi M (2010) Phosphodiesterase 4 inhibitors in inflammatory bowel disease: a comprehensive review. Curr Pharm Des 16:3661–3667
62. Schade AE, Schieven GL, Townsend R, Jankowska AM, Susulic V, Zhang R, Szpurka H, Maciejewski JP (2007) Dasatinib, a small-molecule protein tyrosine kinase inhibitor, inhibits T-cell activation and proliferation. Blood 111:1366–1377
63. Sega EI, Low PS (2008) Tumor detection using folate receptor-targeted imaging agents. Cancer Metastasis Rev 27:655–664
64. Song E, Zhu P, Lee S-K, Chowdhury D, Kussman S, Dykxhoorn DM, Feng Y, Palliser D, Weiner DB, Shankar P et al (2005) Antibody mediated in vivo delivery of small interfering RNAs via cell-surface receptors. Nat Biotechnol 23:709–717
65. Song L, Lee C, Schindler C (2011) Deletion of the murine scavenger receptor CD68. J Lipid Res 52:1542–1550
66. Sugo T, Terada M, Oikawa T, Miyata K, Nishimura S, Kenjo E, Ogasawara-Shimizu M, Makita Y, Imaichi S, Murata S et al (2016) Development of antibody-siRNA conjugate targeted to cardiac and skeletal muscles. J Control Release 237:1–13
67. Thwaites GE, Gant V (2011) Are bloodstream leukocytes Trojan horses for the metastasis of Staphylococcus aureus? Nat Rev Microbiol 9:215–222
68. Tralau-Stewart CJ, Williamson RA, Nials AT, Gascoigne M, Dawson J, Hart GJ, Angell ADR, Solanke YE, Lucas FS, Wiseman J et al (2011) GSK256066, an exceptionally high-affinity and selective inhibitor of phosphodiesterase 4 suitable for administration by inhalation: in vitro, kinetic, and in vivo characterization. J Pharmacol Exp Ther 337:145–154
69. Varghese B, Vlashi E, Xia W, Ayala Lopez W, Paulos CM, Reddy J, Xu L-C, Low PS (2014) Folate receptor-β in activated macrophages: ligand binding and receptor recycling kinetics. Mol Pharm 11:3609–3616
70. Wang RE, Liu T, Wang Y, Cao Y, Du J, Luo X, Deshmukh V, Kim CH, Lawson BR, Tremblay MS et al (2015) An immunosuppressive antibody-drug conjugate. J Am Chem Soc 137:3229–3232
71. Winograd-Katz SE, Fässler R, Geiger B, Legate KR (2014) The integrin adhesome: from genes and proteins to human disease. Nat Rev Mol Cell Biol 15:273–288
72. Yamamoto N, Ikeda H, Tandon NN, Herman J, Tomiyama Y, Mitani T, Sekiguchi S, Lipsky R, Kralisz U, Jamieson GA (1990) A platelet membrane glycoprotein (GP) deficiency in healthy blood donors: Naka- platelets lack detectable GPIV (CD36). Blood 76:1698–1703

73. Yao Y-D, Sun T-M, Huang S-Y, Dou S, Lin L, Chen J-N, Ruan J-B, Mao C-Q, Yu F-Y, Zeng M-S et al (2012) Targeted delivery of PLK1-siRNA by ScFv suppresses Her2+ breast Cancer growth and metastasis. Sci Transl Med 4:130ra48–130ra48
74. Yu S, Pearson AD, Lim RK, Rodgers DT, Li S, Parker HB, Weglarz M, Hampton EN, Bollong MJ, Shen J et al (2016) Targeted delivery of an anti-inflammatory PDE4 inhibitor to immune cells via an antibody–drug conjugate. Mol Ther 24:2078–2089
75. Zhou C, Lehar S, Gutierrez J, Rosenberger CM, Ljumanovic N, Dinoso J, Koppada N, Hong K, Baruch A, Carrasco-Triguero M et al (2016) Pharmacokinetics and pharmacodynamics of DSTA4637A: a novel THIOMAB™ antibody antibiotic conjugate against *Staphylococcus aureus* in mice. MAbs 8:1612–1619

Index

M. Damelin (ed.), *Innovations for Next-Generation Antibody-Drug Conjugates*, Cancer Drug Discovery and Development,
https://doi.org/10.1007/978-3-319-78154-9

Q

R

S

Printed in the United States
By Bookmasters